Concepts of
Occupational Therapy

Kathlyn L. Reed, PhD, OTR, FAOTA, MLIS, AHIP
Visiting Professor, School of Occupational Therapy
Texas Woman's University–Houston Center
Houston, Texas

Sharon Nelson Sanderson, MPH, OTR/L, FAOTA
Professor of Occupational Therapy
College of Allied Health
University of Oklahoma Health Sciences Center
Oklahoma City, Oklahoma

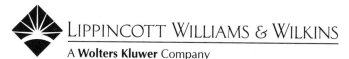
LIPPINCOTT WILLIAMS & WILKINS
A **Wolters Kluwer** Company
Philadelphia · Baltimore · New York · London
Buenos Aires · Hong Kong · Sydney · Tokyo

Editor: Eric Johnson
Managing Editor: Karen Gulliver
Marketing Manager: Chris Kushner
Production Editor: Lisa JC Franko
Design Coordinator: Mario Fernandez

351 West Camden Street
Baltimore, Maryland 21201-2436 USA

227 East Washington Square
Philadelphia, Pennsylvania 19106 USA

Printed in the United States of America

Third Edition, 1992
Second Edition, 1983
First Edition, 1980

Library of Congress Cataloging-in-Publication Data

Reed, Kathlyn L.
    Concepts of occupational therapy / Kathlyn L. Reed, Sharon R.
Sanderson. — 4th ed.
      p. cm.
    Includes bibliographical references and index.
    ISBN 0-683-30454-2
    1. Occupational therapy.   I. Sanderson, Sharon Nelson.
II. Title.
    [DNLM: 1. Occupational Therapy. WB 555 R324c 1999]
    RM735.R4   1999
    616.8'515—dc21
    DNLM/DLC
    for Library of Congress   99-25875
                                     CIP

To purchase additional copies of this book call our customer service department at **(800) 638–3030** or fax orders to **(301) 824–7390**. International customers should call **(301) 714–2324**.

99 00 01 02
2 3 4 5 6 7 8 9 10

This book is dedicated to students and practitioners of occupational therapy and to the clients they will serve.

Preface

This fourth edition of *Concepts of Occupational Therapy* marks a change in format. What was once the single-volume edition of this work will now become two. The first discusses the ideas that shape the conceptual models of practice, and the second describes the management that organizes practice delivery. Whereas the previous three editions focused on an overview of occupational therapy as a profession, the fourth edition will focus on the critical content of the occupational therapy profession. The word concepts is being taken literally in this the first volume to mean the ideas that formed the core knowledge, skills, and attitudes of occupational therapy.

The major focus of the text is on providing students with a basic knowledge of what constitutes occupational therapy information and application. As a profession, occupational therapy presents a unique challenge to its students. The essense of the profession cannot be found in any of the physical tools identified in an occupational therapy clinic or even in the trunk of a practitioner's car. All the physical forms are transitory artifacts and last only as long as people choose to use those particular physical tools in the performance of daily tasks and routines. Occupational therapy is rooted in the occupations of life that people perform every day. Thus, the root concept is at once simple and complex. Occupational therapy is as simple as promoting the doing of everyday things. It is as complex as understanding how the doing is related to health and well-being and how the doing changes within one individual's lifetime in many different environments over the milleniums. The study of doing occupation is not even limited to humans because sometimes the study of other animals brings new insight into human occupation.

Students face the task of trying to understand what is the real occupational therapy and what may masquerade as occupational therapy. They would like the real occupational therapy to please stand up so it can be seen, counted, and described, but the very seeing, counting, and describing become challenges in themselves because the obvious is not always as obvious as it would seem. Understanding how occupation works is much more difficult than seeing occupation done. Occupation evolves; it is not manufactured. The tools are symbols of occupation, but are not the real occupation being performed by the individual in ways both unique to the individual and yet linked to the environmental factors surrounding the individual.

The challenge of writing a textbook in occupational therapy is to convey to students the essence of occupational therapy without entrapping students into a single view of occupational therapy as a practicing discipline. Therefore, this edition of *Concepts of Occupational Therapy* focuses on the basic ideas that in various combinations form conceptual and practice models. An overview of the historical perspective is provided to help the student "ground" the ideas as they were originally envisioned so that similiarities and differences over time, culture, and other contexts can be compared and contrasted.

As always, critique by colleagues is encouraged. Through the sharing of ideas and information better textbooks can be envisioned, written, and published.

Acknowledgments

Both authors acknowledge the collective contribution of our parents, occupational therapy instructors, fellow occupational therapy practitioners, former occupational therapy students, and finally, our clients—who taught us the real value of occupation by applying it to their lives.

Contents

The Philosophical Base

CHAPTER 1

Defining Occupational Therapy

THE MEANING OF WORDS

Occupational therapy can be analyzed by examining the meanings of the words that comprise the professional title. These words are "to occupy," a verb; "occupation," a noun; and "therapy," a noun. As the term is used in the professional title, to occupy means to employ, busy, engage (a person, or the mind, attention, etc.) and to take up, use up, or fill space or time. Occupation means being occupied or employed with, or engaged in something (1). Therapy means treatment of disease or disorder (2). Thus, the name occupational therapy is meant to convey that the practice involves treatment of disease or disorder by employing or engaging a person, the mind, and attention in occupation. Such occupation does by its nature take up, use up, or fill space and time.

Further refinement of these concepts is included in the definitions of occupational therapy as a professional specialty that have evolved over the years.

HISTORICAL DEFINITIONS OF OCCUPATIONAL THERAPY

The first definition of occupational therapy was given by the originator of the term, George Barton, a founder of the profession. In 1914, Barton asked, "if there is an occupational disease, why not an occupational therapy" (3). He hoped to provide a useful occupation for each organ, joint, or muscle of the human body and thus provide an occupational therapy cure for every disease, injury, or dysfunction. Although experience has shown that a specific occupational cure for every disorder does not exist, the name has endured partly because occupation can be used as a therapeutic medium to effect the state of a person's health, quality of life, satisfaction, and sense of well-being.

In 1919, Barton's definition is better formulated (4). He stated the following: "occupational therapy is the science of instructing and encouraging the sick in such labors as will involve those energies and activities producing a beneficial therapeutic effect." This definition illustrates his interests in making occupational therapy a recognized scientific discipline, in teaching and motivating persons with illness and disability, and in using occupations that have a positive effect on the individual.

The first formal definition of occupational therapy was written in 1922 by H. A. Pattison. Dr. Pattison defined occupational therapy as "any activity, mental or physical, definitely prescribed and guided for the distinct purpose of contributing to, and hastening recovery from, disease or injury" (5). This definition explains that the concepts of occupational therapy include the following: 1) a prescribed and guided treatment, 2) mental and physical activity (or occupation), and 3) a contribution to and hastening of recovery. Thus, Dr. Pattison stresses that occupations have a mental as well as a physical component and that treatment using occupation should be viewed as medical therapy and thus prescribed (ordered) and guided (directed) toward hastening the recovery from disease or injury. It can be assumed, therefore, that Dr. Pattison would not have approved of occupations (activities) simply being given to persons to keep them busy without regard for the prescribed therapeutic value to hasten recovery.

These concepts were reaffirmed by Herbert J. Hall in 1923. His definition states that

> occupational therapy provides light work under medical supervision for the benefit of patients convalescing in hospitals or in their homes. The handicrafts are used not with the idea of making craftsmen of the patients, but for the purposes of developing physical and mental effectiveness at a time when courage and initiative are at low ebb. (6)

Dr. Hall's definition adds two more concepts fundamental to occupational therapy. One concept is that occupational therapy uses work (or occupation) to assist in development and recovery of skills needed for tasks. It does not teach people specific job skills for industrial work and does not offer employment services for unemployed workers. The second concept involves helping people gain and regain effective abilities when their emotional and psychological levels are also less than normal. Special attention must be given to the emotional and psychological states while the occupational therapist works with individuals. The total person always must be considered, with the mind and body as an integrated, inseparable whole.

The definition used by the Boston School of Occupational Therapy in 1924 adds still more concepts. This definition says that "occupational therapy aims to furnish a scheme of scientifically arranged activities which will give, to any set of muscles or related parts of the body in cases of disease or injury, just the degree of movement and exercise that may be directed by a competent physician or surgeon" (7). The major addition to the basic concepts in this definition concerns the inclusion of "scientifically arranged activities which will give just the degree of movement and exercise." In other words, occupational therapy should be measured in precise units based on scientific facts that the occupational therapist has learned. Although our ability to measure some tasks, such as muscle strength, is more precise than measuring self concept, every occupational therapist can contribute to the scientific knowledge of occupational therapy. At the same time, occupational therapists must learn that different activities (or occupations) provide different effects on people. The value of occupational therapy is in selecting the just right occupation at just the right level in just the right amount. Analyzing and selecting occupations constitutes a major portion of the learning process in the occupational therapy curriculum.

A new formal definition of occupational therapy did not appear again for nearly 50 years. In 1972, the Council on Standards (8) of the American Occupational Therapy Association (AOTA) proposed the definition that occupational therapy is "the art and science of directing man's participation in selected tasks to restore, reinforce and enhance performance, facilitate learning of the skills and functions essential for adaptation and productivity, diminish or correct pathology and to promote and maintain health." Analysis of this definition shows that the purpose can be identified as "directing man's participation in selected tasks." The focus of participation is on directing but not on controlling the intervention or consultation process. Also, the emphasis on performance, skills, and functions first appears in this definition as does the emphasis on promoting and maintaining health, not just correcting pathology.

In summary, these five historical definitions have stated some important concepts basic to occupational therapy. These are as follows: 1) occupations can be mental and/or physical in nature; 2) occupational therapy should be ordered or written (prescribed), especially if it is part of a medical management plan; 3) one purpose of occupational therapy is to contribute to or hasten recovery from disease or disorder; 4) occupational therapy assists in development and recovery through the use of selected occupations to which the client or consumer is directed; 5) occupational therapy involves the total person, including the mind and attention; 6) occupational therapy has a scientific rationale; 7) occupations can be analyzed and selected according to specific criteria; 8) occupational therapy is concerned with the performance of occupational skills and tasks; and 9) occupations can be used to maintain and promote health, not just to correct pathology.

The same definitions have also ruled out some concepts that do not belong to occupational therapy. These are as follows: 1) occupational therapy should not be used as a means of keeping a consumer busy, with no other objective in mind—it is not "busy work" or "just for fun" activities; 2) occupational therapy is not a substitute for a vocational training service although occupational therapy services may contribute to the preparation for such training; 3) occupational therapy does not provide an employment service for unemployed workers; 4) occupational therapy should not be an unplanned, spontaneous program of activities; and 5) occupational therapy does not control choice of intervention but rather facilitates intervention.

Although the early definitions of occupational therapy provide insight into the thinking that has evolved with the profession, early definitions do not illustrate the major criteria needed in a definition for today's world. The criteria are:

1. A brief account of the *unique feature* of the profession, which distinguishes it from others;
2. Inclusion of the major professional *goals, outcomes, or purposes;*
3. *The population* served;
4. A summary of the service *programs offered;*
5. *The process* model used to deliver service;
6. *The means* through which the results are achieved (media or modalities and methods or techniques); and
7. A concise stating of these elements.

MODERN DEFINITIONS OF OCCUPATIONAL THERAPY

The first modern definition of occupational therapy was accepted by the Representative Assembly of the AOTA in March 1981, for use in state licensure bills. It is as follows:

> Occupational therapy is the use of purposeful activity (unique feature) with individuals who are limited by physical injury or illness, psychosocial dysfunction, developmental or learning disabilities, poverty and cultural differences or the aging process (population) in order to maximize independence, prevent disability and maintain health (outcome). The practice encompasses evaluation, treatment and consultation (processes). Specific occupational therapy services include: teaching daily living skills; developing perceptual-motor skills and sensory integrative functioning; developing play skills and prevocational and leisure capacities; designing, fabricating or applying selected orthotic and prosthetic devices or selective adaptive equipment; using specifically designed crafts and exercises to enhance functional performance; administering and interpreting tests such as manual muscle and range of motion, and adapting environment for the handicapped (means). These services are provided individually, in groups, or through social systems (programs). (9)

This definition fulfills all the stated criteria and, as such, is a positive step in helping identify the elements of occupational therapy. When the Uniform Terminology for Occupational Therapy was revised in 1994, another definition of occupational therapy was written:

> *Occupational therapy* is the use of purposeful activity (unique feature) or interventions to promote health and achieve functional outcomes (generic goals of most health care fields). *Achieving functional outcomes* means to develop, improve, or restore the highest possible level of independence (purpose/goal) of any individual who is limited by a physical injury or illness, a dysfunctional condition, a cognitive impairment, a psychosocial dysfunction, a mental illness, a developmental or learning disability, or an adverse environmental conditions (population served). *Assessment* means the use of skilled observation or evaluation by the administration and interpretation of standardized or nonstandardized tests and measurements to identify areas for occupational therapy services.

Occupational therapy services include, but are not limited to
1. the assessment, treatment, and education of or consultation with the individual family, or other persons (process); or
2. interventions directed toward developing, improving, or restoring daily living skills, work readiness or work performance, play skills or leisure capacities, or enhancing educational performance skills (objectives); or
3. providing for the development, improvement, or restoration of sensorimotor, oral-motor, perceptual or neuromuscular functioning; or emotional, motivational, cognitive, or psychosocial components of performance (objectives). (10)

These services may require assessment of the need for and use of interventions such as the design, development, adaptation, application, or training in the use of assistive technology devices; the design, fabrication, or application of rehabilitation technology such as selected orthotic devices; training in the use of assistive technology, orthotic or prosthetic devices; the application of physical agent modalities as an adjunct to or in preparation for purposeful activity; the use of ergonomic principles; the adaptation of environments and processes to enhance functional performance; or the promotion of health and wellness (means).

A comparison of the two definitions shows the constants and the changes that have occurred over the 13-year span. The unique feature, purposeful activity, remains the same. The goal of achieving independence and health also remains the same. However, the goal of preventing disability, which appears in the 1981 definition, is not included in the 1994 definition in spite of the passage and implementation of the 1990 Americans With Disabilities Act. Why the word or concept of disability was not included in the 1994 definition is not stated. In contrast, the British definition makes disability a central theme.

> The occupational therapist assesses the physical, psychological and social functions of the individual, identifies areas of dysfunction and involves the individual in a structured programme of activity to *overcome disability*. The activities selected will relate to the consumer's personal, social, cultural and economic needs and will reflect the environmental factors which govern his/her life. (11, italics added)

It is also not clear why other worthy goals are not included. For example, the Canadian definition of occupational therapy includes enabling the person to become more productive or live a more satisfying or healthier lifestyle. (12)

> Occupational therapy (OT) is a health care profession which provides services to people whose ability to function in every day living is disrupted by physical illness or injury, developmental problems, the aging process, mental illness or emotional problems. The goal of occupational therapy is to assist the individual in achieving an independent, productive, and satisfying life-style. Occupational therapists use adaptive activities to increase the individual's functioning and productivity.

The description of the population served remains essentially the same between the 1981 and 1994 AOTA sponsored definitions except for the additions of dysfunctional condition, cognitive impairment, and mental illness to the 1994 definition. The phrase "poverty and cultural differences or the aging process," which appears in the 1981 definition, was not repeated in the 1994 one, but the phrase "adverse environmental conditions" may substitute for poverty and cultural differences. Whether the aging process is an "adverse environmental condition" is open to interpretation.

Note that the 1994 definition does not discuss that types of service programs or service models offered. It does not state whether intervention is done individually or in groups, and it does not state whether the intervention is done through medical, education, health, or social service programs. The 1981 definition does include a summary of programs. The lack of reference to programs offered is a serious deficit in the 1994 definition.

The description of the process remains the same except that the word "assessment" is used in the 1994 definition in place of "evaluation." Currently accepted definitions of the two terms suggest assessment refers to the "specific tools or instruments used during the evaluation process" whereas evaluation refers to the "process of obtaining and interpreting data necessary for intervention which includes planning for and documenting the evaluation" (13). Changes in the means also reflects changes in ideas. The term "work readiness" has replaced "prevocational." The phrases "assistive technology" and "rehabilitation technology" have replaced "adaptive equipment." New to the means section is the inclusion of physical agent modalities and the use of ergonomic principles. Both physical and occupational therapists have agreed through their national organizations that media and modalities can not be legislated to one field. The difference and uniqueness are in the explanation and supporting research, not in the application per se. Therefore, occupational therapists are able to use important physical modalities as an adjunct to or in preparation for occupational performance. Likewise, ergonomics has become important to occupational therapy as one means of changing or adapting the environment to facilitate human occupation and reduce discomfort and potential injury.

Some modification of the definition used in the Uniform Terminology might improve the definition as follows:

> Occupational therapy is the analysis and application of selected occupations from everyday life that have meaning and purpose to the consumer (unique feature) and thus enable the consumer to gain, regain, enhance, or prevent the loss of occupational habits, skills, tasks, routines, or roles that the consumer has performed in the past or is learning to perform in order to participate as fully as possible as a contributing member of his or her personal, social, cultural, and economic environment (goals, outcomes, or purposes). Qualified occupational therapy personnel provide the services of assessment, intervention, case management, education, advocacy, and consultation

(process model) to persons of all ages who experience or may experience problems or difficulty in their occupational performance of self-care, home management, work or productivity, work readiness, education, play, or leisure (population served). Such services are provided in cooperation with the individual, the family, or other appropriate persons and are scheduled individually or in groups, though medical, health, education, and social services, facilities, and programs (programs offered). Specific interventions may include but are not limited to the following: analysis, design, fabrication, and training of orthotic and prosthetic devices; analysis, selection, and use of rehabilitation technology; application of physical agent modalities as an adjunct to or in preparation for purposeful occupation; analysis and use of ergonomic and safety principles; application of work readiness and work hardening principles; analysis and training of daily living skills; selected application of sensorimotor, cognitive, and psychosocial skills and tasks; use of therapeutically analyzed crafts, games, and toys; task analysis and development of play, work readiness, and avocation skills; and adaptation of environments to reduce barriers and increase functional performance (the means).

POLITICAL CORRECTNESS

In definitions and descriptions, words must be selected carefully. Preferably, the words should be unambiguous and convey a similar meaning to everyone. Such uniform clarity is more easily attempted than achieved. For example, the word "independence" or word phrase "independent functioning" appear in some definitions of occupational therapy. The concept of independence assumes that the objective of the consumer is to return to independent living in a single-family house or apartment without assistance from anyone other than immediate family members, if any. This view of independence is based on a cultural common in Northern European countries and to much of the Northeastern part of the United States where immigrants from Northern European countries settled. Such independence, however, is not common to consumers for whom extended families interact and live together or nearby. If fact, the reverse concept may apply. Persons with disabilities or limitations in function may be cared for by younger members of the family group. Performing such care is viewed as an honor, not a burden. The responsibility may be welcomed, not rejected, because the job tasks are evidence of growing up or of being a valued member entrusted with the care of a beloved family member. In such families, the therapist's focus on increasing the consumer's independence is seen as interfering with family values—not promoting them. Thus, focus of occupational therapy must be shifted to determine who in the family is going to assume what tasks and roles. The intervention strategies may focus on teaching the caregiver, not the consumer, easy and safe techniques of dressing, transferring, feeding, and performing other daily living tasks important to the individual and family.

The word "exercise" rarely appears in modern definitions of occupational therapy. Exercise has acquired a meaning in occupational therapy folklore that is equated with mindless or endless repetition with little, if any, useful goal-directed behavior. Doodling with a pencil while listening to a boring lecture or turning a paper clip end for end while waiting for appointment are examples of such non-goal-directed behavior. The source of this interpretation remains unclear but the meaning has been passed down by many generations of occupational therapy personnel. Because occupational focuses on purposeful or goal-directed movement and occupation, "mindless and meaningless" exercise is considered antithetical to the purpose and objectives of occupational therapy. Actually, exercise does not need to be mindless, endless, boring, or devoid of meaning especially when paired with a pleasurable occupation such as listening to music or working out with friends. Nevertheless, in the folklore of occupational therapy, the use of the word "exercise" is to be avoided whenever possible.

The phrase "arts and crafts" or even "crafts" by itself infrequently appears in modern definitions. Occupational therapy personnel are reluctant to use the phrase "arts and crafts" for fear of being labeled as "artsy craftsy" persons who supposedly entertain and amuse patients but have no real scientific value to their services. Many arts and crafts used to be full-time occupations such as weaving cloth, making pottery, or making barrels. As machines replaced hands in manufacturing such items, the value of handmade items decreased in society, except in the subculture of the art world. From the Civil War period, 1860, through WWI, 1920, industry increasing manufactured goods that once were made by hand. The value of handcrafts in society decreased. Machines began to make more and sometimes better items than could be handmade, and the prices for these items were less expensive. Arts and crafts went from being full-time occupations to being part-time avocations. Many arts and crafts also changed from being "men's work" to "women's work," such as weaving, spinning, and needlework. Increasingly in today's world, consumers do not place much value on arts or crafts projects. They want to do "real" work such as taking apart a carburetor, cooking meals, or learning keyboard skills. Occupational therapy personnel have responded by reducing or eliminating arts and crafts from many occupational therapy service programs. This three-monkey approach (no see, no hear, no speak) to dealing with crafts is short-sighted at best and may be akin to "throwing the baby out with the bath water." Crafts provide many opportunities for obtaining goal-directed, purposeful actions and tasks. They also have other attributes such as economy of money and space. What is needed in the profession is an objective reevaluation of the role of arts and crafts in the occupational therapy toolkit of media and modalities. There should be less knee-jerk reactions that remove arts and crafts because of their supposed image problem.

SUMMARY

Occupational therapy includes the study of human occupations in relation to personal health, life satisfaction, and sense of well-being and the management of the adaptive behavior or competent performance required to perform these occupations. The study of occupations entails analysis of the kinds of occupations, requirements for their performance, and the meaning or significance of each. Management involves conceptual and practice models, which explain the process of providing occupational therapy services to clients such as evaluation and assessment, occupational therapy diagnosis, planning, intervention, and reevaluation. Thus, the study and management of the purposeful occupations (activities) in which humans engage is the unique feature of occupational therapy that separates its knowledge base from all other professions.

Usually, the purposes of occupational therapy are to do the following: 1) enable each person to achieve optimum function and adaptation in performance of occupations, 2) prevent occupational dysfunction whenever possible, and 3) promote the maintenance of occupational performance. The purposes are applicable to all persons in society, but those persons most likely to need occupational therapy services can be grouped into the following: 1) those with physical illness or injury, 2) those with an emotional disorder, 3) those with congenital or developmental disability, and 4) the elderly.

Services to people with occupational impairment may be offered through medical, health, educational, and social systems. In other words, occupational therapists may be employed and provide occupational therapy in any of the aforementioned systems.

Specific occupational therapy services may include the use of one or more of the following media, methods, and techniques: 1) analysis and training of daily living skills, habits, and routines for the development, restoration, or maintenance of adaptive or competent performance; 2) design, fabrication, and application of orthotic and prosthetic devices to assist or substitute for lack of performance; 3) analysis, selection, and use of rehabilitative and assistive technology or devices to enhance or enable performance; 4) selected application of modified or adapted techniques to develop or redevelop specific performance; 5) use of therapeutically analyzed media such as crafts, games, or toys to promote purposeful actions that can be organized into improved performance; 6) task analysis and development of work, work readiness, play skills, and leisure skills to facilitate the organization of skills into occupations and roles; and 7) adaptation of the environment to improve the health, well-being, and functional performance of all people (environmental barriers).

These specific services are a part of a 12-step problem-solving process of occupational therapy that includes the following stages: 1) acceptance of a consumer for screening assessment (referral, intake); 2) selection of a conceptual model to guide consumer-centered process; 3) completion of the screening evaluation to determine suitability of the consumer as a client for occupational therapy services; 4) completion of the comprehensive evaluation of the client's occupational performance to identify occupational dysfunction or performance problem(s); 5) determination of the occupational therapy diagnosis; 6) selection of a practice model to guide the

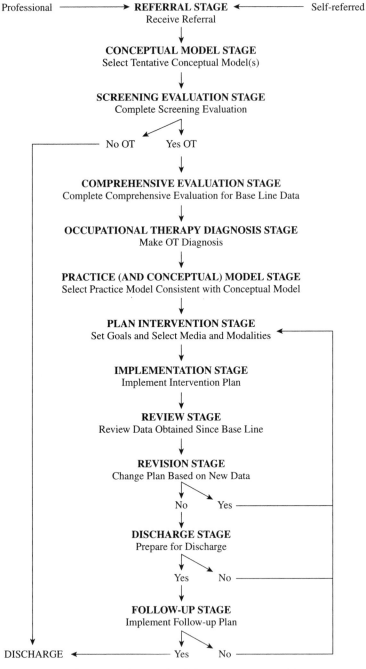

Figure 1.1. Occupational therapy process model.

intervention process; 7) planning of the intervention process with the client including goals to be achieved and the media and modalities to be used to achieve the goals; 8) implementation and management of the intervention program; 9) review and reevaluation of the client and analysis of the results of the program, modification of the program, if needed, and analysis for dismissal (discharge) of the person; 10) revision of the intervention program if necessary; 11) preparation of the client for discharge; and 12) provision of follow-up as necessary. The problem-solving model has been outlined in Figure 1.1.

This chapter has reviewed several definitions of occupational therapy and briefly discussed the relevance of the definitions to occupational therapy as a field of study and a practice discipline. The next chapters will explore aspects of the definition in more detail including the philosophy, concepts and ideas, consumers of occupational therapy services, model development and use, knowledge and skills involved, practice model application, contextual and historical base, and locating occupational therapy literature.

References

1. The Oxford English Dictionary. Oxford: Clarendon Press, 1933.
2. Taylor EJ. Dorland's Illustrated Medical Dictionary. Philadelphia: Saunders, 1988.
3. Barton G. Occupational therapy. Trained Nurse Hosp Rev 1915;54:138–140.
4. Barton G. Teaching the Sick. Philadelphia: Saunders, 1919:62.
5. Pattison HA. The trend of occupational therapy for the tuberculous. Arch Occup Ther 1922;1:19–24.
6. Hall HJ. O.T. A New Profession. Concord, MA: Rumford Press, 1923.
7. Dunton WR Jr. Prescribing Occupational Therapy. Springfield, IL: Charles C Thomas, 1928.
8. AOTA Council on Standards. Occupational therapy: its definition and function. Am J Occup Ther 1972;26:204–205.
9. AOTA Representative Assembly. Minutes. Am J Occup Ther 1981;35:792–802.
10. AOTA Uniform terminology for occupational therapy. 3rd edition. Am J Occup Ther 1994;48(11):1051.
11. College of Occupational Therapists. Core Skills and a Conceptual Foundation for Practice: A Position Statement. London: COT, 1994.
12. OT week guide. Can J Occup Ther 1993;60(3):5.
13. Commission on Practice. Commission on practice clarifies terms. OT Week 9(28):10, 1995 (July 13).

CHAPTER 2

Historical Themes

INTRODUCTION

Occupational therapy derived its founding concepts from many sources. Some had more influence than others but all are useful. Among the historical roots are moral treatment, pragmatism, the arts and crafts movement, the influence of the Quakers, the mental hygiene movement, the settlement house movement, manual training, and rehabilitation equipment. The events and places are summarized in Tables 2.1 and 2.2.

MORAL TREATMENT

Moral treatment began in Europe, particularly in France and England, and was brought to the United States by early leaders in psychiatry who established the Association of Medical Superintendents of American Institutions for the Insane, which later became the American Psychiatric Association. Best-known leaders of the European movement are Philippe Pinel of France and William and Samuel Tuke of York Retreat in England. In the United States, Benjamin Rush (father of American psychiatry), Abraham Brigham (editor, American Journal of Insanity), Isaac Ray (Butler Asylum, Rhode Island), and Pliny Earle (Bloomingdale Asylum, New York) are probably the best-known members of the moral treatment movement.

As Greenblatt (1) states, there was a

> high level of humanism, individual care, and attention accorded the mentally ill patient in hospitals of the early 1800s under the banner of "moral treatment." The dignity of the patient was preserved and enhanced and the conditions of his living were extraordinarily rich and culturally impressive compared with the subsequent era of custodialism . . .

The major assumptions of moral treatment were that persons with mental illness were morally insane and that insanity was a physical disease that could be cured by providing the person with an individualized regimen of work (occupation) and recreation, the services of religion and education, and the support and restrictions of group living (2). Moral treatment involved psychosocial adjustment rather than medical treatment, which at the time relied on ridding the body of poisons by purging using enemas, bloodletting to reduce the pressure in the brain, and using various techniques to rebalance bodily vapors and humors.

Table 2.1.   Influences on the Development of Occupational Therapy
• Philosophy and psychology—humanism, holism, and pragmatism
• Social movements—moral treatment, arts and crafts movement, settlement houses, and the mental hygiene movement
• Education and training—manual training and arts education, learning by doing (from pragmatism), and growth and development
• Religion—humanitarianism and caring
• Business—industrial revolution and work efficiency
• Science and medicine—health and disease, psychiatry (hospitalization of mentally ill), neurology (rest cure), and orthopedics (muscle reeducation and training)

The techniques of moral treatment evolved through a combination of factors occurring during the late eighteenth century (2). Of particular importance was religious humanism, which substituted a rule of love for one's fellow man for the previous fearful relationship of man to God. In the New England states, Puritans believed that wealth should be used to help the less fortunate rather than to show vanity or luxury. Quakers and Unitarians believed that the brotherhood of man under the fatherhood of God ennobled all human beings and made them equal under the eyes of the Lord. As a result, humanitarian service was expected of everyone, especially to those who were less fortunate such as the mentally ill (insane), and humane treatment was extolled.

The scientific community was also increasingly influential through its adherence to study and observation rather than divine retribution or demonic possession. Phrenology was the first systemic study of the brain. Although much of phenomenology would later be discredited, the initial studies suggested that the human brain was malleable and could be changed. Phrenologist believed that the mind was divided into a number of compartments, each of which served a different function such as memory, imagination, passion, will, and morality. Thus, if some compartments were damaged, the rest of the compartments would survive unharmed. Therefore, the old idea of total insanity or total brain damage was not possible under phrenology, and as a result, no person's insanity was hopeless.

The political climate also was favorable to a more humane approach. King George III of England was known to suffer from mental illness. Attempts to treat his illness brought the subject of treatment before many doctors who had previously never considered working with persons who suffered from "nerves" and "bilious conditions" (3). Investigations of insane asylums brought attention to the abusive conditions many inmates suffered; as a result, attempts to improve conditions were initiated.

Table 2.2　Significant Places in the Development of Occupational Therapy
• York Retreat—York, England
• Hart House—University of Toronto, Toronto, Canada
• Devereux Mansion—Marblehead, Massachusetts
• Phipps Clinic at Johns Hopkins Hospital—Baltimore, Maryland
• Sheppard and Enoch Pratt Hospital—Baltimore, Maryland
• Consolation House—Clifton Springs, New York
• Hull House—Chicago, Illinois

Caplan (2) suggests that moral treatment was based on a philosophy then in vogue known as *ideology*, which "emphasized the role of environment in molding personality and mental functioning." The word ideology is attributed to Antoine Destutt de Tracy (1758–1836), a follower of Condillac (4). The concept of ideology was originally set forth by Abbe Etienne de Condillac (1715–1780), a french philosopher, and was based on the ideas of John Locke (1632–1704), an English philosopher. Basically, the philosophy proposed that all operations of the mind are initiated by sensations in the brain. Thus, knowledge and ideas begin with sensation. The sensations transmitted from the outside world become the foundation of all thought and understanding. In insanity, according to Rush, the sensations become disorganized so that the brain does not receive or react appropriately to environmental cues, thus resulting in judgment disorders, delusions, hallucinations, and memory lapses. Rush felt the actual cause of insanity was in the blood vessels of the brain (5).

Treatment requires the understanding that the intellect was viewed as spiritual and aligned with the soul and thus immortal (2). As such, the intellect could not be destroyed, but the brain could be diseased and thus dysfunctional, which would deny the intellect of its power to act on the environment just as paralysis of a limb would frustrate volition. If the brain could be cured, then the intellect would again be able to act. The list of causes of brain damage sometimes stretched imagination including the idea expressed by Rush that booksellers could become deranged because of "frequent and rapid transition of the mind from one subject to another" (5).

Caplan summarizes the idea of moral treatment as:

This malleability of the brain surface was at one its greatest asset and its gravest danger. Proper habits and training and a regular, health life could nurture goodness and sanity. On the other hand, an injudicious upbringing, vicious habits, or injuries and shocks could produce a dissolute or unstable character.

The essence of moral treatment was the belief that, because of this great malleability of the brain surface, because of its susceptibility to environmental stimuli, pathological conditions could be erased or modified by corrective experience. Therefore, insanity, whether the result of direct or indirect injury or disease, or of overwrought emotions or strained intellectual facilities, would be cured in almost every case. (2, p. 9)

Moral treatment was especially strong from approximately 1840 to 1880. After that time, a number of problems arose and doomed the concept (6). The first problem was the expense of building and maintaining asylums. Although ordinally a success story, treating the mentally ill in asylums rather than jails, almshouses, private homes, and the offices of general practitioners became so expensive that local and state governments did not want to provide funds. Second, moral management depended on lay and professional cooperation to provide a "correct" social atmosphere. The ideas of moral treatment in the United States were strongly influenced by middle-class values of persons from Northern European backgrounds. As immigrants from other cultures arrived and criminals, alcoholics, and paupers were placed in the asylums, the mix of patients changed. When these patients did not respond to the existing milieu, regimentation and mechanical restraints began to replace the trust and persuasion used in moral management. Third, the laws designed to help the mentally ill became the instruments against them. Many laws were enacted quickly without their long-range impact considered. The laws resulted in regulations that destroyed the atmosphere and environment necessary to maintain moral management. Fourth, the idea the moral treatment could cure all insanity was oversold to the public. Moral treatment worked when the patient–staff ratio was low. As moral treatment failed under the influx of large numbers of patients, public confidence also failed. New administrators felt the need to try new approaches. Fifth, as insanity was increasing classified as a disease, the role of the medical doctor increased as the role of laypersons decreased. Theories based on medical doctrines overtook nonmedical approaches. Moral treatment had developed as an antimedical approach by laypersons not trained in medicine. As the asylums began to be run by doctor–administrators who had been trained in the "new" medical theories based on physiological causes of mental illness rather than psychosocial causes, the role of laypersons decreased.

In spite of the demise of moral management as a treatment approach, the ideas did not die. Most arose again in the new disciplines of nursing, social work, and occupational therapy. The beliefs and values found in humanitarianism, humanism, holism, habits and order in daily life, environmental influences, and intrinsic motivation all were reassembled into the three new professions. In particular, occupational therapy would focus on the habit and order of daily life occupation.

PRAGMATISM

Pragmatism was developed by Charles Sanders Peirce (1839–1914), an American philosopher, but its best-known theorist was William James (1842–1910), an American philosopher and psychologist. The major assumption of pragmatism is the emphasis on interpreting ideas through their consequences. McGill (7) summarizes Peirce's major assumption as follows: the meaning of any proposition could always be found in some particular sequence of future practical experience. In other words, the meaning of a proposition is its logical (or physical) consequence.

Pragmatism is from the Greek word *pragma* meaning a thing done, an act, or work (8). The term pragmatic was first used by Immanuel Kant (1724–1804), a German philosopher, who tried to distinguish the practical, which relates to the will and action, from the pragmatic, which relates to the consequences.

Pragmatism was a philosophy applied widely to education. Its best-known proponent was John Dewey (1859–1952), an American philosopher and educator. His ideas form much of the basis for public education in the United States. Tracy (9) refers to Dewey (10) regarding the definition and use of occupation in her first chapter "Studies in Invalid Occupations." Pragmatism proposed that knowledge and truth must related to practice, action, and doing. Angeles summarized the key assumptions (8). Knowledge was to be based on experience and practical effort not just from reading books and listening to other people talk. Knowledge should be learned so it could be used to solve the problems of everyday life and to help people adapt to the environment. Ideas must be referenced to their consequences, results, or use to determine their truth and meaning.

Truth was viewed as that which had practical value in our life experiences. Truth was to serve as an instrument or means to attain our goals and to serve our ability to predict and arrange the future for our use. Thus, truth was considered to be changing and tentative as new or different situations and events occurred. The meaning of truth depended on the practical uses to which the idea could be put and the practical consequences stemming from the idea.

Pragmatism is the basis for the concept of "learning by doing" in occupational therapy. Also important is the idea of teaching and learning knowledge and skills useful in the person's living environment. Usefulness is determined by experience, not idealism.

THE ARTS AND CRAFTS MOVEMENT

Hall says the "modern Arts and Crafts idea appealed very strongly, because of the growing interest in the movement and because of the clean, wholesome atmosphere which surrounds such work, and because of the many-sided appeal which such a work as the making of pottery, for instance has to most education minds" (11). The Arts and Crafts Movement began in England with the ideas of John Ruskin, an art and social critic, who felt the Industrial Revolution was not a step forward but a step backwards in civilization because many of the goods made by factories were of poorer quality than those made by hand (12). The psychiatrist Adolf Meyer refers to the problem in 1921: "[t]he man of today has lost the capacity and pride of workmanship and has substituted for it a measure in terms of money; and now his money proves to be of uncertain value" (13).

Although Ruskin stated the philosophy, it was his pupil William Morris who put the ideals into practice. Morris became well-known for his art design and social commentary although his training was in architecture (14). Newton, George Barton's secretary, refers to Morris in reporting a comment made by people as they entered Barton's home: "As people enter they invariably exclaim, 'This looks like home!' And so it does, due to Mr. Barton's belief (and practice) in the tenet of his old master, William Morris, that 'your home should contain only what you know to be useful, and believe to be beautiful' " (15).

In America, the Arts and Crafts Movement was known for eight ideas: design unity, joy in labor, individualism, regionalism, social responsibility, consistency and order, simplicity, and home and hearth (family and fireplace) (16, 17). Design unity refers to the geometric forms based primarily on Gothic design—Ruskin's favorite—which included unembellished structure and natural materials using nature themes of birds and flowers, based on simplicity of function and honest structure. Objects were to be made in which form and structure followed function. Joy of labor was based on the idea that the work of the individual was to be valued. In community living projects work was also expected.

Individualism provided support for diverse attitudes, contradictions in how life should be lived, and originality in design and product. Regionalism shaped the style, image, and use of materials. Social responsibility supported the idea that art and work should benefit the community. Consistency and order are seen in the geometric design and applied to life as a morale principle. Such beatitudes as "cleanliness is next to godliness" were common.

Home and hearth were stressed because the leaders of the Arts and Crafts Movement believed that industrialism, in addition to ruining workmanship, had also shattered the family, bringing rootlessness and loss of traditions. All could be restored or regained by emphasizing family life in which the mother stayed home to care for the children and everyone gathered around the hearth as the center of family life.

The Arts and Crafts Movement was in full bloom during the formative years of occupational therapy in the United States, but the influence of this movement diminished after World War I. Industrialism was recognized as a major factor in providing goods to a growing nation and product quality was rapidly improving.

THE INFLUENCE OF THE QUAKERS

Occupational therapists owe the Quakers a debt of gratitude for promoting many of the ideas and ideals accepted as basic and essential to the practice of occupational therapy. This section is a short review of some of the more relevant ideas the Quakers contributed by their efforts to improve conditions for the treatment and care of the mentally ill.

The Quakers became concerned with conditions in institutions for the mentally ill in 1790 when a member, Hannah Mills, was admitted to the Asylum for the

Insane in York, England and died 6 weeks later. No one had been permitted to visit her, and her sudden death made members of the Yorkshire Friends suspicious about possible mistreatment. As a result of the incident, one member, William Tuke (1732–1822), decided to establish an asylum for the care of Quaker members. He open the York Retreat in 1796.

Tuke wanted the care to encompass more than a medical approach. He viewed mental illness as a disruption of the mind and spirit in addition to the body. The term "moral" was used to refer to emotional and spiritual experiences in the eighteenth and nineteenth centuries. Thus, the treatment became known as moral treatment. Tuke want his staff to recognize that mentally ill persons still retained their spiritual worth and at least some degree of reason in spite of their illness. He felt that treatment should always recognize the person's essential humanity.

The idea of humane treatment resulted in less frequent bleedings and purgings by the medical staff. "Instead they instituted a regime of exercise, work, and amusements that treated patients like sane adults who were expected to behave according to basic societal norms. Patients were to remain neatly clothed, preform chores in a responsible manner, eat politely at the table, and sit quietly at religious services." Tuke and the staff believed that recovery in an atmosphere removed from the stresses of daily life could help a mentally ill person return to normal (18). However, even when a cure was not possible, Tuke and his staff believed that moral treatment was important to help the patients "live at the highest level of humanity possible for them" (19).

In 1813, Samuel Tuke, the founder's grandson, published a book titled *The Description of the Retreat Near York*. The book was published in the United States as well as in England. American Quakers became aware of the care and treatment proposed by Tuke and began visiting the York Retreat. On their return to the United States, the Quakers decided to start a similar institute outside Philadelphia in Frankford, Pennsylvania. The Asylum for the Relief of Friends Deprived of their Reason was established in 1817. The name was usually shorted to the Friends Asylum (Friend is the name Quakers used to refer to all other Quakers), and the concept of moral treatment was adopted. Early advocates of moral treatment felt that if the a mentally ill person could be treated using moral treatment early in his or her illness, the person could be restored to health. Thus, family members were more willing to place a person in the Friends Asylum or a similar institution.

Actually, the Quakers of Philadelphia had been active in providing care for the mentally ill many years before the Friends Asylum opened. As early as 1709, there is a report of the Quakers' interest in helping the insane. This concern, along with a petition drive led by Benjamin Franklin, led to the establishment of the Pennsylvania Hospital for the Insane in 1756 (2). The Asylum was located in the basement of the Pennsylvania Hospital, which had been started in 1751, and the first physician was Benjamin Rush, considered the father of American psychiatry. Gamwell and Tomes state that after the physicians made their rounds, patients could go outside for a walk, read a book, or play games. The hospital provided a bowling alley, a calisthenics room, a miniature railroad, and a museum. After lunch there were carriage rides in the city park, exercise classes, and sporting events. In the evening there were lectures, lantern slide entertainment, concerts, and even dances. Furthermore, patients were trained to work on the farm or in other activities designed to give them a sense of self-worth and permit them to contribute to society (19).

Public institutions for the insane, the term used to refer to the mentally ill in those days, followed the lead of the Quakers and established programs based on moral treatment. Exercise, work, and amusements were included in the daily schedule. By 1850 the use of moral treatment was well established in the institutions serving the mentally ill in the United States. Many of the founders of the Association of Medical Superintendents of American Institutions for the Insane (later the American Psychiatric Association) provided moral treatment in their institutions. One such founder was Pliny Earle at the Bloomingdale Asylum in New York. Unfortunately, in the 1870s, the population in the institutions began to overwhelm the staff.

Another Quaker, Moses Sheppard, was also involved in the care of the mentally ill. In 1857 he left his entire estate of $571,440 to build the Sheppard Asylum (20). Because only the interest was to be used, many years passed by before the hospital was opened in 1891. Five years later, Enoch Pratt left 1 million dollars to the hospital, which then became known by its present name, the Sheppard and Enoch Pratt Hospital. Sheppard specified that "courteous treatment and comfort of all patients" was to given first consideration (20). In 1895, Dr. William Rush Dunton Jr. came to the hospital as a new psychiatrist. Dunton became a founder of the National Society for the Promotion of Occupational Therapy based on his experiences at the hospital.

MENTAL HYGIENE MOVEMENT

The mental hygiene movement formally began on February 19, 1909 when Clifford Beers, a layperson, started the National Committee for Mental Hygiene (NCMH) with the help of Adolph Meyer and William James (21). Beers had been hospitalized for mental illness (probably bipolar disorder), and he felt that patients were mistreated and conditions in the hospitals were poor. The previous year, 1908, he published a book about his experiences titled *A Mind That Found Itself,* which is a classic and has been republished numerous times. Beers wanted the NCMH to work for better conditions in the institutions for the mentally ill, but Meyer suggested that the purpose be broadened to focus on helping people find better ways of living healthy lives, preventing mental illness, and better handling of mental illness that did occur.

Although the NCMH was a national organization with chapters in many states, the primary connection to occupational therapy was through the Illinois chapter.

The Illinois Society for Mental Hygiene began working in 1909 in Chicago but was formally incorporated in the spring of 1910 (22). Its objectives were as follows:

> To cooperate with the public and private agencies in improving the conditions of the insane; to aid in the aftercare of patients discharged from the hospitals for the insane; to secure data regarding social conditions provocative of mental breakdown; to publish and circulate information which may help to avoiding mental disease, and to carry on any other proper work tending to secure and conserve the mental health of men, women, and children, and to enlist the interest and cooperation of others therein.

This wide-ranging mandate provided a number of opportunities but Thompson (22) reported at the founding meeting of the National Society for the Promotion of Occupational Therapy that the primary efforts were toward the prevention of mental breakdown and special attention to social service. In the later capacity, Thomson said that physicians were referring persons and some persons were self-referring for occupation. For example, Thompson quoted a referral in the following: "This patient is not a subject for commitment nor is institutional care of any kind indicated. Patient would doubtless be greatly benefited by congenial employment in a good environment" (p. 397).

Although some persons apparently were placed in regular industry jobs, many could not be placed even though they seemed to have the capacity to work. Thompson said, "it was apparent that what was needed, from both a therapeutic and an economic standpoint, and must be furnished if we were to be of any real help" (p. 397). She then related a case report of an older woman in her sixties who, in 1913, needed employment and through the help of the Illinois Society began making quilts to sell. Thus, the woman became self-supporting. This case sparked the idea of helping other persons with mental or physical handicaps to become independent. Two philanthropic women provided $5,000 to begin a program in 1914. In 1915 Eleanor Clarke Slagle was hired based on her experience at Phipps Clinic, Johns Hopkins Hospital, Baltimore. Slagle had previously lived in Chicago and trained at the Chicago School of Civics and Philanthropy; thus, she was familiar with the Chicago area. Finding a location to carry out the program was initially a constant problem; finally, Hull House, a settlement house in Chicago, provided the use of workshop space. Thus began the relationship of the Illinois Society of Mental Hygiene and the well-known settlement house. Slagle said that to avoid the problem of distinguishing between physical and mental cases, the workrooms were simply called "Workrooms for the Handicapped" (23).

During the first year of operation, 1915/16, 77 individuals were seen and 61 were apparently helped (22). Occupations included needlework, knitting, rug weaving, basketry, decorating word and tin, ornamental cement work, simple cabinet-making, building doll furniture, and making wooden toys. Goods sold amounted to $2,211.51, of which $1,356.95 was paid to the workers.

At the same time, a school for training teachers of occupational therapy was started (23). Originally, the workshop and school were known simply as the Experimental Station, but in 1917 the school became known as the Henry B. Favill School of Occupations (24), named for Dr. Favill, who had been first Vice President of the Illinois Society for Mental Hygiene and an officer in the National Society for Mental Hygiene (25). Also in 1917, the state of Illinois created a Department of Occupational Therapy in the Department of Public Welfare (26) to operate a school of occupations. Because Slagle already had started a school, the state hired her to be the director. The workshop part of the Experimental Station was acquired in the bargain. Thus, the formal connection to the Illinois Society of Mental Health was severed.

The other major connection between occupational therapy and the mental hygiene movement was through physicians who were supporters of occupational therapy and who served in various capacities with the NCMH: Thomas W. Salmon, Frankwood E. Williams, and Adolph Meyer. Dr. Salmon (1876–1927) was hired in 1912 as Director of Special Studies for NCMH and also served as Medical Director. His connection to occupational therapy began in 1917 when he wrote an extensive article (27) on the treatment of war neuroses; this article outlined the need for re-education (pp. 524–525, 534–535).

Dr. Williams was the Associate Medical Director of the NCMH when he wrote about the treatment of mental patients in the Army (28) and discussed the involvement of occupational therapy (pp. 281–282). He gave a more detailed address (29) at the third annual meeting of the National Society for the Promotion of Occupational Therapy.

Dr. Meyer (1866–1950) was an advisor and founding member of NCMH. His major contribution to occupational therapy was his address to the fifth annual meeting, which was published as the first article in the journal *Archives of Occupational Therapy,* started in 1922. Dr. Meyer's article "Philosophy of Occupation Therapy" (30) is considered a classic in occupational therapy literature because it states the first conceptual model of occupational therapy. The second article by Slagle (31) describes a practice model.

THE SETTLEMENT HOUSES

The settlement houses in the United States were patterned after Toynbee Hall in London, England, founded by Canon Samuel A. Barnett. Jane Addams, cofounder of Hull House, is quoted as saying, "It is a community for University men who live there, have their recreation and clubs and society all among the poor people, yet in the same style they would live in their own circle" (32). In other words, settlement houses provided a neighborhood center that included the opportunity for discussion and conversation between two classes of people; such discussion brought rewards to both classes.

In 1889 Hull House was founded in Chicago by Jane Addams and Ellen Gates Starr (32). The stated purpose was "[t]o provide a center for a higher civic and social life, to institute and maintain educational and philanthropic enterprises, and to investigate and improve the conditions in the industrial districts of Chicago" (33).

Although Hull House was not the first settlement house in the United States—the first was in New York City—Hull House rapidly became the most famous. Fame, however, is not the connection between Hull House and occupational therapy. Members of Hull House were involved in four activities that related to the development of occupational therapy. The support of the mental hygiene movement has already been discussed. The Chicago Arts and Crafts Society (34) was formed and met at Hull House.

The third activity was the Hull-House Labor Museum, which started in 1900 so that young people working in neighborhood factories could see through demonstrations provided by their parents and grandparents "a dramatic representation of the inherited resources of their daily occupation . . . Young people could actually see that the complicated machinery of the factory had been evolved from simple tools" (35). Addams hoped the young people could better see the connection between their work and that of their parents, and that the parents or grandparents would feel their knowledge and skills were still of value.

The first curator of the Hull-House Labor Museum was Jessie Luther (36), an arts and crafts instructor. On leaving Hull House, she went to work for Herbert J. Hall at the Delver Mansion in Marble Head, Massachusetts (37), and then she went to the Rhode Island Hospital. In 1918, she enlisted for an overseas position as an occupational therapy aide. Later, she became recognized as an occupational therapist and worked at Butler Hospital in Providence, Rhode Island.

The fourth and most important activity was the participation in the classes offered for training of attendants of the insane. The sponsor of the classes was another settlement house in Chicago called the Chicago Commons, which ran the Chicago School of Civics and Philanthropy (originally Chicago Institute of Social Science) (38). The leader of the Chicago Commons was Graham Taylor. In the summer of 1908, Julia Lathrop, who lived at Hull House, offered a class for attendants of the insane at the Chicago School of Civics and Philanthropy. Lathrop was a member of the Illinois State Board of Charities and had been "appalled at the ignorance of employees in the state hospitals and poorhouse" (38, p. 170). Her training course was designed to teach the attendants that custodial care was not the answer and that they should be using games, arts, crafts, and hobbies. The first course had 24 students. The complete 5-week course is outlined in the 20th Biennial Report of the Board of Public Charities of the State of Illinois (39). Eleanor Clarke Slagle, a founding member of the profession, was a member of the fourth graduating class in 1911 (40).

MANUAL TRAINING

In 1910 Kidner (41), a founder of the NSPOT, in his book *Educational Handwork* wrote:

> The time has passed when the necessary of providing for the training of the hands of the children in our schools has to be insisted on . . . (It) has been found to be of immense benefit as a means of general cultural of the facilities. Eye hand, head and heart are engaged, and the results fully justify the expectations of the advocates of this form of school work.
>
> The acquisition of dexterity and skill of hand; the training of the eye to a sense of form and beauty; the formation of habits of accuracy, order and neatness; the inculcation of a love of industry and of habits of patients, perseverance and self-reliance, are some of the results which may be claimed as peculiarly belonging to work with the hands as a means of education. (p. 9)

Educational handwork was better known as manual training. In the foreword to the book, Robertson states that "Educational Handwork helps to preserve and develop the love of manual labor and to foster the habit of being happy at lessons in school" (41, p. iii). Actually, as Lears (42) states, the rationale was a business proposition. Manual training provided the skills needed in factory work. To businessmen, using the public schools to train workers made good sense.

The arts and crafts proponents were also quick to support the concept of manual training. Students could be taught to appreciate the aesthetics and good taste of well-designed articles while learning the technical skills to produce them. The result would be a complete child who would be a competent worker (43).

John Dewey (44) was also a supporter of manual training. However, he warned:

> [T]hese occupations in the school shall not be mere practical devices or modes of routine employment, the gaining of better technical skill . . . but active centers of scientific insight into natural materials and processes, point of departure whence children shall be led out into a realization of the historic development of man . . . It is through occupations determined by this environment that mankind has made its historical and political progress. It is through these occupations that the intellectual and emotion interpretation of nature has been developed. It is through what we do in and with the world that read its meaning and measure its value. (p. 19)

Dewey saw in manual training the opportunity to teach children about their world and their living environment. This emphasis on intellect rather than on technical skill separated Dewey from the businessmen who wanted a vocational training program in the schools.

Although the manual training movement started with children, it soon was expanded to include adults (42). In 1916, Kidner became Vocational Secretary of the Canadian Military Hospitals Commission (45). His job was to provide occupational work for men being treated in convalescent hospitals. Manual training, re-named as occupational work, became a means of preventing idleness and providing functional or therapeutic re-education and vocational re-education.

Another person knowledgeable about manual training was Rabbi Emil Hirsch. Hirsch was also a member of the State Board of Control in Illinois and, just as Lathrop, was shocked by the idleness he saw on the wards of the state hospitals. According to Dunton (46), he was involved in the course given at the Chicago School of Civics and Philanthropy in 1908. He was also the founder of the Manual Training School of Chicago in 1888 (47) and thus familiar with the concepts of manual training. However, his exact influence on the course of manual training is not clear.

Determining the exact impact of manual training on the development of occupational therapy is difficult to pinpoint because of the overlap with the influence of the arts and crafts movement. The primary focus of manual training was on vocational preparation in spite of Dewey's attempts to focus on intellectual ideas. Skills in mechanical drawing, design, and construction were emphasized in manual training, and these skills do appear in outlines of early educational programs (48, 49).

REHABILITATION EQUIPMENT

The use of occupational therapy in physical rehabilitation started slowly during World War I. The term occupational therapy does not appear until 1918, but the concepts of occupational therapy under the labels of re-education, therapeutic work, and curative workshops began in France in 1914, Great Britain in 1915, Canada in 1916, and the United States in 1918 (50, 51).

Measurement systems including goniometry and dynamometry began during this time. Examples appear in McKenzie (52, 53, 54) and Baldwin (54). McKenzie was a physical educator, and Baldwin was a psychologist who was hired to start occupational therapy at Walter Reed Hospital in Washington, DC. The goniometers MacKenzie used are similar to the ones used today but were called fleximeters (52, p. 187). Those in Baldwin (54) are a bit cumbersome by today's standards but probably just as accurate (54). The dynamometers were either squeeze-bag type (52, p. 189) or strain gauges (54, pp. 24–25). The board for measuring and stretching finger abduction could be used today (53, p. 71). Other equipment such as the arm table were functional but a bit large for most clinics today (53). Baldwin shows several examples of treadle sewing machines adapted for lathes, grinders, and saws (54). Adapted handles made from dental modeling wax are shown for saws and other woodworking tools.

Much of the equipment illustrated in the McKenzie texts and Baldwin monograph was developed at Hart House, a building appropriated by the Military Hospitals Commission for rehabilitation of soldiers at the University of Toronto. Edward A. Bott, the designer and builder, worked in the Department of Psychology of the University of Toronto (55, 56). His work was based on that of Jules Amar (57, 58), a physiologist in Paris who had been developing instruments for the measurement and rehabilitation of war injuries since 1915 and that of Shepard Ivory Franz, a psychologist at St. Elizabeth Hospital in Washington, DC, who was interested in measurement. Franz is mentioned in the writings of Bott (59) and Bowman (60). In the United States, the measurement and treatment of physical disabilities was discussed as metrotherapy (61) and mechanotherapy (59).

Baldwin also provides the first comprehensive analysis of tools and appliances used in various occupations according to the body joints affected (54). Some tools suitable for ward occupations that worked the fingers and thumb include clippers, pliers, scissors, eyelet punch, leather tools, typewriter, carving tools, rake (knitting), knitting needles, braid mat frame, bead loom, belt loom, Persian rug loom, tapestry loom, braid loom, and crotchet hook (p. 54).

As the previous paragraphs illustrate, the concepts of measurement and the equipment used in rehabilitation were developed by persons outside the field of occupational therapy. The concepts of measurement came from psychology while the concepts for equipment came from engineering. Occupational therapy was added to the rehabilitation aspects originally to provide a means of "keeping the patient's mind off himself" (62, p. 188) and to provide vocational training.

SUMMARY

The development and application of occupational therapy has been influenced by many social movements and philosophic beliefs and values. This chapter has reviewed a few of the more significant movements and viewpoints. Beginning with moral treatment in the 1800s through World War I, ideas about using occupation as a therapeutic medium were formed and shaped. These formative ideas continue to provide the base of practice today.

References

1. Greenblatt M. Foreword. In: Caplan RB. Psychiatry and the Community in Nineteenth-Century America: The Recurring Concern with the Environment in the Prevention and Treatment of Mental Illness. New York: Basic Books, 1969:viii.
2. Caplan RB. Background and theory of moral treatment. In: Caplan RB. Psychiatry and the Community in Nineteenth-Century America: The Recurring Concern with the Environment in the Prevention and Treatment of Mental Illness. New York: Basic Books, 1969.
3. Hunter R, Macalpine I. Three Hundred Years of Psychiatry, 1535–1860. London: Oxford University Press, 1963:960.
4. Reese WL. Dictionary of Philosophy and Religion: Eastern and Western Thought. Atlanta Highlands, NJ: Humanities Press, 1980.
5. Rush B. Medical Inquiries and Observations upon the Diseases of the Mind. New York: Hafner Publishing, 1962. (Originally published in 1812.)
6. Caplan R. Factors in the change from moral treatment to custodial care: an overview. In: Caplan R. Psychiatry and the Community in Nineteenth-Century America: The Re-

curring Concern with the Environment in the Prevention and Treatment of Mental Illness. New York: Basic Books, 1969.

7. McGill VJ. Pragmatism. In: Runes DD. Dictionary of Philosophy: Ancient, Medieval, Modern. Totowa, NJ: Littlefield, Adams & Co., 1980.

8. Angeles PA. Pragmatism. In: Angeles PA. Dictionary of Philosophy. New York: Barnes & Noble, 1981.

9. Tracy SE. Methods of teaching. In: Tracy SE. Studies in Invalid Occupations. Boston: Whitcomb & Barrows, 1910:13. (Reprinted by Arno Press, New York, 1980.)

10. Dewey J. The psychology of occupation. In: Dewey J. The School and Society. Chicago: The University of Chicago Press, 1900. (Reprinted in 1990.)

11. Hall HJ. The systematic use of work as a remedy in neurasthenia and allied conditions. Boston Med Surg J 1905;CLII(2):29–32.

12. Ruskin J. The nature of Gothic. In: Ruskin J. The Stones of Venice. New York: DaCapo Press, 1988. (First published in 1853.)

13. Meyer A. The philosophy of occupation therapy. Arch Occup Ther 1922;1(1):8.

14. Stansky P. Redesigning the World: William Morris, the 1880s, and the Arts and Crafts. Princeton, NJ: Princeton University Press, 1985.

15. Newton I. Consolation House. Trained Nurse Hosp Rev 1917;59:321–326.

16. Cummings E, Kaplan W. The Arts and Crafts Movement. London: Thames and Hudson, 1991.

17. Kaplan W. "The Art That Is Life": The Arts and Crafts Movement in America, 1875–1920. Boston: Museum of Fine Arts, 1989.

18. Baxter WE, Hathcox DW. America's Care of the Mentally Ill: A Photographic History. Washington, DC: American Psychiatric Press, 1994.

19. Gamwell L, Tomes N. Madness in America: Cultural and Medical Perceptions of Mental Illness before 1914. Ithaca, NY: Cornell University Press/SUNY, Binghamton, 1995.

20. Forbush B, Forbush B. Gatehouse: The Evolution of the Sheppard and Enoch Pratt Hospital, 1853–1986. Baltimore: The Sheppard and Enoch Pratt Hospital, 1986.

21. Grob GN. The mental hygiene movement. In: Grob GN. Mental Illness and American Society, 1875–1940. Princeton, NJ: Princeton University Press, 1987:144–178.

22. Thomson EE. Occupation and its relation to mental hygiene. The Modern Hospital 1917;8:397–398.

23. Slagle EC. Occupational therapy. New York (State) Conference of Charities and Correction (Proceedings: New York State Welfare Conference) 1919;19:121–135.

24. Monroe AH. Tributes and resolutions: the Henry B. Favill School of Occupations. In: Favill J. Henry Baird Favill, 1860–1916. Chicago: Rand McNally, 1917:87–88.

25. Deaths: Henry Baird Favill, M.D. J Am Med Assoc 1916;LXVI(9):671.

26. Slagle EC. The department of occupational therapy. Institutional Quarterly 1919; 10:29–32.

27. Salmon TW. The care and treatment of mental diseases and war neuroses ("shell shock") in the British army. Mental Hygiene 197;1(4):509–547.

28. Williams FE. Treatment of mental patients in the general hospitals of the United States Army. Proceedings of the American Medico Psychological Association 1919;26:271–286.

29. Williams FE. [Untitled]. In: Proceedings of the Third Annual Meeting of the National Society for the Promotion of Occupational Therapy. Towson, MD: NSPOT, 1919: 101–107.

30. Meyer A. Philosophy of occupation therapy. Arch Occup Ther 1922;1(1):1–10.
31. Slagle EC. Training aids for mental patients. Arch Occup Ther 1922;1(1):11–17.
32. Davis AF, McCree ML. Eighty Years at Hull-House. Chicago: Quadrangle Books, 1969.
33. Davis AF, McCree ML. Hull-House Year Book: Forty-Second Year, 1931.
34. Davis AF, McCree ML. Chicago Arts and Crafts Society. Hull-House Bulletin 1897; II(8):9.
35. Addams J. Twenty Years at Hull-House with Autobiographic Notes. New York: Macmillian, 1945:236.
36. Luther J. The Labor Museum at Hull House. The Commons 1902;7(May):1–12.
37. Luther J. Beginnings of occupational therapy at Rhode Island Hospital. Rhode Island Med J 1943;26(March):47–48.
38. Wade LC. Chicago School of Civics and Philanthropy. In: Wade LC. Graham Taylor: Pioneer for Social Justice. Chicago: University of Chicago Press, 1964:161–185.
39. Wade LC. Nursing and attendance for the insane. In: 20th Biennial Report of the Board of Public Charities of the State of Illinois, July 1, 1906–June 30, 1908. Springfield, IL: Illinois State Journal Co., 1909:56–60.
40. Loomis B, Wade BD. Occupational Therapy Beginning: Hull House, The Henry B. Favill School of Occupations and Eleanor Clarke Slagle. Washington, DC: United States Public Health Service, Allied Health (Grant No. 50579-01), 1973.
41. Kidner TB. Educational Handwork. Toronto: Educational Book Co., 1910.
42. Lears TJJ. No Place of Grace: Antimoderism and the Transformation of American Culture: 1880–1920. New York: Pantheon Books, 1981.
43. Boris E. Schooling taste: art and manual training in the public schools. In: Boris E. Art and Labor: Ruskin, Morris, and the Craftsman Ideal in America. Philadelphia: Temple University Press, 1985:82–98.
44. Dewey J. The school and social progress. In: Dewey J. The School and Society. Chicago: University of Chicago Press, 1990. (Originally published in 1900.)
45. Dewey J. Vocational training for disabled Canadian soldiers. Mod Hosp 1917;8:424.
46. Dunton WR. Historical. In: Dunton WR. Occupation Therapy. Philadelphia: Saunders, 1915:15–16.
47. Hirsch DE. Rabbi Emil G Hirsch: The Reform Advocate. Northbrook, IL: Whitehall Co., 1968.
48. Newman C. Occupation therapy. Manual Train Mag 19:245–247, 1918.
49. Newman C. A forward step in the education of occupational therapists. Occup Ther Rehabil 1931;10:204–206.
50. McKenzie RT. Physical remedies, re-education, and work. In: Fox RF. Physical Remedies for Disabled Soldiers. London: Bailliere, Tindall and Cox, 1917:194–236.
51. Baldwin BT. Helping the wounded soldier to "come back." Mod Hosp 1919; 12:370–374.
52. McKenzie RT. The physical clinic. In: Fox RF. Physical Remedies for Disabled Soldiers. London: Bailliere, Tindall and Cox, 1917:177–193.
53. McKenzie RT. Active movement and re-education. In: McKenzie RT. Reclaiming the Maimed: A Handbook of Physical Therapy. New York: Macmillian, 1918:65–104.
54. Baldwin B. Occupational Therapy Applied to Restoration of Function of Disabled Joint. Washington, DC: Surgeon General of the Army, 1919 (Walter Reed Monograph).
55. Bott EA. Reeducation work for soldiers. Mod Hosp 1917;9:293–294.

56. Bott EA. Functional training. Mod Hosp 1917;9:365–366.
57. Amar J. Organization of vocational training for war cripples. Am J Care Crippled 1916;3:177–183.
58. Amar J. Le psychographe comme instrument de mesure des incapacites de travail. Arch Occup Ther 1922;1(4):255–264. English translation: Amar J. The psychograph as an instrument to measure working capacity. Arch Occup Ther 1922;1(4):265–267.
59. Bott E. Mechanotherapy. Am J Orth Sur 1918;6:441–446.
60. Bowman E. The importance of measurement of movement in orthopedic cases. Arch Occup Ther 1922;1(4):279–280.
61. Albee FH, Gilliland AR. Metrotherapy, or the measurement of voluntary movement. J Am Med Assoc 1920;75(15):983–986.
62. Albee FH. A Surgeon's Fight to Rebuild Men: An Autobiography. New York: EP Dutton & Co., 1943.

CHAPTER 3

Assumptions Inherent in Occupational Therapy

Assumptions are statements of belief that are accepted as true and are necessary to build theoretical and practice models. The assumptions discussed in this chapter are a synthesis of beliefs and values drawn from the models mentioned in section IV and from other models of occupational therapy. Occupational therapy models are drawn primarily from the organismic paradigm, which is further discussed in chapter 13. Therefore, the assumptions center around the ability of humans to take charge and be responsible for individual lives and actions. Occupational therapy is not the only profession based on the organismic paradigm. Nursing and social work, for example, also use the organismic paradigm. Therefore, not all of the assumptions discussed are unique to occupational therapy. In fact, only the assumptions about occupation may be considered unique. The other assumptions are what permit occupational therapy practitioners to work as team members to plan a total program for an individual, not just an occupational therapy program. Unless there are commonalities of thought among team members, working together would be difficult. Certain assumptions must be common, or at least fairly common, to facilitate program development and planning. The most basic assumptions are concerned with the nature of people as human beings.

ASSUMPTIONS ABOUT HUMAN BEINGS

The authors propose that there are six assumptions about people that relate to occupational therapy. First is that a person is a biopsychological and spiritual being; that is, a person functions through the interrelation of biological, psychological, sociological, and spiritual factors. Each of the factors affects the person's being. Biology through the life process affects structure and function, as well as pattern and organization. Further, there is a sequential process of growth and development from birth to death, and it is unidirectional. Growth and development continue to progress regardless of how many problems are encountered along the way. Finally, a person exists in a group of meaningful others. In other words, a person lives in society.

A second assumption is the view that a person is a unified whole. In other words, the person functions as a gestalt whose total is greater than the sum of the parts. Also, the entire person—not just certain parts—functions all of the time. The person's behavior is synergistic or a total response of the whole person, not just a response of a portion of the person. Furthermore, a person interacts in the environment as a total being and not a part. Finally, all behavior of a person is meaningful if the total person and the environment are understood. Conversely then, there is no such thing as meaningless behavior. The person and the person's behavior may be difficult to understand, but it always has some meaning.

The third assumption states that a person is an open system energy unit. As such, a constant interchange of energy occurs between the person and the environment. Because of the interaction, a person is affected by and can change the environment. In turn, the environment is affected by and can cause change in the person. The ability to change, however, permits a person to adapt to different environments and to achieve a balance between using and conserving personal energy in relating to the environment. Thus, a person can learn to conserve energy through organizing the tasks to be done—work simplification —or a person can waste energy through failure to organize, plan ahead, and prioritize tasks.

The fourth assumption is concerned with a person's capacity for thought and sensation. Thought is composed of language, imagery, and abstraction. Sensation in this case refers to perception, feeling, and emotions. The assumption that thought and sensation exist becomes most important when dealing with persons who either have not developed language or have lost it. Language, verbal or non-verbal, is the principal means by which another person can learn about a person's imagery, abstraction, perceptions, feelings, and emotions.

The fifth assumption is that a person has needs. More important, each person develops a unique pattern to meet these needs. Regardless of the pattern, however, each person has a priority for his or her individual needs. The environment, through society, influences the behavior adopted in meeting the needs. At the same time, society attempts to ensure that needs will be met by sanctifying a variety of occupations. Thus, a person's behavior and society can function together to meet the individual's needs, or they can function in conflict. When conflict is involved, the person may find that society will attempt to alter his or her behavior through various means, such as education, correction, rehabilitation, restriction, or some combination of these methods.

That a person has responsibilities is the sixth assumption. Society expects a person to decide what he or she wishes to become and to choose the methods to attain these goals within social sanctions. Each position or role that a person selects or accepts in society has a set of expectations or responsibilities for the person to fulfill. Because a person may occupy several positions and roles at the same time, the responsibilities may be compounded. Furthermore, responsibilities, as well as positions and roles, are inherent in all occupations.

ASSUMPTIONS ABOUT OCCUPATIONAL PERFORMANCE

The next set of assumptions is concerned with how humans use, relate to, and are affected by occupations. Performance is also called competence in some conceptual models.

First, each individual must perform some occupations or have the occupations performed by another in order to survive. The most crucial occupations to survival are those involved in supporting life functions, surviving, and belonging. The occupations, thus, are concerned with the maintenance of the self as an individual entity. Occupational therapy practitioners have referred to such self-maintenance occupations as activities of daily living or self-care skills.

Second, all occupations may be performed by one person, or different persons may perform some occupations (division of labor). A person may try to perform alone all the occupations needed to function and survive as an individual, or some occupations may be shared with others. Some people, such as hermits and loners, try to survive alone. However, most people prefer to divide up the occupations so that some occupations are performed by the individual while others are performed for the individual in the form of goods and services.

Third, a person adapts or adjusts (grows and develops) through the use of and participation in various occupations. Occupations are naturally occurring events for all living organisms because they support life and permit or promote adaptation to the environment. Furthermore, they facilitate growth and development through learning and mastery.

Fourth, through the performance of occupations, a person may adapt to the environment or adapt the environment to him or herself. Occupations provide a person with a choice of changing the self to meet external environmental requirements for adaptive behavior or changing the external environment to accommodate individual requirements for adaptive behavior. The actual choice is influenced by a process of problem-solving.

Fifth, the occupations a person learns and is able to perform or has performed determine the degree to which that person is able to adapt. A person who can perform a number of occupations with mastery and competence increases the opportunity to adapt successfully to the external environment. Adaptation is viewed as related to the ability to perform or have others perform occupations that relate to the maintenance of self.

Sixth, occupations are composed of knowledge, skills, and attitudes. Occupations are considered to be learned as opposed to innate. Learning involves the use of cognitive memory and understanding, sensory motor functioning, and intrapersonal and interpersonal values and judgments. All occupations involve the combining of knowledge, skills, and attitudes in the actual performance of various occupations.

Seventh, occupations may be divided into three major areas: self-maintenance (self-care, activities of daily living), productivity or work, and leisure (play, recreation). Self-maintenance occupations permit a person to maintain individual life-support needs (food, shelter, belonging). Productivity occupations assist society to facilitate each person to meet individual needs by the use of collective resources. Leisure occupations permit the individual or group to express needs for creative outlet and renewal of interest in self-maintenance and productivity occupations.

Eighth, occupations involve positions, roles, and responsibilities that change over the life span. Occupations may be performed as a solo worker, supervisor, participant, or other. The responsibility for acceptable or criterion performance depends on the position or role. Furthermore, the position or role changes over the life span with a concentration of self-maintenance occupations in childhood, productivity in adulthood, and leisure in old age as a general rule.

Ninth, a balance of occupations is facilitating to the maintenance of health and a satisfying life. A person who manages to perform or to have performed those occupations that facilitate health maintenance, provide for basic needs, and permit leisure pursuits is more likely to achieve a state of health than a person who does not. Balance does not imply an equal amount of time in self-maintenance, productivity, and leisure but rather some time in all activities on a regularly occurring basis.

Tenth, occupations permit a person to fulfill individual and group needs. Occupations are designed to fulfill needs for physiological, security, belonging, esteem, and self-actualization needs. Self-maintenance occupations fulfill primarily physiological, security, and belonging needs. Productivity occupations fulfill belonging and esteem needs, and leisure occupations fulfill esteem and self-actualization needs.

Eleventh, all occupations are determined by the environmental needs and demands (physical, biopsychological, and sociocultural). Occupations exist because they serve a need or purpose in human existence. The need or purpose may be related to the physical, biopsychological, or sociocultural environment or may be a combination of these. When an occupation does not serve to meet the needs or demands of the environment, or when another occupation takes its place, the original occupation will decrease in popularity or cease to exist in that particular environment.

Twelfth, occupations must be relevant and useful to the individual in relating to the environment (purposeful). Individuals perform or seek to perform those occupations that have purpose and meaning related to an aspect of usefulness or relevancy in meeting demands from the environment.

Thirteenth, change in an individual's occupations is affected by change in the total environment, including individual skill acquisition, maintenance, and loss, as well as change in adaptive potential. When environmental demands change or the perception of the demands change, occupational performance may be altered. Development is an example of changing environmental demand, which alters the occupations an individual should perform. A change in status, such as marriage, or a change in health also may alter an individual's occupations.

ASSUMPTIONS ABOUT OCCUPATIONAL DISORDER

Occupational disorder, also called occupational dysfunction, is the primary concern of occupational therapy personnel. Therefore, an understanding of how disorder may occur is critical to formulating plans for assessing and intervening in the problems of occupational disorder. The following assumptions outline the problems and possible causes of occupational disorder.

First, occupational disorder may occur whenever an individual's ability to adapt or adjust through occupations changes. Occupational disorder is not an inevitable outcome of change, but it is a possibility. Some people can deal with many changes and continue to perform all occupations satisfactorily, but others cannot deal with even a few changes. Change, therefore, becomes a key element in alerting occupational therapy practitioners to possible problems.

Second, occupational disorder may occur because of sudden changes in the internal or external environments. Sudden changes may include an acute illness, trauma, or injury with which the person cannot cope or adapt. Thus, occupational performance is affected.

Third, occupational disorder may occur because of long-term changes, such as developmental delay, chronic disability, or the aging process, that reduce the person's ability to cope or adapt. These changes may be more difficult to detect because the change is gradual.

Fourth, occupational disorder may result in changing the performance potential in the occupational areas or performance components or both. Occupational disorder may be limited to one or two components or it may involve several components and areas. Assessment should determine the extent of disorder.

Fifth, occupational disorder may result from several different problems. Some examples are failure to develop occupational skills, failure to organize skills into effective patterns, failure to maintain skills, loss of skill components, loss of ability to organize skills, and loss of purpose and goal direction.

Sixth, occupational disorder may result from identifiable problems that can be readily observed or from problems that are felt or imagined as real. Some problems can be easily assessed, such as a missing limb or a paralyzed body. Other problems occur because the person feels or imagines that the problem is present. If so, the problem must be acknowledged as existing and dealt with accordingly.

Seventh, occupational disorder always occurs when the knowledge, skills, and attitudes in occupational performance are inadequate to meet individual's needs and social demands. Because knowledge, skills, and attitudes are the building materials of performance, then insufficient building material, regardless of cause, will result in inadequate performance.

ASSUMPTIONS ABOUT HEALTH—WELLNESS AND ILLNESS

This set of assumptions concerns the beliefs about wellness and illness as these concepts relate to occupational therapy and other professions. First, health is viewed as a dynamic and changing phenomenon. A person is not always well or always ill. By the same token, a person may not be completely well or completely ill. Health status fluctuates. Furthermore, the effect of wellness or illness is different on different persons.

Second, the optimal level of wellness varies owing to factors such as age and genetic inheritance as well as social and environmental factors. Different standards may need to be developed to determine if a given person has or can achieve an optimal level of wellness.

Third, health is a total condition of a biophysiosocial being and cannot be divided into physical, mental, and social health. Occupational therapy practitioners talk of working with the whole person, which speaks to this assumption. A person as a unified whole also has a unified health. If the initial or major health problem occurs to the physical body, mental and social functioning will be impacted as well.

Fourth, illness may interfere with a person's pattern of meeting needs by 1) reducing the energy level available, 2) disrupting the events and persons in the pattern, or 3) changing the ability to perform occupations. Thus, illness may result in a loss of functional capacity and also lead to a decreased ability to meet personal needs.

Fifth, regaining health requires energy, which reduces the available energy for engaging in occupations, fulfilling needs, and accepting responsibilities. In other words, illness reduces the energy level, and regaining health also reduces the available level of energy.

Sixth, illness interferes with a person's ability to meet responsibilities by 1) altering the potential methods of reaching a goal, 2) changing the positions and roles a person occupies, or 3) reducing the number of occupations a person can perform. Illness potentially reduces the individual's ability to meet responsibilities primarily by interfering with occupational performance and by altering the individual's position and role.

ASSUMPTIONS ABOUT RECEIVING HEALTH CARE SERVICES

People seek health care services when illness or the threat of illness directs attention to a health concern. Occupational therapy practitioners believe a person who seeks services has certain rights that should be protected. One right is to decide whether to seek and accept health care services within legal requirements. A person does not have to seek or accept health care services. Health care is not forced upon people but is offered to them.

The second right is to determine the state of health and level of wellness that a person will seek to attain or maintain as long as the decision does not threaten or endanger the health and wellness of other persons. Not everyone wants to expend the energy needed to achieve the maximum level of health that can be obtained.

A third right is for the individual to be consulted in regard to the objectives, goals, and methods to be used in his or her health care plan. The degree to which consultation can be obtained will vary. A 2-week-old child or an unconscious person cannot contribute much to a plan, but an articulate adult can. If the person can participate, that participation should be promoted according to this assumption.

ASSUMPTIONS ABOUT THE DELIVERY OF HEALTH CARE THROUGH OCCUPATIONAL THERAPY

Occupational therapy as a health care profession can deliver certain services, which are based on five assumptions. The first is that occupational therapy can enable a person to meet his or her needs and responsibilities by assisting the individual to perform occupations. Second, occupational therapy practitioners can identify and analyze a person's occupational performance and adaptive behavior to determine the individual's assets and liabilities in meeting those needs and responsibilities. Third, an occupational therapy practitioner can establish a management program, with the person's active involvement, which will enable the person to attain or maintain a level of occupational performance and adaptive behavior. Fourth, the management program should begin at the point in the sequential level of the client's current functioning and maintain the existing level or increase the level to progressively higher or more advanced levels. Fifth, the management program should be oriented toward enabling the client to do the following: 1) achieve the highest level of occupational performances and adaptive behavior consistent with the client's goal; 2) return to a normal living environment in the community, if possible; 3) increase independent adaptive behavior and decrease dependent, maladaptive behavior; and 4) increase successful occupational performance and decrease nonproductive performance.

ASSUMPTIONS ABOUT OCCUPATIONAL THERAPY

Occupational therapy as a professional discipline is based on certain assumptions. First, therapy, as used in occupational therapy, is the use of directed purposeful occupations or activities to influence positively a person's sense of well-being and, thus, the person's state of health and level of functional independence. Second, the use of directed, purposeful occupations encourages and enables a person to assume responsibility for meeting his or her needs. Third, the use of directed, purposeful occupations can orient a person toward meeting responsibilities through increasing occupational performance levels and improving adaptive behavior. Fourth, active doing or involvement encourages the person to develop, redevelop, or maintain performance in the areas of self-maintenance, productivity, and leisure occupations. Fifth, selected occupations can benefit a client by preventing loss of skills, developing skills, increasing the level of skills, restoring or reintroducing weakened or lost skills, permitting altered or adapted methods of performing skills, and maintaining skills at an established performance level.

ASSUMPTIONS ABOUT THERAPEUTIC USE OF OCCUPATIONS

Occupations are the tools of occupational therapy as a therapeutic process. There-fore, occupational therapy practitioners should have some idea as to why occupa-tional tasks and activities are considered to be therapeutic. The following as-sumptions provide some rationale for the use of occupations in promoting health and wellness.

First, if occupations are useful in facilitating normal development, they should also be useful in helping a person with abnormal development to experience more normal development. Occupations are natural vehicles for facilitating development; that is, they provide the environmental stimulus that creates an opportunity for an individual to respond. Occupations are naturally occurring development nurturers.

Second, if occupations facilitate initial learning, they should be useful also with persons who need to relearn various skills. Occupations are useful in the promo-tion of learning through exploration, repetition, practice, and problem solving. In-teraction with occupations through play, work, and leisure teaches a person use-ful skills whether the person is learning or relearning the skills.

Third, occupations can be graded from simple to complex to meet a variety of human learning needs. Occupations are often more involved than they may ap-pear; that is, an occupation may be observed to be a simple task, such as making a pot holder, but actually is more complex when all factors are analyzed.

Fourth, occupations can be selected to promote performance of cognitive, sen-sorimotor, and psychosocial skills. Occupations can be selected based on which certain tasks or skills they require. Analysis of specific occupations ascertains the requirements of the activity.

The fifth assumption is that occupational performance provides the opportunity for a person to develop a sense of competency through knowing that he or she can perform the task or activity. Competency and mastery are the results of practice and repetition of successful performance. Competency indicates the person is able to perform the occupations needed to cope successfully in the environment.

Sixth, performance of occupations permits a person to meet the individual needs and demands of society. Occupations are associated with people who are able to perform and function in the environment. A person who can perform a va-riety of occupations is considered to be a capable individual.

Seventh, the performance of occupations can facilitate orientation to reality be-cause occupations require attention to the here and now in order to be performed correctly. Occupations also increase attention when they are of interest to the in-dividual and serve a purpose in his or her life.

Eighth, chosen occupations can increase the level of responsibility a person must accept to perform at the expected level of performance. The person begins with structured tasks that minimize the chance of failure and moves to tasks that require individual judgment and attention to detail to ensure successful completion.

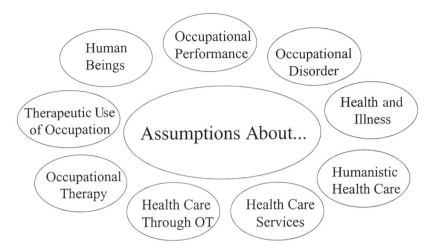

Figure 3.1. Assumptions underlying occupational therapy conceptual and practice models.

In summary, the assumptions included in this chapter are a start toward the process of identifying the basic beliefs in occupational therapy. They provide an initial attempt to develop concepts, principles, and theories that substantiate and develop the practice of occupational therapy as a worthwhile and significant service to consumers. Summarizing all the assumptions in this chapter is difficult. Figures 3.1 and 3.2 provide visual diagrams of some pertinent assumptions involved in the occupational therapy process.

OUTLINE OF ASSUMPTIONS UNDERLYING THE CONCEPTUAL AND PRACTICE MODELS OF OCCUPATIONAL THERAPY

Assumptions About a Human Being

1. A person is a biopsychosocial and spiritual being.
   A. The life force has structure, function, pattern, and organization.
   B. There is a sequential process of growth and development from birth to death, which is unidirectional.
   C. The person exists in a group of meaningful others.
2. A person is a unique whole.
   A. A person's behavior is synergistic.
   B. A person interacts in the environment as a total being.
   C. All behavior is meaningful (although the meaning may not be immediately apparent).

Unity of	In consideration of	In relation to	In support of	Through the use of	Results in ability to	Which is recognized by	Achieves the outcome of
mind functions/skills	internal environment (biopsycho-social self)	cross-sectional time (immediate present)	doing (performing, mastering)	purposeful oc-cupations	meet social demands	functional in-dependence	improved state of health and wellness
and	and	and	and	and	and	and	and
body functions/skills	external envi-ronment (human and nonhuman)	longitudinal time (past and fu-ture)	attaining (sense of competence, achievement)	guided practice	satisfy individ-ual needs	community liv-ing	a better quality of life

Figure 3.2. Occupational therapy view of humans in the occupational therapy process.

3. A person is an open system energy unit.
   A. There is a constant interchange of energy between the person and the environment.
   B. A person can adapt to many environments.
   C. A person dynamically affects the environment and is affected by it.
   D. A person can achieve a balance between using and conserving energy in the environment.
4. A person has the capacity for thought and sensation.
   A. A person is capable of abstraction, imagery, and language.
   B. A person is capable of perception and feeling and has emotions.
5. A person has needs.
   A. Each person develops a unique pattern to meet these needs.
   B. The needs are met on a priority basis within the pattern.
   C. The environment through society influences the patterned behavior of meeting needs.
   D. Society attempts to ensure that needs will be met by sanctifying a variety of occupations.
6. A person has responsibilities.
   A. A person must decide what he or she wishes to become and the methods to be used to attain the goals.
   B. A person assumes positions/roles in the society, each with its set of expectations.
7. A person has potential.
   A. Potentials are, in part, biologically determined.
   B. Potentials can be hindered and facilitated by the environment.
   C. Every person has the potential for continuous growth.
8. A person is the sum total of his or her life experiences.
   A. Current behavior is the result of past experiences.
   B. Current experiences will influence future behavior.
9. A person has basic rights.
   A. A person has the right to maximize individual potential.
   B. A person has the right to have physiological, security, and belonging needs if he or she is unable to provide them.

Assumptions About Occupational Performance

1. Each individual must perform some occupations or have the occupations performed for him or her in order to survive.
2. All occupations may be performed by one person, or different persons may perform some occupations (division of labor).
3. A person adapts or adjusts (grows and develops) through the use of and participation in various occupations.
4. Through the performance of occupations, a person may adapt to the environment or adapt the environment to him or herself.
5. The occupations a person learns and is able to perform or has performed determine the degree to which he or she is able to adapt.
6. Occupations are composed of knowledge, skills, and attitudes.
7. Occupations may be divided into the following three major areas: self-maintenance, productivity, and leisure.
8. Occupations involve positions, roles, and responsibilities that change over the life span.
9. A balance of occupations facilitates the maintenance of health and a satisfying life.
10. Occupations permit a person to fulfill individual and group needs.
11. All occupations are determined by environmental needs and demands (physical, biopsychological, and sociocultural).
12. Occupations must be relevant and useful to the individual in relating to the environment (purposeful).
13. Change in an individual's occupations is affected by change in the total environment—external and internal.

Assumptions About Occupational Disorder and Dysfunction

1. Occupational disorder may occur whenever there are changes in the individual's ability to adapt or adjust through the use of occupations.
2. Occupational disorder may occur because of sudden changes in the internal or external environment, such as acute illness, trauma, or injury.
3. Occupational disorder may occur because of long-term changes, such as developmental delay, chronic disability, or the aging process.
4. Occupational disorder may result in changing the performance potential in the occupational areas, or performance components or both.
5. Occupational disorder may result from several different problems that occur singly or in combination.
6. Occupational disorder may result from identifiable problems or from problems that are felt or imagined as real.
7. Occupational disorder always occurs to some degree when the knowledge, skills, and attitudes in occupational performance are inadequate to meet individual needs and social demands.

Assumptions About Health—Wellness and Illness

1. Health is a dynamic and changing phenomenon.
2. The optimal level of wellness varies due to factors such as age and genetic inheritance as well as social and environmental factors.
3. Health is a total condition of a biopsychosocial being; it cannot be divided into physical health, mental health, and social health.
4. Illness may interfere with a person's pattern of meeting needs by:
   A. Reducing the energy level available;
   B. Disrupting the events and persons in the pattern; and
   C. Changing the ability to perform occupations.
5. Regaining health requires energy that reduces the available energy for engaging in occupations, fulfilling needs, and accepting responsibilities.
6. Illness interferes with a person's ability to meet responsibilities by:
   A. Altering potential methods of reaching a goal;
   B. Changing the positions/roles a person occupies; and
   C. Reducing the number of occupations that a person can perform.

Assumptions About Humanistic Health Care

1. A person is more than a disease state or injury condition (the pneumonia case or fractured leg).
2. A person is more than just a body; a person is a unique, interdependent relationship of body, mind, emotions, culture, and spirit.
3. Each person has the capacity to define and be increasingly responsible for his or herself, regardless of the nature and degree of disease or injury.
4. A professional is more than a scientifically trained mind using technical skills; a professional has a body, emotions, culture, and spirit that can also be useful in providing health care services.
5. The professional seeks to assist the person in taking and fulfilling responsibility for the self.
6. Health and disease are not matters of the moment but have an intricate past, present, and future.
7. Physical disease, pain, suffering, aging, and even death can frequently be valuable, meaningful events in an individual's life.
8. Effective practice of health care requires not just conventional skills but also effective development and use of human qualities such as intuition, inventiveness, and empathy.
9. Both the person receiving care and the professional are whole human beings interacting in the healing effort.

Assumptions About Receiving Health Care Services

1. A person has the right to decide whether to seek and accept health care services, within legal limitations.

2. A person has a right to determine the state of health and level of wellness that he or she will seek to attain or maintain as long as the decision does not threaten or endanger the health and wellness of other persons.
3. A person has a right to be consulted regarding the objectives, goals, and methods to be used in his or her health care plans.

Assumptions About Delivering Health Care Through Occupational Therapy

1. At times, a person may need assistance from occupational therapy to meet individual needs and responsibilities to perform occupations.
2. A person's occupational performance and adaptive behavior can be identified and analyzed to determine his or her assets and liabilities in meeting those needs and responsibilities.
3. A management program can be developed with the person's active involvement, which will attain or maintain his or her occupational performance and adaptive behavior.
4. A management program is most useful to the client if it begins at the sequential level of the client's current functioning and maintains the existing level or increases the functional level to progressively higher (advanced) levels.
5. A management program should be oriented toward enabling the client to:
   A. Achieve the highest level of occupational performance and adaptive behavior consistent with the client's goal;
   B. Return to a normal living environment in the community, if possible;
   C. Increase independent adaptive behavior and decrease dependent, maladaptive, or nonadaptive behavior; and
   D. Increase successful occupational performance and decrease nonproductive occupational performance.

Assumptions About Occupational Therapy

1. Therapy (in occupational therapy) is the use of directed, purposeful occupations to influence positively a person's sense of well-being and, thus, his or her state of health.
2. Directed, purposeful occupations encourage the person to assume responsibility for meeting needs.
3. Directed, purposeful occupations are useful in orienting a person toward meeting responsibilities through increasing occupational performance levels and improving adaptive behavior.
4. Active doing (involvement) encourages the maintenance, development, and redevelopment of occupations, specifically, self-care, work, and leisure-time skills.
5. Selected occupations can:
   A. Increase the level of specified development skills;

B. Prevent loss of skills;

C. Reintroduce or restore weakened or lost skills;

D. Permit altered methods of performing skills; and

E. Maintain skills at an established level of performance.

Assumptions About the Therapeutic Use of Occupations

1. If occupations are useful in facilitating normal development, they should also be useful in helping a person with abnormal development to experience more normal-like development.

2. If occupations facilitate initial learning, they should be useful also with persons who need to relearn various skills.

3. Occupations can be graded from simple to complex to meet a variety of human learning skills.

4. Occupations can be selected to promote performance of sensorimotor, cognitive, and psychosocial skills.

5. Performance of occupations provides a person with the opportunity to develop a sense of competency through knowing that he or she can perform the task or activity.

6. Performance of occupations permits a person to meet individual needs and the demands of society.

7. The performance of occupations can facilitate the orientation to reality because it requires attention to the here and now in order to perform the occupation correctly.

8. Occupations can be selected that increase the level of responsibility a person must take to perform at the expected level of performance.

CHAPTER 4

Value of Occupational Therapy

The value of occupational therapy may be examined from the following four perspectives: 1) the individual occupational therapy practitioner's contribution, 2) the cumulative knowledge and skills of the profession, 3) the effects on the individual client, and 4) the gains achieved by the community. These values are illustrated in Figure 4.1.

INDIVIDUAL OCCUPATIONAL THERAPY PRACTITIONER'S CONTRIBUTION

Occupational therapy's value is determined by the practitioner's ability to examine the total occupational performance (also called occupational functioning and occupational competence) output of an individual in terms of identifiable skills, competencies, strengths, and weaknesses and to make suggestions or recommendations to solve any problems observed in the tasks, routines, or habits of daily living. The occupational performance is viewed as an interacting system in which a number of components or subsystems must be functioning to produce satisfactory results. The components have different names in different models, but the interactive aspect appears. Thus, the major occupational performance of a person can be examined using the six W's in relationship to each other. The six W's are: what, why, when, who, how, and where.

The focus of occupational therapy permits an examination of how a person uses performance potential by assessing *what* skill areas the individual uses. Good performance skills will enable a person to do a task with efficient use of energy and time. Poor performance may require too much energy and too much time.

The next focus is on *why* the person performs certain occupational behaviors. The analysis of why is important because the acceptance or nonacceptance of behavior by society is determined, in part, by the type of occupation the person does. Because behavior is a product of a combination of performance skills, the type of occupation can vary. The professional golfer and the weekend golfer are using similar performance skills, but the occupational areas are different.

Another focus of occupational therapy is *when* performance is accomplished, which implies the concept of time. Occupational therapists can analyze the

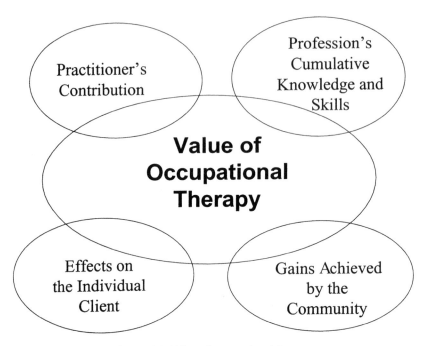

Figure 4.1. Value of occupational therapy.

amount of time a behavior occurs, the frequency of occurrence, and the time of day during which behavior occurs. "When" also involves a measurement in relation to the value judgment of too much, too little, or just the right amount. This aspect is important because society expects a person not only to perform but also to perform whenever skill is needed to accomplish the task. Too little or too much performance may be viewed as a problem just as important as poor performance.

Next, the occupational therapist may examine *who* does the behavior. Although the emphasis is on the client, that individual may not be performing all of the behaviors needed to complete the occupational performance. A family member, a friend, or an employee may be doing some behavioral units of an occupational area. This information becomes important in assessing the individual's independence. If the spouse is dressing the client, the client is not independent in dressing. Thus, if the spouse becomes ill, the client may be unable to go to work.

How performance occurs can be examined to determine how best to perform occupational skills. A client may be accustomed to standing to take a shower and using a wash cloth. However, if balance and range of motion are limited, a shower chair may be used to sit instead of stand and an extension shower head may be used to spray rather than wash. How performance occurs may make performance safer, easier, more efficient, and less time-consuming.

Where performance occurs can be examined to select the best place for occupations to occur. A person may be accustomed to getting dressed in a walk-in closet. However, this closet space may restrict movement. Changing where performance occurs may result in improved performance potential without any change in skill level. Where performance occurs also affects safety, efficiency, ease of performance, and time consumption.

Personal Values

In addition to professional values, the occupational therapy practitioner has personal values that contribute to the therapeutic environment. A personal value is defined as a belief or an ideal to which an individual is committed (1). Seven basic concepts have been described by the American Occupational Therapy Association as core values that occupational therapy personnel should express and implement in occupational therapy service programs. The seven concepts are altruism, equality, freedom, justice, dignity, truth, and prudence (Figure 4.2). Altruism is the unselfish concern for the welfare of others. Altruism is concerned with the action and attitudes toward commitment, caring, dedication, responsiveness, and understanding. Occupational therapists show altruism by commitment to caring for others, through dedication to their work and profession, by being responsive to the needs of their clients and community, and by taking the time to try to understand each client's special circumstances.

Equality is based on the concept that all individuals are perceived as having the same fundamental human rights and opportunities. Equality is demonstrated

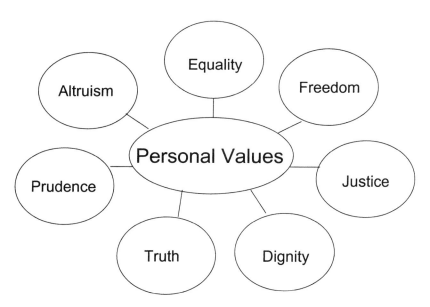

Figure 4.2. Personal values of a practitioner.

through fairness, impartiality, and respect toward clients, their families, and other health care professionals. In a multicultural society, there are values, beliefs, and lifestyles that are different from those of the individual occupational therapists. Occupational therapy services are provided because the services are needed without judgment of the client's value system or living arrangements.

Freedom describes the exercise of choice, independence, initiative, and self-direction. Freedom implies that each individual should be given the opportunity to choose between options, live as independently as health and social obligations will permit, use individual initiative to get things done that is satisfying to the person, and direct personal actions whenever possible. Total freedom is not realistic, however. Each person must find a balance between autonomy and social roles and responsibilities. Humans can be both independent and interdependent with other humans and their nonhuman environment. Adaptation through the use of occupation and purposeful activity is considered by occupational therapists to be critical to developing and exercising the freedom to pursue goals that have personal and social meaning.

Justice is a moral and legal principle involving fairness, equality, truthfulness, and objectivity.

Occupational therapists must be knowledgeable about the legal rights of each individual whether the individual is receiving occupational therapy services or is a citizen in the community. Because occupational therapists frequently work with individuals who do not necessarily know their rights or how to act to secure these rights, it is important not to take advantage of the situation and to be an advocate whenever a situation arises in which someone else is abusing or denying others' rights. In addition, occupational therapists must be knowledgeable about legal obligations such as laws and regulations governing occupational therapy services whether the legal obligations are local, state, or federal.

Dignity is based on the belief that each person is unique and has inherent worth. Dignity is demonstrated through empathy and respect for self and others. When dignity is nurtured, a person gains a sense of competence and self-worth. Occupational therapy contributes through the use of occupation and activities that help the individual build personal attributes and resources.

Truth is a commitment to facts and reality. Truth is demonstrated by being accountable, honest, forthright, accurate, and authentic. Occupational therapists have an obligation to be truthful to ourselves, our clients, our colleagues, and our society. One major way occupational therapists show commitment to truth and veracity is through dedication to lifelong inquiry and commitment to maintain and upgrade professional competence.

Prudence is grounded in reason, rational thinking, and intelligent reflection. Prudence is demonstrated through judiciousness, discretion, vigilance, moderation, care, and circumspection in the management of personal and professional situations. Through prudence, judgment prevails over temper and discretion overcomes indiscretion.

Summary

In summary, both attitudes and values are shaped by individual behavior and professional practice. As a professional in the field of occupational therapy, each therapist needs to know and practice the attitudes and values that underlie the core of the profession and govern the interactions of occupational therapists with clients and other professionals. Attitudes and values provide insight into the profession's philosophy, act as a basis for defining the profession's purpose, and empower the profession through shared commitment.

CUMULATIVE KNOWLEDGE AND SKILLS OF THE PROFESSION

The cumulative knowledge and skills of occupational therapy enable practitioners to be of value to clients in at least seven aspects.

1. The occupational therapy practitioner can suggest to the client a greater variety of solutions that may be more useful in solving problems than the person or his or her family might have been able to conceive.
2. The practitioner can identify, acquire, or better utilize the needed resources to solve problems than an individual may be able to do alone.
3. The practitioner can assist the client in accomplishing the outcomes or goals identified in the problem-solving process in less time than the client alone could be expected to accomplish the same outcomes or goals.
4. A practitioner has access to a wider variety of media and methods, which have been developed over the years, from which to select those that may best assist the individual client.
5. The practitioner is able to provide a graduation of environments in which the client can develop and practice skills. The graduation ranges from the structured and safe environment of a clinic to the unstructured and normal-risk environment of the community.
6. The practitioner can analyze a task, activity, or job into as many or as few steps as the client needs in order to learn or relearn the performance requirements. The analysis may indicate the need for splints or other specialized equipment that the therapist can make or have purchased.
7. The practitioner can provide feedback in terms of constructive criticism as well as praise for performance and accomplishment during and after the doing of a task, activity, or occupation.

EFFECTS ON THE INDIVIDUAL CLIENT

As a result of occupational therapy service, a person may see the value of occupational therapy in terms of the following: 1) increased ability and capacity to do and perform various daily tasks; 2) change in the organization of when and how tasks are done, which permits more to be accomplished or leaves more time for self-selected activities; 3) increased sense of accomplishment, satisfaction, and control over one's own life and less feelings of dependence and hopelessness; 4) increased ability to get around the house, yard, and community safely because architectural barriers have been removed or because specialized equipment has been installed; 5) improved level of physical and mental health and sense of well-being resulting from the increased ability to perform, organize, and fulfill those social demands and individual needs that occur in the process of living; and 6) increased sense of dignity and self-worth through the knowledge that ability, not disability, is important to the quality of life.

COMMUNITY GAINS FROM OCCUPATIONAL THERAPY SERVICES

A community gains from occupational therapy services some or all of the following: 1) a greater number of individuals who are more able to perform daily tasks for themselves and thus require less expensive help from others; 2) increased productive potential because the injured or ill person is able to return to work, is able to work for the first time, or is able to contribute in unpaid service, such as volunteer work; 3) a decrease in the number of individuals who feel hopeless or helpless and may have been using many hours of a physician's or other service person's time for very little constructive purpose; 4) a safer community, which is accessible to all, because barriers have been reduced or eliminated; 5) a healthier community because more people are aware of the relationship of performance capacity to physical and emotional well-being; and 6) an increased sense of commitment to the quality of life as well as the quantity of life through recognition that dignity and self-worth are part of the rights of each individual regardless of individual limitations.

Summary

In summary, the value of occupational therapy encompasses the ability to solve problems of daily living associated with disability, deficits, dysfunction, and limitations in occupational performance. Through the problem-solving process, the occupational therapy practitioner assists the client by replacing feelings of hopelessness and helplessness with the feeling of being able to perform (mastery and competence) at least some of the daily living tasks independently or in a manner acceptable to the client's society and culture. Occupational therapy sometimes has been described as the art and science of making "doing" (performance, mastery, competence) possible. Much of the value of occupational therapy is related to the doing and performing potential inherent in occupations.

Reference

1. Kanny E. Core values and attitudes of occupational therapy practice. Am J Occup Ther 1993;47(12):1085–1086.

CHAPTER 5

Purpose of Occupational Therapy

Through the years, three general purposes of occupational therapy have evolved: diversion, expression, and skill building. These purposes provide the framework for more specific and more individualized goals and objectives. The purposes, however, are what most people think about when they describe occupational therapy. Dictionary definitions often describe one of the purposes without reference to the others. Thus, the initial understanding of occupational therapy is based on a limited view of the potential of occupational therapy.

DIVERSION

Diversion, also called distraction, was the first to be described. Used primarily with chronic conditions such as mental illness, tuberculosis, and rheumatic heart disease, the primary objective was to divert or distract attention away from the disease or disorder toward more healthful ideas and positive thinking. Dr. Dunton began a column in the *Maryland Psychiatric Quarterly* called "Occupations and Amusements" (1). The column discussed ideas that could be used to distract patients in mental institutions away from mental aberrations such as hallucinations or destructive behavior toward useful tasks or occupations such as painting, weaving, pottery, sewing, or woodworking. Amusements included playing games, listening to music, playing music, watching or performing plays, participating in physical exercises and sports, as well as doing a variety of arts and crafts.

There was an understanding that the tasks provided different responses and should be applied with attention to the desired result. Thus, if the person were manic, the tasks should be soothing, but if the person were depressed, the tasks should be brighter and more cheerful. During the 1920s, several articles were devoted to analyzing the characteristics of various handicrafts to classify and describe the inherent values of the handicraft.

Dunton states the purpose of diversion as follows: "The first mental objective to be attained is usually improvement of the patient's mental attitude, of his morale, as if is often expressed" (2). He continues by saying that "the production of a well-made, useful, and attractive article, or the accomplishment of a useful task, requires healthy exercise of mind and body, gives the greatest satisfaction, and thus produces the most beneficial effects."

Although diversion or distraction is usually not recognized as therapeutic goals in the United States, other countries continue to publish articles about the effective use of such programs. In 1991, Westbrook, Skropeta, and Legge published an article in the *Australian Occupational Therapy Journal* about a survey of diversional therapists (3). The therapists were asked to report their experiences with planning programs for clients with diverse ethnic backgrounds. The survey was sent to 750 people, of which 563 were members of the Australian Diversional Therapy Association. A majority of respondents agreed that developing programs to accommodate the needs of ethnic clients was difficult.

Radziewicz and Schneider, nurses in Cleveland, reported using diversional activity to enhance coping skills as part of treating diversional activity deficit, which is a recognized nursing diagnosis (4). They used such activities for patients with cancer, and the results were published in an article in *Cancer Nursing*. The nursing diagnosis is described as "the state in which the individual experiences, or is at risk for experiencing, an environment that is devoid of stimulation or interest." Use of music, art, wit, and humor are described in the article although the assessment instrument lists many more available activities.

Miller, Hickman, and Lemaster, nurses in Cincinnati, reported using distraction for the control of burn pain when changing burn dressing (5). The distraction they used was viewing one of four video programs composed of scenic beauty accompanied by music. A significant reduction in pain and anxiety was reported.

Finally, Badry, Robins, and Forestier, Canadian nurses at the University of Alberta Hospitals, reported developing a diversional program for long-term residents to provide needed stimulation, to increase social interaction, to develop a more positive outlook in patients, to enhance self-esteem, to boost morale, and to prevent boredom (6). The program involved outings, games, crafts, and special projects. Patients became more vocal about their surroundings, abusive language and aggressive behavior decreased, conversion increased, table manners improved, and some patients were able to eat without using bibs.

Clearly, diversional therapy does have a place in the delivery of health care. The difficulty is justifying such therapy in a reimbursement system oriented to dramatic results. Diversional therapy adds to the quality of life, but direct reduction of symptoms related to disease or disorder is more difficult to present in convincing research. Most reimbursement agencies will not pay for "happier" or "better-adjusted" patients. In the United States, diversional therapy exists only to the extent that it costs little.

EMOTIONAL EXPRESSION

Emotional expression, also called creative expression, became important to occupational therapy during the years of Freudian psychology. Through the use of the creative arts and crafts patients could express attitudes, feelings, and ideations—

according to Fidler and Fidler who wrote the best-known textbook (7). They could express hostility, dependency, and infantile oral and anal needs. They could also develop better self-concepts, improve personal identities, and build more healthy egos. Creative arts and crafts provided opportunities of reality testing as well. The objects and processes offered sensory contact, shared values, and consensual validation.

Emotional expression was sometimes taken to extreme. Psychiatrists Azima and Wittkower felt that too much emphasis had been placed on the diversional and occupational aspects of activities at the expense of psychodynamic problems (8). They organized a theory of occupational therapy based totally on expression of unconscious needs at the anal and oral level. The media used to meet anal needs were mud, brown clay, coca powder, cocoa mud, plasticine, and finger paints. For meeting oral needs, baby bottles filled with milk were offered along with other liquids; gradually, meals were incorporated in the treatment sessions.

The use of expression dominated occupational therapy in psychiatry in the 1960s and 1970s. As the influence of psychodynamic psychiatry decreased, the use of expression in occupational therapy also decreased, but its use still continues today. The difficulty today is in separating expression of psychodynamic ideas of the unconscious from the use of creativity as a means of understanding how materials in the environment can be used constructively in daily life. Artwork, for example, can be done because the person enjoys the process of drawing and painting. The product does not have to be psychoanalyzed for subconscious meanings.

SKILL BUILDING

Skill building has been a part of occupational therapy from the beginning, but its purpose has expanded in recent years as reimbursement has become tied to functional performance and outcomes. Terms such as occupational behavior, occupational performance, occupational competence, and occupational adaptation are associated with skill building. Initially, skills were primarily honed in relation to work situations. Hall, for example, called occupational therapy the "work cure" (9). He used work in 15-minute intervals to improve the mental health of people diagnosed with neurasthenia. Neurasthenia is similar to chronic fatigue syndrome and other stress disorders diagnosed today. Barton used work to help convalescent patients regain strength and endurance (10). Haas states that the first mission of the occupational therapy department is "to create a modified normal atmosphere in which the sick man may spend a certain percentage of his time. The normal atmosphere of the average man is that of work activity" (11). Sometimes, the emphasis on work got a little out of hand as is illustrated by the Hayworth and MacDonald's statement that the "aim of an occupational therapy department in a mental hospital should be to employ every patient in the hospital who is capable of, or can be made capable of, employment" (12).

During the 1950s, the concept of activities of daily living (ADLs) was added to the purpose of skill building. Initially, activities of daily living were assessed and managed primarily in children, but the purpose was quickly added to adult rehabilitation. Activities of daily living, also called self-care, included such tasks as dressing, grooming, walking, and eating. Instrumental activities of daily living were first described by Katz and colleagues who felt the concept of ADLs needed to be expanded to include dialing the telephone, preparing meals, doing light housekeeping, and shopping in the community (13).

In the 1970s, skill building began to be described in three or four areas and three to five components. The descriptors varied but usually the areas were called self-care or daily living skills, work or productivity, and play-leisure or recreation. The components may be called physical, motor, sensory, sensorimotor, cognitive, intrapersonal, psychological, interpersonal, social, psychosocial, or cultural. Gradually, the term performance became a key concept. In the first Uniform Terminology for Reporting Occupational Therapy Services, skill and performance components were divided into independent living/daily living skills and performance, sensorimotor skill and performance components, cognitive skill and performance components, and psychosocial skill and performance components (14).

Skill building was and still is being used as a general term. Some people would probably prefer to called this third purpose function building, task building, or role building. Others would want to add the words such as developing, attaining, achieving, mastering, organizing, rebuilding, reintegrating, maintaining, and sustaining. Skill building is short and makes the point that skill plus building form the central purpose.

The importance of skill building to occupational therapy today can be appreciated in the comments of Munich and Lang (15). According to them, the view of occupational therapy in mental health by fields outside of psychiatry may be negative and counterproductive. Occupational therapy has been viewed as an expressive, creative, or diversional therapy along with art, music, and recreation. It is not viewed as concerned with building and strengthening skills, habits, and functional performance.

Another example by Jackson follows:

> There is also the deep-seated belief that the mentally ill can't work at any meaningful task, and it is therefore inappropriate to ask them to do so. Instead their time is to be filled with group therapy, *occupational therapies heavily dependent on arts and crafts that have little practical value,* and "skills training" for situations in which clients may or may not find themselves, since skills training is not expected to relate to utilization. (16, italics added)

As the articles by Munich and Lang and by Jackson suggest, occupational therapy would do well to continue to focus on the skill concept in mental health as in other areas of occupational therapy practice. The current emphasis on functional outcomes also supports the skills focus. The economic and political climate today supports the skills-based approach.

SUMMARY

Occupational therapy has evolved around three different purposes as illustrated in Figure 5.1 and Table 5.1. Diversion of attention came from the heritage of working with chronic conditions that required long periods of bed rest and/or confinement in an institutional setting. Emotional expression came from the changing ideas about mental illness based on dynamic psychiatry. Skill building developed initially from the attempts to enable clients to establish or reestablish work skills, but the scope enlarged over the years to include all aspects of daily living roles including self-care, home management, child care, education, independent living, community living, play, and leisure. The skills are usually combined to form the habits, routines, and roles necessary to perform activities, tasks, and occupations that the person wants to perform and the environment expects or demands to be performed. The primary focus of occupational therapy practice today is on skill building and subsequent processes.

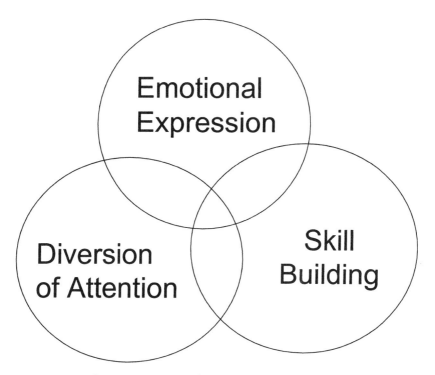

Figure 5.1. Purposes of occupational therapy services.

Table 5.1.   Uses of Occupation in Occupational Therapy
• To divert the mins from boredom, idleness, or undesirable symptoms such as hallucinations or acting out behavior
• To facilitate expression of mood, feelings, or behavior through the use of creative activities such as arts and crafts
• To improve and organize the actual performance of skills, tasks, routines, or roles—especially those that are useful and appropriate in daily living or facilitate adaptive responses.

References

1. Dunton WR. Occupations and amusements. Maryland Psychiatric Quarterly 1923; 2(1):19–20.
2. Dunton WR. Prescribing Occupational Therapy. Springfield, IL: Charles C Thomas, 1928:10,14.
3. Westbrook MT, Skropeta M, Legge V. Ethnic clients in diversional therapy programmes. Australian Occup Ther J 1991;38:251–258.
4. Radziewicz RM, Schneider SM. Using diversional activity to enhance coping. Cancer Nursing 1992;15(4):293–298.
5. Miller AC, Hickman LC, Lemaster GK. A distraction technique for the control of burn pain. J Burn Care Rehabil 1992;13(5):576–580.
6. Badry E, Robins M, Forestier M. Diversional therapy. Can Nurse 1990;86(2):33–35.
7. Fidler GS, Fidler JW. Occupational Therapy: A Communication Process in Psychiatry. New York: Macmillan Co., 1963:81.
8. Azima H, Wittkower ED. Gratification of basic needs in treatment of schizophrenics. Psychiatry 1956;19:122.
9. Hall HJ. The work cure. J Am Med Assoc 1910;LIV:12–14.
10. Newton IG. Consolation House. Trained Nurse Hosp Rev 1917;59:321–326.
11. Haas LJ. Occupational Therapy for the Mentally and Nervously Ill. Milwaukee: Bruce Publishing Co, 1925:22.
12. Hayworth NA, MacDonald EM. The Theory of Occupational Therapy. London: Bailliere, Tindal & Cox, 1948.
13. Katz S, Ford AB, Moskowitz RW, et al. The index of ADL: a standardized measure of biological and psychosocial function. JAMA 1963;185:914–919.
14. Representative Assembly. Uniform terminology for reporting occupational therapy services. In: Hopkins HL, Smith HD. Willard and Spackman's Occupational Therapy. 6th ed. Philadelphia: Lippincott, 1983:899–907.
15. Munich RL, Lang E. The boundaries of psychiatric rehabilitation. Hosp Comm Psychiat 1993;44(7):661–665.
16. Jackson R. How work works. Psychosoc Rehabil J 1992;16(2):63–67.

CHAPTER 6

Uniqueness and Outcomes
of Occupational Therapy

Every profession should offer the customer (client, patient, resident, student, etc.) a service that is unique and different from the services offered by other professions. Occupational therapy does provide a unique service. The unique aspects of occupational therapy are:

1. Focus on a person's skills, habits, and routines necessary to perform the occupations of everyday life throughout the life span;
2. Study and synthesis of knowledge on the development, integration, interrelatedness, role, and context of occupation in everyday life and throughout the life cycle;
3. Application of the knowledge of occupation to assist persons to develop, learn, and maintain occupational performance (also called occupational competence, occupational function, or occupational mastery); and
4. Application of methods (called also techniques or approaches) of adapting and changing a person's occupational behavior to meet the demands of the human and nonhuman environments (environmental press) or adapting and changing the environment to a person's occupational needs.

Occupational therapy as a profession grew out of the concern that people must be able to do and perform certain skills, habits, routines, tasks, and roles, at a certain time, with a certain level of performance or criterion, to meet certain personal needs or environmental demands. Persons with mental health problems, for example, often do not do what is expected of them, or they do it at the wrong time. They may also underexceed or overexceed the performance criterion. In short, their behavior does not measure up to social expectations and/or personal needs; thus, such persons are viewed as candidates for mental health services.

Historically, occupational therapy practitioners tried to develop programs to help each person learn or relearn collective occupational activities and individual skills to achieve a role that would be acceptable to society and be satisfactory to the individual. Examples included scheduling each 24-hour day and assigning each person selected occupations based on individual interests and abilities.

Such concern for occupations requires considerable knowledge. Occupational performance is assumed to be the result of developmental maturation and of learning many skills to be performed in a certain context. Furthermore, combinations of skills and application of these skills need to be learned and applied at the right time and place, in the right amount needed, and for the right purpose. Thus, occupational therapy practitioners must know also how component or subsystem skills are integrated into a single pattern or interrelated into a total pattern, such as a role that involves many separate skills. Such skills may include motor abilities, sensory and cognitive functioning, psychological and emotional behavior, social awareness, work adjustment, avocational interests, leisure activities, and other skills.

Through the application of knowledge about occupations, occupational therapy practitioners assume that a person's health, wellness, life satisfaction, and need fulfillment will be positively affected and changed. Occupational therapy practitioners further assume that the positive effects occur when a person has achieved a basic level of occupational performance and can balance the need for occupation into a lifestyle that is acceptable to the individual, community, and society, as well as in the political, economic, and cultural environment.

In addition to knowledge about occupation, occupational therapy practitioners are also expected to know how the environment affects performance. Human and nonhuman environments can facilitate or impede performance of occupations. Occupational therapy practitioners have developed methods both to modify the individual's behavior and to change the environmental response to the individual. Education of clients about assistive technology, consultations with the family about attitudes and expectations, and meetings with community members about environmental barriers are examples of how occupational therapy practitioners attempt to change the environment to meet individual needs.

In summary, it is the breadth of concern and the depth of concern for occupation and its application in daily life and throughout the life span that are the distinguishing features of occupational therapy. Occupational therapy includes the theory and application of occupation to health, wellness, and satisfaction. The individual may gain a sense of well-being, self-efficacy, mastery, competence, fulfillment, achievement, and balance. The wide variety of choices reflects the focus of occupational therapy practice on individual choice rather than predetermined professional perspectives. Also included are the purpose and function of occupations in daily life; the activities and tasks that comprise occupations; the development of skills; the organization of skills into roles; the work habits that contribute to productivity; the individual's interests in work and leisure; the individual's values toward self-care, work, and play; and the individual's beliefs about how occupations and roles are learned. All of these aspects are the concern of occupational therapy.

OUTCOMES OR GOALS OF OCCUPATIONAL THERAPY SERVICE PROGRAMS AND PRACTITIONERS

All professions must state what will happen to the consumer as a result of the profession's intervention. Intervention is a service provided by the professional to the consumer for which payment is expected whether in cash, insurance reimbursement, or barter. Thus, the consumer usually wants to know what results can be expected for the money. The results are usually stated as outcomes or goals. The major outcomes or goals of occupational therapy service programs for the individual consumer are to do the following: 1) assess human function and behavior in terms of occupations, occupational performance, the components of that performance, and the required adaptive behavior; 2) support the optimum occupational performance of each person based on the individual's needs and the community demands for occupational performance; 3) develop, improve, reestablish, promote, or maintain normal occupational functions and performance in daily life and throughout the human life span; and 4) prevent, remedy, or minimize problems (disorder, dysfunction, disease, injury, etc.) in occupational performance and adaptive behavior in daily life and throughout the life span.

Occupational therapy practitioners can provide six major outcomes through occupational therapy intervention: 1) help individuals learn or relearn the performance of occupation necessary to adapt to daily life and to the life cycle; 2) help individuals to plan, organize, and balance the sequence of occupational performance within daily life and throughout the life cycle; 3) provide suggestions for alternative ways of performing occupations, which can facilitate performance for persons with temporary or chronic disability; 4) provide the methods and resources for practicing and trying out different ways of performing occupations for a person with disability or a person who is at risk for disability; 5) assist in identifying, through evaluation and assessment, the specific problems a person is experiencing in performing occupations of daily life; and 6) determine the need for and arrange provision of assistive technology needed for performance of daily occupations.

Adaptation, health, and wellness are viewed in the occupational therapy discipline as dealing with the performance of daily life occupations and of achieving a balance between individual needs and skills in relation to community or environmental demands (requirements or rewards) for occupational performance. When a person has the occupational skills, habits, and routines and is able to use them to fulfill needs and meet demands, that person can achieve a state of adaptation, health, or wellness.

Conversely, when a person does not have the occupational skills, habits, or routines and/or is unable to use the them to fulfill needs and meet demands, that person has not achieved a state of adaptation, health, or wellness. The effect of the lack of adaptation, health, or wellness may be observed in the performance of everyday occupations. For example, a person may have forgotten how to get dressed or may lack the fine coordinated motor skills of the hand needed to button. In either situation, the person does not have the occupational skills to get dressed; thus, adaptation, health, or wellness may be compromised. Individual analysis is always important because the level of performance in dressing skills changes across the life span. An 6-month-old infant is not expected to have dressing skills; therefore, the lack of skills is not viewed as negatively impacting adaptation, health, or wellness. An 25-year-old adult has such expectations, and therefore, lack of such skills is more likely to be viewed negatively. Loss of dressing skills in older individuals is also viewed as a problem that must be solved by having someone assist the individual or by avoiding all situations in which dressing is an expectation. The later solution significantly alters adaptation, health, and wellness by reducing quality of life.

Another example is work or productive occupation. If a person does not have an employable set of skills related to an occupation or cannot perform a specific work skill because of weak muscles, an employment agency is not of assistance. Placing the want ads section of a newspaper before the person will not help either. Lack of opportunities in productivity also negatively influences adaptation, health, or wellness.

Lack of leisure skills has negative connotations in two dimensions. One is the "disuse effect." A person who does not use the occupational skills regularly tends to lose the ability to perform. Performance capacity tends to be correlated to adaptation, health, and wellness. For example, good performance, good health; poor performance, poor health. The second dimension concerns motivation. Opportunity to engage in leisure activity encourages some people to engage in dressing and productivity tasks. Leisure activity is a reward to such persons. Others fear leisure time because they have no leisure skills and thus continue to engage in dressing or work tasks to fill in the time available for leisure pursuits. Using leisure activity to reward the self is regarded as having a positive effect on health whereas avoiding leisure activity may decrease health by permitting the individual to overdo routine maintenance and productive tasks.

Occupational therapists can use a variety of assessment techniques and evaluation strategies to determine if a person is experiencing difficulty in the performance of daily skills, habits, or routines. Based on the outcome of the evaluation, an occupational therapy practitioner may further assess the individual to determine if assistive technology may be helpful.

Goals and outcomes must be carefully coordinated with the client and often with family members as well. Occupations may be grouped into general categories but they are practiced individually. Each person has selected occupations that are being acquired, in the case of a child or adolescent, or have been acquired, in the case of an adult. Most often, clients prefer to continue to perform familiar occupations. When adaptations or changes must be made, for whatever reason, understanding and cooperation of the person and family are critical to integration of the adaptations and changes into daily life habits and routines. Unless the individual and family agree the adaptation or change is acceptable and are willing to make the effort to adapt or change, the new occupation or new method of performing the old occupation is unlikely to be integrated into daily life. Goals and outcomes in occupational therapy are dependent on acceptance and cooperation of the client and usually also the family. The best-designed goals and outcomes specified by the occupational therapy practitioner are mere words on paper if the client and his or her family do not understand the rationale or chose not to follow the recommendations in daily life. For example, quality of life is very specific. One person's idea of quality of life is not the same as another as illustrated in Figures 6.1 and 6.2.

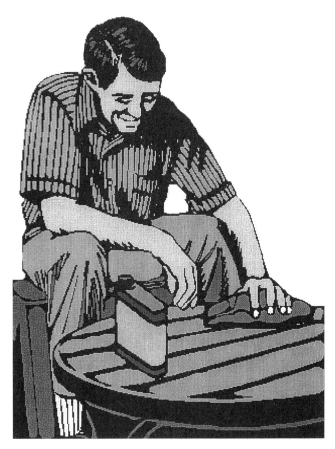

Figure 6.1. Quality of life.

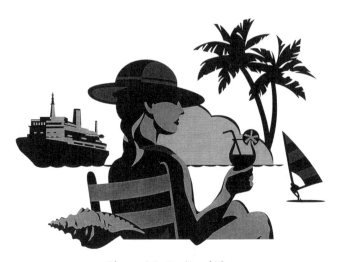

Figure 6.2. Quality of life.

In summary, the outcomes of occupational therapy services relate to occupation and how occupation is used in daily life and through the life cycle. The specific outcomes depend on the individual preference and on the demands of the environment in which the person lives. The outcomes also depend on the position of the person within the life span.

The Conceptual Base

CHAPTER 7

Introduction to Major Concepts

A *concept* is an idea or notion (1). Concepts are formed by mentally combining the characteristics or particulars of an object or thing. In conceptual models, concepts form the basic building material. Conceptual models are graphic or schematic representation of concepts and assumptions that act as a guide for theory development (2). Assumptions are broad, general statements that are taken for granted for the sake of the argument (3) which suggest the relationship between two or more concepts. When concepts are combined to form a relationship as stated in assumptions, concepts form the basic structure of the theory. A theory explains phenomena by specifying which variables (concepts) are related; how these variables are related to each other permits prediction about the phenomena (4). The theory level is rarely reached in applied disciplines because of the number of potential variables and their interactions.

Most conceptual models have three major or central concepts to which all other concepts are related. Often, groups of three concepts will be connected to the major ones so the theoretical model has twelve concepts—three major concepts and three more attached to each of the major ones. In examining the concepts found in conceptual models of occupational therapy, a three-plus-one arrangement allowed a simple figure, a venn diagram, to be drawn and an outline to be constructed. For example, the three-plus-one structure includes outcome, doing process, tools, and context, which become the major categories for organizing the concepts identified in occupational therapy (Figure 7.1, Table 7.1).

Outcomes are the perceived goals, final end point, or desired results of applying the doing process and tools to a problem situation described in the conceptual model. The doing process is the mechanism of individual action that will permit the outcomes to be obtained using selected tools. The tools are the media through which the doing process is used to achieve the outcomes. Finally, all three central concepts occur with a given context that facilitates or constrains the final output.

Outcomes or goals come in two varieties: those with two dimensions and those with multiple dimensions. Outcomes with two dimensions are either attained or not attained. Four concepts identified in the conceptual models fit the two-dimensional format balance of occupations, health in medicine, cure, and survival. Balance of

Table 7.1. Organization of Concepts in Occupational Therapy Models

OUTCOMES/GOALS (desired results, functional outcomes, and states of being that are measured in absolutes or levels)

*Balance of occupation (Absolute)

Cure (Absolute)

Health as Defined in Medicine (Absolute)

Survival (Absolute)

Achievement Level

*Adaptation (Level)

Autonomy (Level)

*Competent/Competence (Level)

Coping (Level)

*Health Through Occupation (Level)

Health Promotion (Level)

*Independent/Independence (Level)

Mastery (Level)

*Occupational Competence (Level)

*Occupational Performance (Level)

*Occupational Role Performance (Level)

Quality of Life (Level)

Prevention (Level)

Satisfaction (Level)

Wellness (Level)

DOING PROCESS (of individual action using mechanisms, methods, techniques, and approaches)

Activity (of occupation) Process

Adaptive Process

Coping Process

(Doing) Meaningful Activity

*(Doing) Purposeful Activity

(Doing) Rituals

*(Doing) Routines

(Doing) a Series of Steps

*(Doing) Tasks

Educating Process

(Following) a Sequence

continued

Table 7.1.   Organization of Concepts in Occupational Therapy Models
*Functioning Process
Group Process
*Habit Training
Instructional Process
Learning Process
Mastering Process
Role-playing Process
Simulation
*Skills Practice
Teaching Process
Training Process
TOOLS (Media)
*Occupation
*Activity
*Activities (Occupations) of Daily Living
*Instrumental Activities (Occupations) of Daily Living
*Interest (in Occupations)
*Leisure Occupations
Productive Occupations
*Play Occupations
Rest and Sleep (Occupations)
Routine Tasks (of Daily Living)
Self-care Occupations
Self Maintenance (Occupations)
*Work Occupations
Work Readiness Occupations
CONTEXT (situation in which action occurs and tools are used)
*Environment (biological, social, cultural, physical, organic, inorganic, human, nonhuman, physiologic, temporal, spacial, medical, health care, political, or economic)
Order ("natural" rhythm, harmony, cycles, oscillating, equals, repetition, rules, norms, mores, laws, or organization)
*Discussed in chapters 8, 9, or 10.

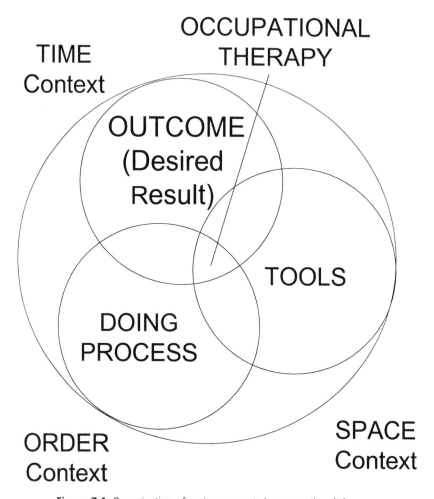

Figure 7.1. Organization of major concepts in occupational therapy.

occupations, for example, is either attained or it is not. To say a person's balance of occupations is more or less in balance is not a clearly stated outcome. The desired balance either has or has not been obtained. Health as a medical concept can be explained in the same way. According to the biomedical or pathology model, a person is either free of disease (pathology) or is not. In other words, a person has either attained health or is sick. A person is not sort of healthy or sort of sick. The same logic applies to cure and survival. A person is either cured or not cured and either survives or dies.

The other form of outcome tends to have levels although the exact number of levels is not always specified. Rather, inherent in the model is a scale comprised of various positions on a line (visual analog) or a sequence to follow. The levels may be organized according to chronological age, a known sequence of physiologic recovery from injury, or a series of steps that must be accomplished to attain the goal. For example, independence is often measured in several levels. A widely known assessment, Functional Independence Measure (FIM), uses a seven-level scale to determine the degree of care and supervision a person may require from a caregiver. Therefore, the term *moderately independent* is a variable which can be described and illustrated within the guidelines of the assessment. Many other outcomes have been described including achievement, autonomy, competence, maintenance of health, mastery, occupational competence, occupational performance, quality of life, role attainment, survival, and wellness.

The doing process requires action on the part of the individual that enables him or her to do something better than before, to do something for the first time, or to do something again. These doing processes are not mutually independent of each other. Similar subprocesses may be the same. The labels have simply come from different sources. These doing processes provide one of the criteria that separates occupational therapy from other professions. The doing action must be done by the individual. Occupational therapy personnel can help, guide, and facilitate, but the doing process only succeeds when the individual does the doing. For example, the individual must adapt (a doing action) to his or her context. Occupational therapy personnel can not do the adapting for the individual or to the individual. There are numerous doing processes including education, function, habits, learning, mastery, performing, role performance, skill, and training.

Tools are the media through which action and doing occur. The major tools are grouped according to the type of occupation involved. Various conceptual models use self-care, activities of daily living, routine tasks, instrumental activities of daily living, homemaking, or self-maintenance occupations to form one major area of occupation in a person's life. Another area is usually referred to as work, productivity, or work-play. A third area may be called play, leisure, or play–leisure. Other possibilities include rest, sleep, or tasks. In addition, the major concepts in occupations can be subdivided into many components. Table 7.2 shows some of possible subdivision of occupational components.

Finally, the context usually includes the concepts of time, space, and order. The actual concepts often use the term environment such as temporal environment; spacial environment; or social, cultural, political, or economic environment. The concept of order has many variations. Older conceptual models sometimes referred to the natural rhythms and harmony with nature. Conceptual models developed in the 1960s and 1970s often use hierarchy, levels, or stages based on human physiology to present the concept of sequential order. New conceptual models consider a variety of factors related to order—especially those related to the physical, social, and cultural environment.

The concept of order is a particularly important one in conceptual models for occupational therapy because it usually sets the stage for the discussion of disorder

Table 7.2. Subdivisions of Occupational Components

Sensorimotor	Cognitive–perceptual	Psychosocial
Sensory	*Cognitive*	*Intrapersonal*
Auditory	Attention	Achievement
Gustatory		Affect
Kinesthesia	Concentration	Competence
Olfactory	Concept Formation	Emotions
Pain	Decision Making	Feelings
Pressure	Orientation	Interests
Proprioception	Problem Solving	Mastery
Temperature	Time Management	Motivation
Touch		Self-concept
Vestibulation	*Perceptual*	Self-efficacy
Vibration	Hearing	Self-esteem
Vision	Kinesthetic	Will
Cross-modal	Mechanical	
Multisensory	Pain Awareness	*Interpersonal*
Sensory Integration	Proprioceptive	Beliefs
	Smell	Community
Motor	Tactile	Country
Accuracy	Taste	Dyad
Coordination	Vestibular	Groups (Small, Large)
Dexterity	Vibratory	Neighborhood
Gestures		Roles
Joint Range of Motion		Values
Muscle Strength		World
Perceptual (Motor)		
Reflex/Reaction		
Speech		
Speed		
Developmental		
Milestones		
Synergy		

Table 7.3. Terms and Definitions of Disorder

Disorder: a derangement or abnormality of function; a morbid physical or mental state

Abnormality: the quality or fact of being abnormal or a malformation or deformity

Deformity: distortion of any part or general disfigurement of the body; malformation

Derangement: mental disorder or disarrangement of a part or organ

Development, Arrested: cessation of the developmental process at some stage prior to its normal completion.

Deviation: a turning away from the regular standard or course

Disease: any deviation from or interruption of the normal structure or function of any part, organ, or system (or combination thereof) of the body that is manifested by a characteristic set of symptoms and signs and whose cause, pathology, and progress may be known or unknown

Dysfunction: disturbance, impairment, or abnormality of the functioning of an organ

Injury: harm or hurt; a wound or maim, which is usually applied to damage inflected to the body by an external force

Maladjustment: failure to fit one's inner needs to the environment

Retardation: delay; hindrance; delayed development

Delay or Delayed: not defined in Dorland's

Impaired or Impairment: not defined in Dorland's

Definitions from: Dorland's Illustrated Medical Dictionary. Philadelphia: Saunders, 1994.

in the practice model. A practice model organizes one or more concepts from the conceptual model or theory so that the concept(s) can be applied to a real world problem such as a client being seen in an occupational therapy service. Occupational therapy practitioners work with people who have disorder in their lives or are at risk for disorder. For example, if a child should be able to perform certain occupational tasks at a certain age and cannot, the child is behind or delayed in development. Developmental delay is a type of disorder. If an adult is unable to perform the tasks in role such as parent or worker because of a disease (which is itself a disorder), the person experiences role dysfunction. Dysfunction is also a disorder. Most practical models in occupational therapy address how assessment and intervention, through the use of tools in occupational therapy, can correct or reduce the impact of disorder in the performance of human occupations. Table 7.3 defines some of the types of disorder seen by occupational therapy practitioners.

Table 7.4.   Concepts in Context

Concept	Characteristics	Focus	Relevance for Occupational Therapy
Achievement	Measured by external environment demands	Society and professional	Used to justify therapy programs
Adaptation (personal)	Coping and adjustment skills	Society and professional	Used with therapy programs
Autonomy	Individual choice	Client, society, and professional	Central
Competence or occupational competence	Decision making and skilled performance	Society and professional	Used to justify therapy programs
Coping	Adjustment skills	Society and professional	Used to justify therapy programs
Health through occupation	Must be explained to client	Professional	Used to justify therapy programs
Health promotion	Designed to maintain good health	Society	May be important to client
Independence	Community living out of an institution	Client	Central
Independent	Able to do occupations without assistance	Profession	Used to justify therapy program
Mastery	Decision making and skilled performance	Society and professional	Used to justify therapy programs
Occupational performance	Completion of tasks and roles	Society and professional	Used to justify therapy programs
Occupational role performance	Performance of role expectations	Society and professional	Used to justify therapy programs
Quality of life	Able to do what is important to the client	Client	Central
Prevention	Avoiding disorder	Society and professional	Used to justify therapy programs
Satisfaction	Agreeable to client	Client	Central
Well-being	Feeling good	Client	Central

continued

Table 7.4. Concepts in Context

Concept	Characteristics	Focus	Relevance for Occupational Therapy
Wellness	Achievement of better health and life	Society	May be important to client
Occupational balance	Changing degree or type of tasks and roles	Society and professional	Used with therapy programs
Cure	Get well; get rid of sickness	Client and professional	Client accepts therapy professional justifies
Health (medicine)	Absence of disease	Professional	Used to justify therapy programs
Survival	To live	Client and professional	Client accepts therapy; professional justifies
Activity process	Meaning and relevance to client often absent	Professional	Minimal, adjunctive
Adaptive process	Meaning and relevance difficult for client to understand	Society and professional	Used to justify therapy programs
Coping process	Able to do what is important to the client	Client	Central
Meaningful activity	Meaning and relevance difficult for client to understand	Society and professional	Used to justify choice of therapy program
Purposeful activity	Purposefulness to client absent or unclear	Society and professional	Used to justify choice of therapy program
Rituals			
Routines			
Doing series of steps			
Tasks			
Educating process			

continued

Table 7.4. Concepts in Context

Concept	Characteristics	Focus	Relevance for Occupational Therapy
Following a fixed sequence			
Functioning process			
Group process			
Habit training			
Instructional process			
Learning process			
Mastering process			
Role-playing process			
Simulation			
Skills practice			
Teaching process			
Training process			
Occupation	Meaningful and purposeful to client	Client	Central
Activity			
Activities of daily living			
Instrumental activities of daily living			
Interests			
Leisure occupations			
Productive occupations			
Play occupations			
Rest and sleep occupations			
Routine Tasks			

continued

Table 7.4.	Concepts in Context		
Concept	Characteristics	Focus	Relevance for Occupational Therapy
Self-care occupations			
Work occupations			
Work readiness occupations			
Context and environment	Doing what is important to client where it is important to the client	Client	Central

Expanded from: Golledge J. Distinguishing between occupation, purposeful activity and activity, part 1: review and explanation. Br J Occup Ther 1998;61(3):104.

Blanks intentional for reader to complete.

CONCEPTS IN CONTEXT

Golledge suggests that terms, which are actually concepts, should be examined in relation to the characteristics, the focus, and the relevance for occupational therapy (5). Table 7.4 is based on the idea presented by Golledge and expanded to include other concepts to provide a summary of the concepts discussed in the chapters that follow.

References

1. Webster's New Universal Unabridged Dictionary. New York: Barnes & Noble, 1996.
2. Wolman BP. Dictionary of Behavioral Science. 2nd ed. New York: Van Nostrand Reinhold, 1989.
3. Reese WL. Dictionary of Philosophy and Religion: Eastern and Western Thought. Atlantic Highlands, NJ: Humanities Press, 1980.
4. Kerlinger N. Foundations of Behavioral Research. 3rd ed. New York: Holt Rinehart & Winston, 1986.
5. Golledge J. Distinguishing between occupation, purposeful activity and activity, part 1: review and explanation. Br J Occup Ther 1998;61(3):100–105.

CHAPTER 8

Concepts Related to Outcomes and Goals

This chapter reviews five concepts usually associated with outcomes and goals. The concepts are presented in alphabetical order to avoid the appearance that one concept is inherently better than another. Each has been used in models several times. As yet there is no clear indication of which one is the best—if there is one best—concept to explain outcome in occupational therapy practice.

ADAPTATION OF THE INDIVIDUAL

The concept of adaptation has been borrowed from biological science where traditionally it has had two different meanings. One meaning is biological or evolutionary adaptation and refers to the changes in structure and function of total organisms or parts of organisms that affect the process of natural selection and thus the survival of a species over successive generations. Steen defines biological adaptation as the "modification of an organism in structure of function in adjusting to a new condition or environment" (1). King defines evolutionary adaptation as a change in the structure or function of an organism or any of its parts that result from the process of natural selection (2).

The other meaning refers to individual adjustment or change made by a person to enhance his or her survival and potential. Individual adaptation is defined as "adjustments made by the individual that primarily enhance personal rather than species survival, and secondarily contribute to actualization of personal potential" (2). Tinbergen, a biologist, states that "adaptedness is a certain relationship between the environment and what the organism must do to meet it" (3). *Webster's New Universal Unabridged Dictionary* defines individual adaptation as a sociological term in which "a slow, usually unconscious modification of individual social activity in adjustment to cultural surroundings" occurs (4). Individual adaptation focuses on the relationship between what the environment demands and what the person must do to meet those demands. The individual is seen as adapting when the person is able to organize data and make a response that meets the demands. Occupational therapy is interested primarily in individual adaptation.

Use of Adaptation in Occupational Therapy

The term adaptation began appearing in the occupational therapy literature in 1922 when Meyer stated that diseases seen in psychiatry are "largely problems of adaptation" and that psychiatry was among the first disciplines to recognize the need for adaptation and the value of *work* as a help in the problems of adaptation (5). Wood suggests that three assumptions are derived from Meyer's work: 1) life demands an ongoing process of adaptation; 2) disease and disability often disrupt this process; and 3) people solve problems of adaptation through engagement in occupation and thereby influence their health favorably (6).

Since 1922, the concept of adaptation has been incorporated into the occupational therapy literature in multiple uses. Some uses can be easily identified. The source of others has not been clearly identified although current use can be identified. The following uses are known: adaptation to activity, adapted device(s), adapted equipment, adapted environment, adapted technique(s), adapted technology, adaptive approach, adaptive behavior, adaptive process, adaptive repertoire, adaptive response(s), adaptive skill(s), adaptive state, adaptive techniques, adaptive technology, occupational adaptation, spatial temporal adaptation, and temporal adaptation. Definitions of these usages often overlap; therefore, clear delineation is not possible.

Adaptation to activity, also called adapted activity or adaptive techniques, is the modification of features such as sequence, complexity, positioning, location, use of tools, construction of equipment, et cetera, to meet objectives or goals in the intervention process such as improved performance (7).

An *adapted device or adapted equipment* involves altering a tool, utensil, or machine to permit the item to be used by a person who is disabled or to improve the use by a normal person (8). An *adapted environment* is one specially designed to aid an individual in performing necessary daily tasks (9). These three uses of adaptation can be called *adapted techniques,* which means using alternative methods to accomplish a task. The alternative methods permit a person to accomplish the same objective but the procedures, sequences, or tasks are changed to permit performance of a part or all of the task in a different manner.

Adapted, adaptive, or *assistive technology* is "any item, piece of equipment, or product system, whether acquired commercially off the shelf, modified or customized, that is used to increase, maintain, or improve functional capabilities of individuals with disabilities (10)." Smith, however, has made a useful distinction between two types of technology used in occupational therapy practice. One is the technology used to rehabilitate or educate such as software for cognitive rehabilitation programs, biofeedback instruments, and electrical stimulation units. This technology is not actually adaptive or assistive technology but rather rehabilitation or education technology. True adaptive or assistive technology substitutes for impaired function and allows the individual to perform an occupation more independently (11).

An *adaptive approach* involves the use of skills that are relatively intact that are used to develop compensatory methods for deficit areas. Pedretti stresses that adaptive approaches usually involve making the person aware of a problem such as neglecting items in the left field of vision (left-field neglect)—which may occur in a person who had a stroke (12). Occupational therapy practitioners cannot correct the perceptual processes but can assist the person to take compensatory actions. Adaptive approaches are thus internal, usually cognitive, strategies. Therefore, adaptive approaches are considered a subcategory of adapted activity or a separate category.

Adaptive behavior is a term borrowed from psychology. Adaptive behavior means behavior that is functioning to facilitate adaptation. It is appropriate and useful in aiding adjustment. Reber points out that, increasingly, the term adaptive behavior is used to mean normal or sane behavior (13). Reed and Sanderson stress that adaptive behavior involves the integration of the skills areas with the socially accepted values to accomplish occupations and tasks (8).

Closely related are the terms *adaptive process* and *adaptive responses*. King defines adaptive process as the means that are involved in a person's active acquisition of knowledge and techniques whereas an adaptive response is the means of eliciting goal-directed or purposeful behavior. These two terms are further illustrated in the discussion of King's model of the adaptive process.

According to Spencer, Davidson, and White, an adaptive repertoire is the accumulated set of occupational forms a person uses to organize memories of past experiences that a person is accustomed to performing (14). The term is borrowed from music: a person learns to play or sing a number of musical compositions, which becomes his or her repertoire. Adaptive repertoires are an accumulation of knowledge about how occupations are performed and where they occur. This knowledge is learned over a lifetime.

Adaptive skills have been defined by Creek as learned patterns of behavior that assist a person to function adequately within the individual's environment (15). Turner, Foster, and Johnson expand the definition by stating that adaptive skills are those required and acquired to undertake adaptation (16).

Occupational adaptation, spatial–temporal adaptation, personal adaptation through occupation, temporal adaptation, and adaptive response model are models developed by occupational therapists based on the concept of adaptation. Occupational Adaptation was developed by Schkade and Schultz (17). Spatial–Temporal Adaptation was developed by Gilfolye, Grady, and Moore (18). Personal Adaption Through Occupation was developed by Reed and Sanderson (8). Temporal Adaptation was developed by Kielhofner (19). The adaptive response model was developed by King (2). Schkade and Schultz further expanded the terminology derived from adaptation by adding terms such as adaption energy, adaptive response behavior, adaptive response evaluation, adaptive response mechanism, adaptive response mode, and adaptive state.

Disadaptation, Maladaptation, and Sensory Deprivation

In contrast to adaptation, a person may experience disadaptation when there is failure to organize and respond, and maladaptation when there is incorrectly organized data to a response that does not meet the situation's. The cause of both disadaptation and maladaptation is reduced or missing sensory input and information, which is called sensory deprivation. Adaptive behavior requires sensory input.

Reduced or missing input may result in insufficient data to organize and respond correctly to sensory stimulation, which may be considered disadaption. Examples include confusion and disorientation.

If sensory data are received but organized incorrectly, the response is likely to be incorrect or inappropriate. Examples of maladaptation are hallucinations and delusions. Maladaptation may also occur from sensory information that is not patterned such as the constant hum of a motor on a machine dispensing intravenous fluids or other "white noise" such as the test pattern on the television set or the all-white environment of an intensive care unit.

Missing sensory input such as occurs in sensory deprivation also may result in maladaptation. An example is immobilization in bed resulting in loss of proprioception and kinesthetic input. Sensory deprivation may also cause loss of motivation that may last long after sensory stimuli have been restored.

The Process of Adaptation

King has suggested that the process of adaptation involves four characteristics (2). First, the person must adjust to different conditions or environments. In doing so the person must be an active participant, not a passive recipient on which action is imposed. Second, adaptation is a response to the demands of the internal or external environment. The individual is challenged because of something the person needs or wants to change in the self or the external environment. An adaptive response, however, is not truly adaptive until it is incorporated into recurring or daily life. Third, adaptation is most effective when the individual operates in an automatic fashion that requires little, if any, conscious attention. The adaptive response needs to become habitual to be effective. Fourth, adaptation provides its own reward; thus, an adaptive response is self-reinforcing.

Occupational therapy, King feels, can facilitate adaptation through involving the person in active participation and response, selecting purposeful activities that will meet demands, promoting purposeful behavior which can be integrated subcortically, and encouraging self-reinforcing experience. The adaptive process and facilitating characteristics of occupational therapy are summarized in Figure 8.1.

Individual adaptation is an attractive concept to occupational therapists. The model King proposes is consistent with the organismic view that a person can maintain a locus of control in the environment and has some chance through ac-

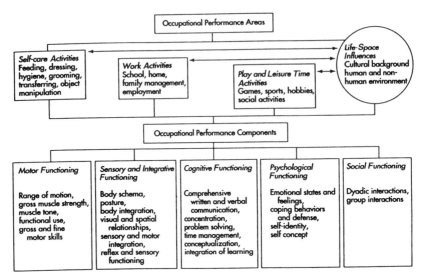

Figure 8.1. Occupational performance areas and componenets. (From: American Occupational Therapy Association. A curriculum guide for therapy educators. Rockville, MD: The Association, 1974.)

tive participation, as in the change process of intervention. In addition, the model supports the selection of purposeful occupations and activities as the primary tools (medium) of achieving individual adaptation through the method or technique of promoting purposeful behavior, which the individual can repeat. Furthermore, individual adaptation is seen as a developmental process that begins in childhood and continues throughout the life span. Although individual adaptation is attractive, it requires careful application. Occupational therapists must clarify the concepts of purposeful activity and purposeful behavior. These terms need to be seen through the individual's eyes, not the therapist's or society's. It is easy to select activities that are purposeful to the therapist because the knowledge base is readily available in the therapist's mind. It is harder to help others select activities that have purpose to them. Good skills in assessment and analysis are important to learn how to facilitate the selection of purposeful activities and to promote the development of purposeful behavior through these activities.

Adaptation As a Life-change Process

In terms of life changing events Spencer, Davidson, and White suggests that two aspects of adaptation are particularly important (14). The first is the idea that "adaptation is an interactive process that occurs between an organism and its environment." Thus, life-changing events involve not only the individual but the relationships with other people, with the environment, or with both. An example is moving to a new home in a new city. There will be new neighbors, old friends are probably a greater distance away, and a new physical and community environment must be learned.

Second, "adaption is an inherently cumulative process in which the past shapes the future." In the human species, the past includes both the genetic transmission of successful traits and the cultural transmission of successful adaptive strategies learned from previous generations. An individual has the inborn physiological mechanisms and the capacities for memory (hindsight) and intention (foresight). Therefore, occupational therapy practitioners should be aware of both continuity and change in clients' lives.

Summary

Adaptation is a central concept in occupational therapy literature and practice. The number of terms based on adaptation and the number of models built using the concept of adaptation attest to its importance. Frank suggests that adaptation is also a foundation for the academic discipline of occupational science (20). She suggests the following definition of adaptation be considered: "Adaption is a process of selecting and organizing activities (or occupations) to improve life opportunities and enhance quality of life according to the experience of individuals or groups in an ever-changing environment."

COMPETENCE AND OCCUPATIONAL COMPETENCE

Webster's New Universal Unabridged Dictionary defines competence as: a) the quality of being competent; adequacy; possession of required skills, knowledge, qualification, or capacity; b) sufficiency; a sufficient quantity; c) an income sufficient to finish the necessities and modest comfort of life; and d) other definitions dealing with law, embryology, linguistics, immunology, and geology (1).

Reber defines competency as the "ability to perform some task or accomplish something" (2).

White is the acknowledged guru on the concept of competence (3). His article in the *American Journal of Occupational Therapy* is widely quoted in the occupational therapy literature. Equally important are two of his other articles (4, 5). White defines competence as "fitness or ability to carry on those transactions with the environment which result in its maintaining itself, growing, and flourishing"(4).

Reilly used the concept of competency in her model of play development (6). She borrowed White's definition, which was sufficient or adequate behavior to meet the demands of the situation (5). She was concerned with competency behavior, which she characterized as a drive to deal with the environment and influence the environment through feedback. Competency behavior was the middle stage between exploratory behavior and achievement behavior.

Kielhofner and Miyake suggest there are four essential elements to competence: 1) the abilities of the individual; 2) individual self-assessment; 3) the objective or collective experiences of others for task performance in the persons' environment; and 4) the range of opportunities and resources available to an individual in the environment (7). Competence requires an interaction between the self and the environment and the ability or willingness to learn and adapt to the information provided. Furthermore, the four essentials suggest that if a person is unable or unwilling to learn or adapt to the information in the environment, difficulty or problems in achieving or maintaining competence are likely to occur.

Hagedorn suggests that competence is linked to the performance of roles and that persons who are dysfunctional often have difficulty sustaining roles because their performance is incompetent (8). In other words, competence and performance of roles are linked together. Problems in competence may lead to poor or inadequate performance of roles and problems in performance threaten a person's competence.

Mocellin is a strong advocate of the concept of competence (9). He feels it is not occupation, per se, that is therapeutic but rather the achievement of competence, which he describes as "the experience of efficacy, control and of self-determination."

Polatajko borrows her definition of competency from the nursing literature (10). Competencies defined as "adequacy or sufficiency, answering all the requirements of an environment" (11). Polatajko discusses occupational competence and describes it as "the result of a goodness of fit between the person, the occupation and the environment" (10). In other words, occupational competence "is determined by the interaction of the individual and the environment" (12). She states that occupational therapy personnel must adopt many roles and use many tools to help their clients to achieve occupational competence. In Palotajko's opinion, occupational therapy is a discipline concerned with enabling occupational competence (12). To illustrate, she uses a Rubik's Cube puzzle to show the three dimensions of the occupational competence model: the individual, occupational, and environmental. Within each dimension are three domains. The individual includes cognitive, affective, and physical domains. Occupational includes self-care, productivity, and leisure domains, and the environmental includes physical, social, and cultural domains. Occupational competence is therefore a product of the dynamic interaction between the environment, the individual, and the changes made responding to the other.

Summary

Competence and occupational competence have become important concepts in models of occupational therapy. These concepts are being used more in models outside the United States. It is unclear whether occupational performance and occupational competence are synonymous terms and are tapping the same information or whether competence and occupational competence are tapping information not included in the defintion of occupational performance.

HEALTH THROUGH OCCUPATION

Health has been defined in many ways. Surprisingly, the dictionary only refers to two descriptions: the general condition of the body or mind with reference to soundness and vigor or freedom from disease or ailment (1). The biomedical model health focuses on the idea that health is the absence of pathology or disease. Occupational therapy has focused more on the idea that health is related to a interactive focus on mind, body, and spirit, which taken together form the whole person or—more accurately—the person as a whole.

The focus of health in this discussion is limited to the relationship of health to occupation. As Mocellin points out, the views regarding the relationship of health to occupation has changed over the years (2). Originally the primary contribution was to keep clients occupied in normal (according to Northern European culture) occupations and amusements of everyday life. For persons confined to bed or to a hospital, the occupations and amusements were handicrafts, reading, or playing quiet games. For persons able to leave the hospital, there were jobs farming the land owned by the institution, working in the kitchen or laundry, going for walks or rides, and watching groups of entertainers.

Meyer with the help of Slagle began a program called habit training to help clients regain health because he believed that schizophrenia, and perhaps other disorders, resulted from disorganized habits of living (3, 4). Habit training focused on organizing the tasks of daily living into a time schedule. The schedule included all aspects of daily living including the performance of daily self-care and productive occupations as well as amusements and other leisure pursuits. All clients followed a schedule considered best-suited to their current stage of health.

Occupation was also used to divert clients from their florid symptoms, especially for those with psychotic disorders. As Dunton said: "When attention is directed (focused) upon some occupation or task the patient cannot think of his illness or discomfort as two objects cannot occupy the focus of attention at the same time" (5). By engaging the person in occupation, the occupational therapists could focus the person on reality and thus reduce the degree of dysfunction the person displayed while hallucinating or acting delusional. Occupation could replace the abnormal behaviors with more normal ones. Occupation could also be used to divert attention away from pain and psychological stress. Diverting attention away from illness or discomfort should be distinguished from diversional activity. Diverting attention is a direct approach to treating a specific problem. Diversional activity is primarily providing a means of passing the time pleasantly rather than doing nothing or being bored.

Dunton also discusses the use of occupation as a means of improving clients' mental attitude or morale (5). The objective was to improve clients' contentment because a positive attitude is known to have a positive effect on regaining health. Dunton cautions that an occupational therapist is skilled in determining the correct balance between amusing through diversion and overfatiguing clients whereas a nurse or family member may overstress or fatigue clients.

Similar ideas are expressed by Hall in his discussion of equivalents, immunities, and substitution (6). Hall suggests that clients who cannot pursue their customary work may "be able to make an effort equal to that which will later be needed in [their] life outside the hospital." Hall felt the need to learn to concentrate was the most important result of equivalent work within the hospital. Others might suggest that the person was maintaining or increasing work tolerance and health fitness for work tasks (7). Hall felt that equivalent work should be novel but at a low level with frequent rest breaks.

Hall's concept of immunity is to increase the person's tolerance to noise because so many clients had been protected from noise by their families and health care workers during their illness. In order to function in a work environment, the person must be able to tolerate a certain amount of noise. Hall suggests that initially the client should be making the noise because such self-created noise did not seem to bother the client. Gradually, the noise made by others was introduced until the person could tolerate the normal level of noise associated with the type of work the client did. As the noise sensitivity decreased, the person's potential for returning to normal work activities increased. Being able to return to work is often equated by clients and their families as evidence of returning health.

Substitution is the process of incorporating "successful achievement in a small way for failure in a large way" according to Hall. He wanted clients to find "a new interest, a new belief in self, which is an excellent substitute for the old sense of inadequacy and the old worries." Through occupation, persons replace unhappy thoughts and feelings for feelings of accomplishment and belief in personal health.

Hall also conceptualized the work cure, which he developed for clients who had neurasthenia, a stress disorder (8). He would introduce a client to work while the client was still in bed and encourage the person to work for a few minutes once a day in the morning. For example, a woman might work on embroidery for 5 minutes for 5 days. After a few days, Hall would ask the person to sit on the side of the bed and increase the duration, perhaps to 10 minutes. Later he would ask the person to sit in a chair beside the bed and again increase the time to 15 minutes. Next, the person would be asked to sit in the day room for perhaps 5 minutes in the afternoon while still continuing the 15 minutes of activity in the bedroom. Other clients might join the person, and work time would be increased to 15 minutes in the afternoon as well as the morning. Still later, the person would be encouraged to work in another building or outside. The time would increase to half a day with rest periods throughout. Finally, the person would be able to work a normal day and will have regained personal health.

Hall was not the first to see the relationship of work and labor to health. Kirk-bride wrote the following in 1854: "Labor then is one of our best remedies; it is as useful in improving the health of the insane, as in maintaining that of the sane. It is one of the best anodynes for the nervous, it composes the restless and excited, promotes a good appetite and a comfortable digestion, and gives sound and re-freshing sleep to many who would without it pass wakeful nights" (9).

Barton also discusses the use of occupation to directly influence health (10). He hoped that the administration of occupation could be given in dosages like phar-maceuticals were given. The dosage approach was tried by Licht who wanted oc-cupational therapists to record the number of repetitions a client did such as beats on the loom to tighten the woven threads (11). Unfortunately, the exact number of repetitions of a movement do not easily translate into observable changes in health. Furthermore, a given occupation cannot be performed to decrease the symptoms of a specific disease as Barton had hoped.

Barton also saw occupation as a means of teaching or educating people about healthful living. In his workroom he had a sign bearing the phrase "Happiness through Occupation. " He also wrote a book in which he defined occupational therapy as "the science of instructing and encouraging the sick in such labors as will involve those energies and activities producing a beneficial therapeutic effect" (12). For several years, he organized a group of convalescent men to teach them how to organize their lives and develop vocational pursuits.

Using occupation to promote health and to cure was also the idea behind the curative workshops in which clients with physical disabilities were seen (13). The curative workshop primarily cured unemployment because most were operated as sheltered workshops for person with physical limitations owing to industrial ac-cidents, fractures, polio, arthritis, cerebral palsy, or cardiac disease. Curative workshops were often community organization sponsored by the Junior League for Woman, a woman's social organization. Gradually, the workshops were fi-nanced by insurance companies and/or state workers compensation departments. All were interested in helping clients find employment or return to previous em-ployment.

In 1962 Reilly made one of the most famous statements in the occupational therapy literature regarding health through occupation when she stated that "man, through the use of his hand as they are energized by mind and will, can influence the state of his own health" (14). She suggested that there is a reservoir of sensi-tivity and skill in the hand which can be tapped to foster health. Basically, Reilly believed humans have a basic need for occupation and thus occupation is central to establishing, maintaining, and regaining health.

Yerxa suggests a relationship between health and skills exists (15). Specifically, "occupation that develops skills can prevent illness and influence health by de-veloping competency and making life worth living." She envisions health "as the possession of a repertoire of skills to achieve one's own purposes." Skills that lead to mastery and competence can be attained regardless of pathology or impairment. Thus, health through occupation is related to skill acquisition and use, not freedom from disease.

Common to all of these ideas of health through occupation is the theme that health can be influenced positively by the occupation one does. Order, in this case health, can be achieved by doing occupation as part of daily life. Implicit is the subtheme that mind, body, and spirit need to function and be focused together for the best results.

INDEPENDENT AND INDEPENDENCE

Webster's New Universal Unabridged Dictionary provides 23 definitions of the word independent. The first six seem most relevant:

1. not influenced or controlled by others in matters of opinion, conduct, etc.; thinking or acting for oneself; an independent thinker;
2. not subject to another's authority or jurisdiction; autonomous; free; an independent business man;
3. not influenced by the through or action of others; independent research;
4. not dependent; not depending or contingent on something else for existence, operation, etc.;
5. not relying on another or others for aid or support; and
6. refusing to be under obligation of others. (1)

The concept of independence goes back to the beginning of this century. The earliest reference found was by Hall in 1905 (2). He states that "to encourage a feeling of independence" patients who turn out valuable work should have their products sold through an agency of the workshop and the proceeds credited to the maker. The idea of selling patients' products for profit was not successful. The pottery works at Marblehead was separated because patients could not make the detailed designs on the pottery (3). The medical workshop at Massachusetts General Hospital was discontinued after only 2 years. It should be clear that the use of independence is associated with economic independence and not specifically to independence in self-care although independent self-care may have been implied. Thus, the concept of independence was not identified in the early literature.

Occupational therapists and the concept of independence appear to have joined forces and emerged sometime after World War II. The first reference located in an occupational therapy textbook is in 1950. Dr. Licht speaks of independence as a goal for persons with traumatic paraplegia (4). He is not specifically referring to independence as the goal of occupational therapy but rather for the patient. He states that the "ultimate objective for all patients with traumatic paraplegia is independence. Physical independence is the foundation of all other aspects of independence and for the paraplegic this means great strength in the muscle of the upper extremities and shoulder girdle which will facilitate crutch walking."

There appears to be a correlation between the concept of independence and the rise of physical medicine and rehabilitation. The first article written by an occupational therapist appears in 1957. Zimmerman begins her article saying that the "word independence, besides a universal interpretation of freedom, has as many meanings as there are individuals" (5). To the physically disabled it is a keynote word. But even then, all too frequently it is apt to mean independence through sheer physical strength. She then illustrates the need for special tools and equipment (adapted devices and equipment) to accomplish tasks in everyday living. Her article ends by stating that it is "the right of every disabled person to seek independence through the use of whatever tools or devices will assist him in his efforts to make use of his inherent skills and abilities to become a productive and useful member of society."

Hightower continues the theme of independence through activities of daily living by stating that the

> use of adaptive equipment will sometimes give your patient added independence, a feeling of fulfillment through achievement and free the family members of some responsibility. . . In achieving independence, training in the use of the residual ability is always necessary and training in the use of self-help devices or specialized equipment is often indicated. (6)

She then proceeds to describe and illustrate several self-help devices.

By 1980 the concepts of independent and independence were well established in the collective minds of occupational therapists. Baum extends those concepts to the government plan to facilitate independent living through the passage of the Rehabilitation Act of 1973 Amendments of 1978 (PL 95–602) (7). She begins her presentation by stating that "independent living is a concept occupational therapists have long valued" and that services in occupational therapy have been directed toward developing the skills to "function as an independent person in work, leisure, and maintenance activities."

In spite of the general support, little is written about the concept of independence as it applies to occupational therapy. Mostly, the word just appears. For example, the 1981 definition of occupational therapy includes the phrase "in order to maximize independence" (8). What is meant by maximizing independence is not stated. Apparently "everybody knows" what is meant.

The 1979 Uniform Terminology document uses the term independent living, which refers to the "skills and performance of physical and psychological/emotional self-care, work, and play/leisure activities to a level of *independence* appropriate to age, life-space, and disability" (italics added) (9). Once again, the word independence is neither defined nor described.

Rogers states that "independence connotes self-reliance, self-determination, self-directedness, and a perspective of personal control" (10). Occupational therapists regard persons who can do things for themselves as independent. In addition, she suggests that functional independence is a core concept of occupational therapy and is the goal of the occupational therapy process. Furthermore, functional independence results from the interaction between the person and the environment.

Baum briefly discusses independence in relation to resources such as assistive technology (11). She states that independence "means having access to and using the necessary devices and human helpers in order to perform the tasks of daily living." She is referring to the problem of whether a person is or is not considered independent if the person uses assistive technology such as adapted devices. The problem occurs when physicians and perhaps other professionals view a person as a patient unless or until the person becomes "normal" or cured. As a result, some assessments of independence such as the original version of the Functional Independence Measure (FIM) did not rank a person as fully independent if assistive devices were required (12). On the FIM Level 4 was Complete Independence and Level 3 was Modified Independence, which was described as follows: "Activity requires any one of the following: an assistive device, more than reasonable time, [or] safety consideration." The FIM was later changed to the seven-level code now used, and Levels 6 and 7 are both considered independent but Level 6 indicates that devices (extra time or safety consideration) are used to achieve the independence (13). Independence is defined as follows: "Another person is not required for the activity."

The problem of whether assistive technology reduces the level of independence prompted the American Occupational Therapy Association to prepare a paper titled "Broadening the Construct of Independence" (14). The essence was to state the belief that there are a variety of ways for individuals to achieve independence and all should be recognized and accepted. Among these ways are hiring persons to perform certain tasks, using assistive devices or technology, or using adapted methods of performing tasks. Furthermore, an individual should not be stigmatized by the use of devices or strategies to accomplish daily living tasks. The example given is the use of a date book to keep appointments.

Hagedorn suggests there are two concepts rather than one (15). The other is the individual as an autonomous person. She suggests that therapists describe a person as autonomous when they mean a person is "capable of exercising choices and control over one's personal life" and as independent when they mean "able to do what is required to remain health, without needing someone else to help." In other words, autonomy relates to individual choice and independence relates to self-maintenance. To achieve autonomy, a person would need to be capable of making choices and decisions about how do direct his or her life. To achieve independence, a person would need to be able to perform the tasks necessary to maintain some minimum level of health and well-being.

OCCUPATIONAL PERFORMANCE

Occupational performance first appeared in the literature in the 1970s. In 1973 the American Occupational Therapy Association published *The Roles and Functions of Occupational Therapy Personnel,* which defined occupational performance as:

. . . the individual's ability to accomplish that tasks required by his or her role and related to his or her development stage. Roles include those of a "preschooler," student, homemaker, employee, and retired worker. Occupational performance includes self-care, work and play/leisure time performance. (1)

The model of occupational performance appearing in Figure 8.1 was first published in 1974 (2). Occupational performance included the areas of self-care, work, and play/leisure time activities, which interacted with the life space influences. The performance components that supported the occupational performance areas include motor, sensory–integrative, cognitive, psychological, and social functioning. The performance components were defined as "the learned developmental patterns of behavior which are the substructure and foundation of the individual's occupational performance."

In April 1974 a report on target populations for occupational therapy defined occupational performance "as the ability to accomplish the tasks related to a developmental stage; it includes the ability to develop and sustain a lifestyle that is equally balanced among goal-directed activities—toward self-care, independence, contributions to others, and gratification of personal needs" (3). The goal of occupational therapy services based on the occupational performance model is to improve the occupational performance of the individual but also to seek "removal of social, architectural education, psychological, or economic barriers which interfere with a person's ability to fulfill an occupational role and achieve an equitably balanced life style."

Changes in the Concept

By 1976 the definition of occupational performance had already begun to change. Llorens defines occupational performance as including the concerns of work, education, play, self-care, and leisure (4). The problem of deciding how to categorize the performance areas has been addressed by Christiansen (5). Table 8.1 expands Christiansen's table. Christiansen suggests and the author concurs that disagreement about categories and contents within the categories hinders both practice and research within the field. Without agreement, a true taxonomy is not possible.

In 1986 the definition changed to active engagement in life tasks related to self-maintenance, leisure, and play (6). Because the subject of the position paper is children, perhaps the authors felt self-maintenance, leisure, and play were the appropriate life tasks for young people and thus no mention is made of a work or productivity task.

In 1991, Christiansen and Baum state that occupational performance

refer(s) to the day-to-day engagement in occupations that organize our lives and meet our needs to maintain ourselves, to be productive, and to derive enjoyment and satisfaction within our environment. Occupational performance includes engagement in tasks as routine and necessary as bathing and dressing and those more involved and complex that are related to one's work requirements. (7)

Table 8.1. Classification of Occupations

Meyer (1)	Work	Play	Rest	Sleep
Mosey (2)	School/work	Play/leisure recreation	ADL	Family interaction
AOTA (3)	Work	Play and leisure	Self-care	
AOTA (4)	Work and productive	Play or leisure	ADL	
CAOT (5)	Productivity	Leisure	Self-care	
Reed (6)	Productivity	Leisure	Self-maintenance	
Kielhofner, Burke, Heard-Igi (7)	Work	Play	Self-maintenance	
Clark (8)	Work	Play	Self-maintenance	
Hagedorn (9)	Work	Leisure	ADL	
Katz (10)	Work	Play/recreation and leisure	Daily living tasks	
Llorens (11)	Work	Education	Play	Self-care	Leisure

Expanded from: Christiansen C. Classification and study in occupation: a review and discussion of taxonomies. J Occup Sci: Aust 1994;1(3):3–20.

1. Meyer A: A theory of occupation therapy. Arch Occup Ther 1922;1(1):1–10.

2. Mosey AC. The Psychosocial Components of Occupational Therapy. New York: Raven Press, 1986.

3. American Occupational Therapy Association. A Curriculum Guide for Occupational Therapy Educators. Rockville, MD: The Association, 1974.

4. American Occupational Therapy Association. Uniform terminology for occupational therapy. 3rd ed. Am J Occup Ther 194;48(10):1047–1054.

5. Canadian Association of Occupational Therapists. Intervention Guidelines for the Client-Centred Practice of Occupational Therapy. Ottawa: Ministry of National Health and Welfare, 1986.

6. Reed KL. Concepts of Occupational Therapy. Baltimore: Williams & Wilkins, 1980.

7. Kielhofner G, Burke J, Heard-Igi CA. Model of human occupation: part four: assessment and intervention. Am J Occu Ther 1980;34:777–788.

8. Clark NH. Human development through occupation: a philosophy and a conceptual model for practice. Am J Occup Therapy 197933:505–514.

9. Hagedorn R. Occupational Therapy: Foundations for Practice. Edinburgh: Churchill-Livingstone, 1992.

10. Katz N. Occupational theray's domain of concern: reconsidered. Am J Occup Ther 1985;39(8):521.

11. Llorens LA. Application of a Developmental Therapy for Health and Rehabilitation. Rockville, MD: American Occupational Therapy Association, 1976:3.

Llorens changed her concept of occupational performance between 1976 and 1991 (8). In her chapter of the Christiansen and Baum text, she describes occupational performance as "the accomplishment of tasks related to self-care/self-maintenance, work/education, play/leisure, and rest/relaxation, [and] is critical to the assumption of social or life roles, the functional positions that people hold in the society—worker, parent, mate, peer, etc."

According to Levine and Brayley (9), occupational performance can be categorized as follows:

1. Achievement: demonstration of knowledge, skills, and attitudes needed to perform an occupational role.
2. Competence: adequate performance that can be improved and organized into consistent habits and patterns.
3. Exploration: manipulation of objects, skills, and communication tools that provides an opportunity for learning; can be playful and entertaining with little serious commitment. (10,11)

In 1995 Baum and Law wrote a position paper for the American Occupational Therapy Association (12). In that paper they state that " occupational performance reflects the individual's dynamic experience in daily occupations within the environment." Also, occupational performance can be described as occupational function or as function. They state that "occupational therapy uses the word *function* interchangeably with performance and occupational performance because occupational therapy's domain is the function of the person in his or her occupational roles."

Pedretti states that occupational performance refers to the ability to perform those tasks that allow one to carry out occupational roles in a satisfying manner appropriate to the individuals' developmental stage, culture, and environment (13).

Assumptions

Pedretti and Pasquinelli suggest that the assumptions of the occupational performance model are as follows:

1. Occupational roles of human beings can be categorized into areas.
2. Development, performance, and maintenance of occupational roles are influenced by elements from both the intrapersonal and extrapersonal realms.
3. An appropriate balance of occupational roles is critical to the maintenance of health.
4. Appropriate balance changes with chronological/developmental age, life stage, and life circumstances.
5. Failure in development of occupational roles or loss, disruption, or change of occupational roles can be caused by intrapersonal and/or extrapersonal elements.

6. Adequate performance of occupational roles depends on the integrated functioning of the (performance component) subsystems of the individual.
7. Defect, disease, or injury affecting a performance component causes a failure of integration of the performance components subsystem. This results in a failure or disruption in the performance skills and, thus, of occupational role performance.
8. The role of the occupational therapist is to facilitate both an appropriate balance and optimal performance of occupational roles.
9. The occupational therapist is concerned with remediation of and compensation for deficits in performance components and performance skills.
10. Primary tools of the occupational therapist for the remediation of performance skills and performance components are purposeful and enabling activities.
11. The occupational therapist also prepares the patient for performance of purposeful activity. The therapist may use adjunctive methods, such as exercise, facilitation and inhibition techniques, splints, and sensory stimulation in the treatment continuum toward the development of the ability to master the performance skills and to engage in functional activities appropriate to the patient's occupational roles.
12. Exclusive use of preparatory methods out of the patient's occupational performance context is not considered occupational therapy.
13. A human is defined as an individual with an intrinsic need to deal with the environment. (13)

Application

The first attempt to use the model of occupational performance was proposed by two students and their instructor to outline occupational therapy's role in assisting a person with terminal illness (14). The authors defined occupational performance as "a process in which a client relearns old skills, learns new skills, and modifies or maintains present skills as necessary for satisfactory performance of his or her occupational therapy." To plan an intervention program, the occupational therapist "begins at the client's present level of function." With the treatment program, "adaptive behavior is demanded and motivation is stimulated." Alternate roles must also be considered with role models available as well as opportunities to practice new roles and adaptive skills.

The model of occupational performance has been assured a place in the history of occupational therapy practice models because the concept of occupational performance has been incorporated within the model of human occupation as revised by Fisher and Kielhofner and within the model of person–environment occupational performance by Christiansen and Baum (15, 16). In the 1997 discussion of their model, Christiansen and Baum define occupational performance as "the doing of occupation." Nelson further developed the concept of occupational performance as the "action elicited, guided, or structured by the preexisting occupational form" (17).

Assessments

Kielhofner and Henry developed the first assessment specifically designed to measure occupational performance; they called this the Occupational Performance History Interview (18). The instrument was latter published by the American Occupational Therapy Association (19). Other instruments that measure occupational performance are the Occupational Case Analysis Interview and Rating Scale (OCAIRS) by Kaplan and Kielhofner (20), the Assessment of Motor and Process Skills (AMPS) by Fisher (21), and the Canadian Occupational Performance Measure (COPM) by Law and colleagues (22).

Other Applications

The first edition of "Uniform Terminology for Occupational Therapy", published in 1979, does not use the model of occupational performance (23). Beginning with the second edition, which was published in 1989, the organization of the occupational performance model is used although the term occupational performance is not (24). The concepts of occupational performance areas and occupational performance components are described but not defined. The third edition, published in 1996, still does not define or describe occupational performance, but it does describe performance areas, performance components, and performance contexts (25). Performance areas are described as "including activities that the occupational therapy practitioners emphasizes when determining functional abilities" such as activities of daily living, work, and other productive activities as well as play or leisure. "Performance areas are broad categories of human activity that are typically part of daily life" and constitute both the major concern of occupational therapists and the ultimate treatment outcome, which is to enable a person to attain and maintain function in the performance areas. Performance components "are the elements of performance that occupational therapists assess and, when needed, in which they intervene for improved performance." Performance components include sensorimotor, cognitive, psychosocial, and psychological aspects. "Performance components are fundamental human abilities that . . . are required for successful engagement in performance areas." Performance contexts "are situations or factors that influence an individual's engagement in desired and/or required performance areas." Performance contexts include temporal aspects such as chronological age, development age, place in the life cycle, and heath status as well as environmental aspects such as physical, social, and cultural considerations. The model is seen in Figure 8.2.

Summary

The concept of occupational performance has become a mainstay in the development of models of occupational therapy. It operates as a means of connecting the individual to roles and to the sociocultural environment.

I. Performance Areas	II. Performance Components	III. Performance Contexts
A. Activities of Daily Living	A. Sensorimotor Component	A. Temporal Aspects
B. Work and Productive Activities	B. Cognitive Integration and Cognitive Components	B. Environment
C. Play or Leisure Activities	C. Psychosocial Skills and Psychological Components	

From: Am J Occup Ther 1994, 48(11):1050.

Figure 8.2. Outline of the Uniform Terminology for Occupational Therapy

One problem with occupational performance and similar concepts that focus on doing and motor behavior is how to assimilate the cognitive processes of thinking, planning, organizing, and even rehearsing when no evidence of motor action exists. Occupational therapy practitioners recognize the importance of cognitive skills especially in problem solving and decision making but do not prove much credit for cognitive performance by itself.

OCCUPATIONAL ROLE

In the occupational therapy literature, both the terms role and occupational role appear. The term role has three meanings in *Webster's New Universal Unabridged Dictionary,* which are as follows: 1) a part or character played by an actor or actress; 2) proper or customary function; such as the teacher's role in society; and 3) from sociology, the rights, obligations, and expected behavior pattens associated with a particular social status (1). The last two definitions are those primarily used in occupational therapy literature.

The concept of role is derived from sociology, social psychology, and anthropology. The word is derived from the early French theater, where a role was the roll of paper upon which an actor's part was written (2).

The concept of role appears first in Reilly's work on occupational behavior (3). In 1969 she proposed a change in the educational model used to guide the occupational therapy program at the University of Southern California. Part of the proposed change was to add role theory to the theoretical framework. Reilly states that role theory suggests that roles are learned in the process of socialization (3, p. 302). Heard, a student of Reilly's, wrote about occupational roles (4). She based her classification of roles from Katz and Kahn, which were personal–sexual, familial–social, and occupational roles (5). Only occupational roles were considered to be part of the domain of concern to occupational therapy. In 1986 Oakley and colleagues suggested that the viewpoint of occupational roles should be changed to recognize that personal–sexual and familial–social roles might have a relationship to occupational roles and thus should be considered as well (6).

Pedretti defines occupational roles as "the life roles that the individual holds in society. These may include roles such as preschooler, student, parent, homemaker, employee, volunteer, or retired worker" (7, p. 3).

Christiansen and Baum define role as "a set of behaviors that have some socially agreed upon function and for which there is an accepted code of norms." Role competence is defined as the "achievement of the behaviors which have some socially agreed-upon function and for which there is an accepted code of behavioral norms or expectation" (8, p. 603).

According to Kielhofner, roles provide a means for individual needs to be met, and by engaging in the occupational role behaviors, the individual derives a sense of purpose, identity, structure, and regularity (9). Furthermore, roles can organize occupational behavior by influencing manner and style within the content of interaction with others, can influence the set or groups of tasks that are part of the role performance routine, and can partition or divide the occupational behaviors into temporal dimensions. Kielhofner lists the following roles as having occupational dimensions: student, worker, volunteer, caregiver, home maintainer, friend, family member, religious participation, hobbyist or amateur, and participant in an organization (5, p. 74).

Hagedorn suggests the occupational roles "identify the person as a 'doer' of particular jobs, arts, crafts or techniques. . . while. . . social roles identify relationships" (10). She states that "roles imply required actions, knowledge, skills, attitudes, duties or responsibilities." The importance to occupational therapy practitioners is " the ways roles are acquired, retained, changed, exchanged, owned, or rejected" because of the effects on the person. Role acquisition simultaneously brings occupation, which in turn defines or characterizes a role. Hagehorn states that role acquisition is an example of which comes first, the chicken or the egg. Knowledge, skills, and attitudes form the information on what and how to perform an occupation while duties or responsibilities entail the actual doing. Role performance is probably related to competence.

Assessments

The concept of occupational role has helped to develop several assessment instruments. Among the instruments are the following: Adolescent Role Assessment by Black (11); Role Activity Performance Scale by Good-Elis, Fine, and Spencer (12); Role Change Assessment by Jackoway, Rogers, and Snow (13); Role Checklist by Oakley and colleagues (6); and Worker Role Interview by Velozo discussed by Biernacki (14).

Summary

The concept of role is probably attractive to occupational therapy because of its strong relationship to occupation. In particular, the concept has lead to the development of several assessment instruments. One caution is the problem of conceptualizing role as identical across cultures. Roles and the expectations of roles change from one culture to another. Can assessments developed in one culture be used successfully in another culture without bias?

BALANCE

The word balance appears frequently in the occupational therapy literature and is usually related to a discussion of different types of occupation in relation to time such as 24 hours in a day. Balance is another word with multiple definitions that allow various interpretations as to what the founders or early leaders of occupational therapy meant when they used the term. *The Oxford English Dictionary* lists 22 definitions for the word balance as a noun and 17 as a verb (1). A summary follows:

1–4. An apparatus for weighing or any apparatus used in weighing, whether acting by leverage or by the resistance of a spring; one scale of a balance or a flat dish resembling a scale.
  5. One of the zodiacal constellations (more commonly called Libra).
  6. Watchmaking, a mechanical contrivance that regulates the speed of a clock or watch.
  7. *Nautical.* The operation or result of reefing with a balance-reef.
  8. The metaphorical balance of justice, reason, opinion, by which actions and principles are weighed or estimated.
  9. The wavering balance of fortune or change in which issues hang in suspense.
 10. Subjective or objective uncertainty or suspense, hesitation, wavering doubt, risk, or hazard.
 11. Power to decide or determine; authoritative control.
 12. A weight put into one scale to equal the prepondering weight in the other; a counterpoise.
 13. A condition in which two (or more) opposing forces balance each other: equilibrium.
 14. General harmony between the parts of anything, springing from the observation of just proportion and relation; especially in the art of design.
 15. Stability or steadiness due to the equilibrium prevailing between all forces of any system.
 16. The prepondering weight; the net result of estimating conflicting principles, forces, etc.

17–21. The process of finding the differences, if any, between the debit and credit sides of an account. The sum of money remaining over after realizing all assets and discharging all liabilities.
22. Combined words such as balance beam, balance step, etc.

To discover which meaning the theorists had in mind, it is necessary to locate the sources containing the word. The word is most often quoted in Meyer's paper on the philosophy of occupation therapy (2). Meyer used the word balance or balances four times in three separate sections of his paper. They are as follows:

1. ". . . Miss Wright was chosen to attend it (Chicago School of Civics and Philanthropy training course) and she returned to organize the work throughout the institution—with a wise **balance** between organized shopwork and more individual work on the wards." (p. 3, boldface added)
2. "Our conception of man is that of an organism that maintains and **balances** itself in the world of reality and actuality by being in active life and active use, i.e., using the living, and acting its *time* in harmony with its own nature and the nature about it. " (p. 5, italics in original, boldface added)
3. There are many other rhythms which we must be attuned to: the *larger rhythms* of night and day, of sleep and waking hours, of hunger and its gratification, and finally the big four—work and play and rest and sleep, which our organism must be able to **balance** even under difficulty. The only way to attain **balance** in all this is *actual doing, actual practice,* a program of wholesome living as the *basis* of wholesome feeling and thinking and fancy and interest. (p. 6, italics in original, boldface added).

Although the term balance is the one most often cited from Meyer's paper, two other words concerning order are also included: harmony in the phrase "acting its time in harmony" and rhythm in the phrase "[t]here are many rhythms to which we must be attuned to: the larger rhythms of night and day." The significance of these two terms has received little attention in the occupational therapy literature.

Another view of organizing life is provided by Hall (3). Although he does not use the term balance, he does discuss organizing occupation into segments of clock time, a concept that Meyer also mentioned. He states: "A division of the twenty-four hours into changeable periods of work, rest and recreation" (p. 13).

The concept of balance as stated by Meyer and Hall is actually related to the concepts of rhythm, harmony, and changeability—not to the concept of equal measure of equal sums of weight, value, or time. Note that the phrase "equal division of time" does not appear in either Meyer's writing or Hall's writing. The use by Meyer and Hall is consistent with dictionary definition number 6—a harmonious or satisfying arrangement or proportion of parts of elements, as in a design—and number 14—general harmony between the parts or any portion and relation; esp. in the Arts of Design. This usage would be consistent with the ties of occupational therapy to the arts and crafts movement, which Meyer mentions by its anti-industrialism themes stated as the following: 1) "Present day humanity seems to suffer from a deluded craze for finding substitutes for actual work"; 2) "Out industrialism has created the false . . . idea of success in *production* . . . bringing with it a kind of nausea to the worker . . . "; and 3) "The man of today has lost the capacity and pride of workmanship and has substituted for it a measure in terms of money; and how his money proves to be of uncertain value" (p. 8).

McHenry, in *The New Encyclopedia Britannica,* states that rhythm and balance result from the three-dimensional arrangement of elements and materials on the site (4). Rhythm is a sequence or repetition of similar elements, for example, a double row of trees. Balance is the sense one gets looking in any direction that the elements to one's left balance those to one's right and the feeling one has that the view is in equilibrium. Thus, balance is related to rhythm, harmony, and symmetry.

Therefore, balance does not mean equal amounts of time as Mocellin suggests when he says that the "concept of activity balance has been borrowed from ideas which have derived from changes in work practice during the last century" (5). There is no mention in Meyer's or Hall's work of creating the day's division into 8 hours of work, 8 hours of play, and 8 hours of sleep. Besides, Meyer divided the natural rhythms into four categories—work, play, rest, and sleep—so the hours would have to be 6 work, 6 play, 6 rest, and 6 sleep. This notion of equal amounts of time does not fit the essence of Meyer's statements but rather the modern interpretation of them. Mocellin is reflecting on Australian society and culture. Meyer and Hall were talking about rhythms of interchangeable units, not fixed units. Nowhere do they say that each day, or even each week, must be perfectly balanced in terms of hours spent in certain activities. The emphasis of balance in the works of the early theorists was on order and organization, not on division and equal segments.

Christiansen suggests there are three perspectives on balance that should be considered by occupational therapy practitioners (6). One is the historical view of balance represented by Meyer and the contemporary extensions of the historical view represented by Reilly in the occupational behavior model and Kielhofner in the temporal adaptation model (7, 8). The second is the patterns of time use and individual characteristics as represented by time budgets (9), logs, diaries, or perhaps more correctly, activity budgets. Time budgets much more closely relate to the interpretation of balance as equal units. Christiansen summarized several studies and found the average percentages of time use were 15% (approximately 4 hours) in activities of daily living, 25% (6 hours) in work, 30% (approximately 7 hours) in discretionary or leisure, and 30% (7 hours) in sleep. Thus, the "balance" becomes 4, 6, 7, and 7. Even if ADL and work are combined as "obligatory" time versus discretionary time, the "balance" is still unequal at 10 hours obligatory, 7 hours of discretionary time, and 7 hours of sleep.

The third perspective is chronobiological balance based on biological rhythms. Best-known of the biological rhythms are circadian rhythms controlled by physiologic systems. Physiologic systems appear to follow cycles such as sleep–wake or rest–activity cycles. Internal mechanisms are known as oscillating systems, in which external mechanisms such as light, heat, and socialization patterns are called Zeitgebers (time givers). Meyer may have been suggesting the concept of chronobiology when he discussed rhythms.

Cynkin suggests the use of an activities clock to represent "bands of time allocated to specific activities over a designed period" to depict patterns of activity (10). She feels such an approach allows for individual idiosyncracies as well as cultural variations. She does not suggest a specific balance or rhythm.

Simpson has proposed that the phrase occupational balance be used to organize the concept of balancing occupations within the practice of occupational therapy (11). He proposed 14 premises or belief statements (assumptions) in three conceptual frameworks: function–dysfunction continuum, evaluation, and intervention. The practice frame of reference is outlined in the following.

The four statements on the function–dysfunction continuum are: 1) humans are occupation-oriented beings, and the balance of occupation (or performance areas) including self-care, work and productivity, and leisure is essential for health functioning; 2) the term balance in this context describes managing occupational participation in a way that is personally fulfilling (or meaningful) and meets role demands; 3) occupational balance is different for each person—each person has an individual occupational balance schema that suits his or her health; and 4) often, a psychosocial, cognitive, or sensorimotor impairment (performance components) upsets occupational balance and may affect one, two, or all three performance areas. In other words, the person is no longer able to participate in occupations in a way that is meaningful to him or her or in a way that adequately meets previous role demands. Such an imbalance is unhealthy and constitutes occupational dysfunction.

Three statements on evaluation follow:

1. To facilitate change, the occupational therapist must first evaluate the person's current function level in each occupational performance area.
2. For those occupational performance areas that are out of balance, the occupational therapist must evaluate which skills (performance components) are insufficient to meet the demands of the performance area.
3. If it is impractical or unfeasible to evaluate a performance area, the therapist must instead evaluate performance components and use clinical reasoning to project the impact of disabilities on performance areas.

The seven statements on intervention are as follows:

1. The treatment planning process in guided by three types of treatment goals: remediation of occupational schema imbalance, compensation for occupational schema imbalance, and occupational rescheming. Remediation of occupational schema imbalance means that performance component deficits are treated di-

rectly, with the aim of correcting deficits so that the person can carry out former activities as he or she previously had. Compensation for occupational
schema imbalance means that the performance component deficit will be cir-
cumvented so that the client learns adaptive methods, uses adaptive equipment,
or benefits from environmental compensation. Occupational rescheming is
used for a client who is no longer able to participate in former occupational activities and must therefore develop new occupational balance schema.
2. The building of skills (sensorimotor, cognitive, psychosocial) is essential to the
   restoration of occupational balance.
3. Specific skill-building techniques are drawn from existing knowledge within
   the field of occupational therapy. These techniques include remedial approaches (e.g. , neurodevelopment, biomechanical) as well as compensatory
   approaches. The approach used depends on the goal.
4. The means through which skills are built is through purposeful activities. The
   treatment activities should match the demands of the actual occupational activities as closely as possible; the selection of treatment activities is known as activity matching.
5. There are three levels of activity matching from which the therapist may choose:
   a) same activity, same environment; b) same activity, different environment; or
   c) different activity, different environment.
6. These levels of activity matching are placed on a continuum, from the most generalized to the least generalized.
7. The levels of activity matching also fall on a continuum from most targetive to
   least targetive.

Summary

The concept of balance in occupational therapy is poorly understood and often
misinterpreted. The issue is whether balance is tied to equal amounts of clock
time, which is external to the person, or to physiological rhythms of the internal
body. If control is centered in the individual, then internal rhythms would be more
consistent with a view of the individual as the source of action.

References

ADAPTATION OF THE INDIVIDUAL
1. Steen EB. Dictionary of biology. New York: Barnes & Noble, 1971.
2. King LJ. Toward a science of adaptive responses. Am J Occup Ther 1978;32(7):
   429–437.
3. Tinbergen N, Hall E. A conversation with Nobel prize winner Niko Tinbergen. Psychol
   Today 1974;March:66,74.
4. Webster's New Universal Unabridged Dictionary. New York: Barnes & Noble, 1996.
5. Meyer A. Philosophy of occupation therapy. Arch Occup Ther 1922;1(1):1–10.

6. Wood W. Legitimatizing occupational therapy's knowledge. Am J Occup Ther 1996;50(8):626–634.
7. Hagedorn R. Foundations for Practice in Occupational Therapy.2nd ed. New York: Churchill Livingstone, 1997.
8. Reed KL, Sanderson SN. Concepts of Occupational Therapy. Baltimore: Williams & Wilkins, 1992.
9. Pumwar AJ. Occupational Therapy: Principles and Practice. 2nd ed. Baltimore: Williams & Wilkins, 1994.
10. Congressional Report on PL 100–407. The Technology-related Assistance for Individuals With Disabilities Act. Washington, DC: U. S. Government Printing Office, 1988, section 3.
11. Smith RO. Technological approaches to performance enhancement. In: Christiansen C, Baum C. Occupational Therapy: Overcoming Human Performance Deficits. Thorofare, NJ: Slack Inc., 1991:746–786.
12. Pedretti LW. Evaluation of sensation and treatment of sensory dysfunction. In: Pedretti LW. Occupational Therapy: Practice Skills for Physical Dysfunction. 4th ed. St. Louis: Mosby, 1996:232.
13. Reber AS. Dictionary of Psychology. 2nd ed. London: Penguin, 1995.
14. Spencer JC, Davidson HA, White VK. Continuity and change: past experience as adaptive repertoire in occupational adaptation. Am J Occup Ther 1996;50(7):526–534.
15. Creek J. Occupational Therapy and Mental Health. 2nd ed. New York: Churchill Livingstone, 1997.
16. Turner A, Foster M, Johnson SE. Occupational Therapy and Physical Dysfunction: Principles, Skills and Practice. 4th ed. New York: Churchill Livingstone, 1996.
17. Schkade JK, Schultz S. Occupational adaptation: toward a holistic approach for contemporary practice, part 1. Am J Occup Ther 1992;46:829–837.
18. Gilfoyle E, Grady A, Moore J. Children Adapt. Thorofare, NJ: Slack Inc., 1981.
19. Kielhofner G. Temporal adaption: a conceptual framework for occupational therapy. Am J Occup Ther 1977;31:235–242.
20. Frank G. The concept of adaptation as a foundation for occupational science research. In: Zemke R, Clark F. Occupational Science: The Evolving Discipline. Philadelphia: FA Davis, 1996:47–55.

COMPETENCE AND OCCUPATIONAL COMPETENCE

1. Webster's New Universal Unabridged Dictionary. New York: Barnes & Noble, 1996.
2. Reber AS. Dictionary of Psychology. 2nd ed. London: Penguin Books, 1995.
3. White R. The urge toward competence. Am J Occup Ther 1973;25:273.
4. White R. Motivation reconsidered: the concept of competence. Psychol Rev 1959;66:297–333.
5. White R. Sense of interpersonal competence. In: White R. The Study of Lives. New York: Atherton Press, 1964.
6. Reilly M. Play as Exploratory Learning. Beverly Hills: Sage, 1973:146–147.
7. Kielhofner G, Miyake S. Rose-colored lenses for clinical practice: from a deficit to a competency model in assessment and intervention. In: Kielhofner G. Health Through Occupation: Theory and Practice in Occupational Therapy. Philadelphia: FA Davis, 1983:257–266.

8. Hagedorn R. Occupational Therapy: Perspectives and Processes. Edinburgh: Churchill Livingstone, 1995:57–59.
9. Mocellin G. An overview of occupational therapy in the context of the American influence on the profession: part 2. Br J Occup Ther 1992;55(2):55–60.
10. Polatajko HJ. Dreams, dilemmas, and decisions for occupational therapy practice in a new millennium: a Canadian perspective. Am J Occup Ther 1994;48(7):592–593.
11. Pridham KF, Schutz ME. Rationale for a language for naming problems from a nursing perspective. Image. J Nurs Scholarship 1985;17(4):122–127.
12. Polatajko HJ. Naming and framing occupational therapy: a lecture dedicated to the life of Nancy B. Canadian Journal of Occupational Therapy 1992;59(4):196–197.

HEALTH THROUGH OCCUPATION

1. Webster's New Universal Unabridged Dictionary. New York: Barnes & Noble, 1996.
2. Mocellin G. Occupational therapy: a critical overview, part 1. Br J Occupy Ther 1995;58(12):504–505.
3. Meyer A. Remarks on habit disorganization in the essential deteriorations, and the relations of deterioration of the psychasthenic, neurasthenic, hysterical and other constitutions. In: Winters E. The Collected Papers of Adolf Meyer. v II. Psychiatry. Baltimore: John Hopkins Press, 1951:421–431.
4. Slagle EC. Training aids for mental patients. Arch Occup Ther 1922;1(1):11–20.
5. Dunton WR. Prescribing Occupational Therapy. Philadelphia: Saunders, 1928:38.
6. Hall HJ. OT equivalents, immunities, and substitutions. In: Hall HJ. OT: A New Profession. Concord, MA: Rumford Press, 1923.
7. Licht S. The principles of occupational therapy. In: Dunton WR, Licht S. Occupational Therapy: Principles and Practice. Springfield, IL: Charles C Thomas, 1950:13.
8. Hall HJ. The work cure. JAMA 1910;CIV:12–13.
9. Kirkbride TS. On the Construction, Organization and General Arrangements of Hospitals for the Insane. Philadelphia: Lippincott, 1880.
10. Barton GE. Occupational therapy. Trained Nurse Hosp Rev 1915;54:138–140.
11. Licht S. Dosage in kinetic occupational therapy. Occup Ther Rehabil 1947;26:167–171.
12. Barton GE. Teaching the Sick: A Manual of Occupational Therapy and Reeducation. Philadelphia: Saunders, 1919.
13. Faulkes WF. The curative workshop from the viewpoint of industrial accident compensation. Occup Ther Rehabil 1927;6(4):253–264.
14. Reilly M. Occupational therapy can be one of the great ideas of 20th century medicine. Am J Occup Ther 1962;16:1–9.
15. Yerxa EJ. Dreams, dilemmas, and decision for occupational therapy practice in a new millennium: an American perspective. Am J Occup Ther 1994;48(7):586–589.

INDEPENDENCE

1. Webster's New Universal Unabridged Dictionary. New York: Barnes & Noble, 1996.
2. Hall HJ. The systematic use of work as a remedy in neurasthenia and allied conditions. Boston Med Surg J 1905;CLII(2):29–32.
3. Hall HJ. The out-patient workshop: a new hospital department. Transactions of the American Hospital Association 1913;15:349–355.
4. Licht S. Kinetic occupational therapy. In: Dunton WR, Licht S. Occupational Therapy: Principles and Practice. Springfield, IL: Charles C Thomas, 1950.

5. Zimmerman ME. Ideas for independence. Crippled Child 1957;34(5):7.
6. Hightower MD. Independence through activities of daily living. Delaware Med J 1966;38:238.
7. Baum CM. Nationally speaking: Independent living: A critical role for occupational therapy. Am J Occup Ther 1980;34(12):773.
8. AOTA Representative Assembly. Minutes. Am J Occup Ther 1981;35(12):792–803.
9. AOTA Representative Assembly. Uniform terminology for reporting occupational therapy service. Am J Occup Ther 1979;33:780–813.
10. Rogers JC. The spirit of independence: the evolution of a philosophy. Am J Occup Ther 1982;36(11):709.
11. Baum C. Identification and use of environmental resources. In: Christiansen C, Baum C. Occupational Therapy: Overcoming Human Performance Deficits. Thorofare, NJ: Slack Inc., 1991:790.
12. Hamilton BB, Laughlin JA, Fiedler RC, Granger CV. Interrater reliability of the 7-level Functional Independence Measure (FIM). Scan J Rehab Med 1994;26:116.
13. Keith RA, Granger CV, Hamilton BB, Shersin FS. The Functional Independence Measure: a new tool for rehabilitation. In: Eisenberg MG, Grzesiak RC. Advances in Clinical Rehabilitation. Vol 1. New York: Springer Publishing Co., 1987:12.
14. AOTA. Broadening the construct of independence. Am J Occup Ther 1995;49:1014.
15. Hagedorn R. Occupational Therapy: Perspectives and Processes. Edinburgh: Churchill Livingstone, 1995:53.

OCCUPATIONAL PERFORMANCE
1. American Occupational Therapy Association. The Roles and Functions of Occupational Therapy Personnel: Rockville, MD: The Association, 1974:1,37.
2. American Occupational Therapy Association. A Curriculum Guide for Occupational Therapy Educators. Rockville, MD: The Association, 1974:12.
3. American Occupational Therapy Association. Task force on target populations. Association report II. Am J Occup Ther 1974;28:231–232.
4. Llorens LA. Application of a Developmental Theory for Health and Rehabilitation. Rockville, MD: American Occupational Therapy Association, 1976.
5. Christiansen C. Classification and study in occupation: a review and discussion of taxonomies. J Occup Sci Aust 1994;1(3):3–20.
6. Morroni K, Hickman L. Early childhood intervention: position paper. Am J Occup Ther 1986;40(12):834.
7. Christiansen C. Occupational therapy: intervention for life performance. In: Christiansen C, Baum C. Occupational Therapy: Overcoming Human Performance Deficits. Thorofare, NJ: Slack Inc., 1991:27.
8. Llorens LA. Performance tasks and roles throughout the life span. In: Christiansen C, Baum C. Occupational Therapy: Overcoming Human Performance Deficits. Thorofare, NJ: Slack Inc., 1991:46–66.
9. Levine RE, Brayley CR. Occupation as a therapeutic medium:a contextual approach to performance intervention. In: Christiansen C, Baum C. Occupational Therapy: Overcoming Human Performance Deficits. Thorofare, NJ: Slack Inc., 1991:622,624.
10. Reilly M. Play as Exploratory Learning. Beverly Hills: Sage, 1974:47,146.
11. Kielhofner G. The human being as an open system. In: Kielhofner G. The model of Hu-

man Occupation: Theory and Application. Baltimore: Williams & Wilkins, 1985: 64,66–67.

12. Baum C, Law M. Occupational performance: occupational therapy's definition of function. Am J Occup Ther 1995;49(10):1019.
13. Pedretti LW, Pasquinelli S. A frame of reference for occupational therapy in physical dysfunction. In: Pedretti LW, Zoltan B. Do Occupational Therapy: Practice Skills for Physical Dysfunction. 3rd ed. St. Louis: Mosby, 1990:3.
14. Gammage SL, McMahon PS, Shanahan PM. The occupational therapist and terminal illness: Learning to cope with death. Am J Occup Ther 1976;30(5):296.
15. Fisher A, Kielhofner G. Mind–brain–body performance subsystem. In: Kielhofner G. A Model of Human Occupation: Theory and Application. 2nd ed. Baltimore: Williams & Wilkins, 1996:83–89.
16. Christiansen C, Baum C. Occupational Therapy: Enabling Function and Well-being. Thorofare, NJ: Slack, Inc. 1998:54.
17. Nelson NL. Occupation: form and performance. Am J Occup Ther 1988;42(10): 633.
18. Kielhofner G, Henry AD. Development and investigation of the Occupational Performance History Interview. Am J Occup Ther 1988;42(8):489–498.
19. Kielhofner G. Henry AD. A User's Guide to the Occupational Performance History Interview. Bethesda, MD: American Occupational Therapy Association, 1995.
20. Kaplan K, Kielhofner G. Occupational Case Analysis and Interview Rating Scale. Thorofare, NJ: Slack Inc., 1989.
21. Fisher AG. Assessment of Motor and Process Skills. Fort Collins, CO: Department of Occupational Therapy, Colorado State University.
22. Law M, Baptiste S, McColl MA, et al. The Canadian Occupational Performance Measure. 2nd ed. Toronto: Canadian Association of Occupational Therapists, 1994.
23. AOTA. Uniform Terminology for Occupational Therapy. Am J Occup Ther 1979.
24. AOTA. Uniform Terminology for Occupational Therapy—Second Edition. Am J Occup Ther 1989;43:817–831.
25. AOTA. Uniform Terminology for Occupational Therapy—Third Edition. Am J Occup Ther 1996;43(10):808–815.

OCCUPATIONAL ROLE

1. Webster's New Universal Unabridged Dictionary. New York: Barnes & Noble, 1996.
2. Reber AS. Dictionary of Psychology. 2nd ed. London: Penguin, 1995.
3. Reilly M. The educational process. Am J Occup Ther 1969;23(4):299–307.
4. Heard C. Occupational role acquisition: a perspective on the chronically disabled. Am J Occup Ther 1977;41:243–237.
5. Katz D, Kahn RL. The Social Psychology of Organization. New York: John Wiley & Sons, 1966.
6. Oakley F, Kielhofner G, Barris R, Reichler RK. The role checklist: development and imperial assessment of reliability. Occup Ther J Res 1986;6(3):157–169.
7. Pedretti LW. Occupational performance: a model for practice in physical dysfunction. In: Pedretti LW. Occupational Therapy: Practice Skills for Physical Dysfunction. 4th ed. St. Louis: Mosby, 1996:3.
8. Christiansen C, Baum C. Occupational Therapy: Enabling Function and Well-being. Thorofare, NJ: Slack Inc., 1997.

9. Kielhofner G. A Model of Human Occupation: Theory and Application. 2nd ed. Baltimore: Williams & Wilkins, 1995:70–75.
10. Hagedorn R. Occupational Therapy: Perspectives and Processes. Edinburgh: Churchill Livingstone, 1995:73–74.
11. Black M. Adolescent role assessment. Am J Occup Ther 1976;30(2):73–79.
12. Good-Ellis MA, Fine S, Spencer JH. Developing a role activity performance scale. Am J Occup Ther 1985;41(4):232–241.
13. Jackoway I, Rogers J, Snow T. Role change assessment. Occup Ther Mental Health 1987;7(1):17–37.
14. Biernacki S. Reliability of the worker role interview. Am J Occup Ther 1993;47(9): 797–803.

BALANCE
1. The Oxford English Dictionary. Oxford, England: Claredon Press, 1933.
2. Meyer A. The philosophy of occupation therapy. Arch Occupl Ther 1922;1(1):1–10.
3. Hall H. The work cure. Boston Med Surg Jour 1910;LIV(1):13–15.
4. McHenry R. Rhythm and balance. In: The New Encyclopedia Britannica. (Online verson). Chicago: University of Chicago, 1995.
5. Mocellin G. Occupational therapy: A critical overview, Part 1. Br J Occup Ther 1995;58(12): 505.
6. Christiansen C. Three perspectives on balance in occupation. In: Zemke R, Clark F. Occupational Science: The Evolving Discipline. Philadelphia: FA Davis, 1996:431–451.
7. Reilly M. A psychiatric occupational therapy program as a teaching model. Am J Occup Ther 1966;20(2):61–67.
8. Kielhofner G. Temporal adaptation: a conceptual framework for occupational therapy. Am J Occup Ther 1977;31(4):235–242.
9. Converse PE. Time budgets. In: Sills EL. International Encyclopedia of the Social Sciences. New York: Macilliam, 1968:42–47.
10. Cynkin S. Occupational Therapy: Toward Health Through Activities. Boston: Little, Brown & Co., 1979:24–25.
11. Simpson PL. Occupational balance: a holistic frame of reference for physical disability practice. J Occup Ther Students 1997;4:7–12.

CHAPTER 9

Doing Process

PURPOSEFUL ACTIVITIES AND OTHER USES
OF THE TERM PURPOSEFUL

The earliest reference in the occupational therapy literature to the term purposeful activity occurred in 1922. Dr. Bowman discusses the role of psychology in the field of occupational therapy (1). Her perspective is that the "fundamental principle of occupational therapy is a psychological principle; the substitution of a coordinated *purposeful activity,* mental or physical, for scattered activities or the idleness which comes with weakened body or mind" (italics added). Unfortunately, she does not elaborate on the definition of "purposeful activity." Later in the address, she does discuss the idea of purpose, or "aufgabe," the German term. Her point is that in mental processes, the purpose, the task, and the instructions often convey the essence of what the person does and remembers. She uses the example of a research study in which one group of subjects were instructed to look at the letters in some nonsensical groupings. Another group was instructed to look at the colors. Some subjects who were instructed to look at the letters did not remember seeing the colors while some subjects who were instructed to look at the colors did not remember seeing the letters.

There may have been instances of the term purposeful activity being used in literature between 1922 and 1949, but the next identified use was in 1949. Alessandrini uses the term in her discussion of play (2). She stated: "Play is not folly. It is purposeful activity, the result of mental and emotional experiences." She was trying to convey that play is serious business and not just diversion or idle use of time.

In 1950, Bunnell discussed the need to use the splinted handed because "there is revivification of tissues on voluntary use and the will to do (3). Here-in lies the superiority of occupational therapy over physiotherapy. Occupational therapy is *purposeful activity* with interest a goal ahead" (italics added). Bunnell also did not elaborate on the term "purposeful activity." Thus, the term appeared in the early literature but was stated as an understood "given" without needing explanation.

In 1958, Ayres was the first person located in the literature of occupational therapy to offer an explanation (4). She stated that:

[the] use of *purposeful activities* . . . based on motor demands of a normal human existence, constitutes the common element and distinguishing feature of occupation.

Any procedures which are intimately associated with purposeful activity and which are essential to maximally therapeutic utilization of the activities are likewise necessarily the concern of occupational therapy. (Italics added)

She continued with the following:

[I]t must be recognized that purposeful activity while the distinguishing feature of occupational therapy is not limited to that profession. Speech therapy involves the purposeful use of speech. Physical therapists use walking as an end as well as a means. Likewise, purposeful activity has long been providing a large part of the foundation of modern educational procedures.

However, in occupational therapy, the objective (of purposeful activity) is focused on the pathological condition with the learning objective evolving from this condition.

In 1979, the Representative Assembly adopted a statement on the philosophical base of occupational therapy that individual development and adaptation are facilitated through purposeful activity (5). At the same time, the individual is able to influence physical and mental health and the social and physical environment through purposeful activity. In addition, occupational therapy is based on the belief that purposeful activity and occupation can be used therapeutically to prevent and mediate dysfunction while eliciting adaptation through intrinsic motivation.

Clark stated that purposeful activities were "the goal-directed use of a person's resources, time, energy, interest, and attention." She philosophized a view of man based on human adaptation in which man is distinguished by the capacity to purposefully effect the world of self, culture, and environment. Furthermore, man is aware of two abilities: to formulate and symbolize concepts, and to use the human hands to translate concepts into action. "Man's awareness of the abilities promotes the will for purposeful activities" (6, p. 579).

Gilfoyle, Grady, and Moore in 1981 suggested that "activity becomes purposeful when the nature of and participation with the activity/event facilitates meaningful responses for the nervous system. Responses become meaningful when the feedback associated with actions provides directions and efforts that are more mature or at a higher level than those previously experienced. Thus, purposeful activity augments neural mechanisms and sensorimotor–sensory integration" (7, p. 135).

Mosey defined purposeful activities as "doing processes that involve investigating, trying out and gaining evidence of one's capacities for experiencing, responding, managing, creating and controlling" (8). Thus, purposeful activity involves both the human and nonhuman environments. During the maturation process, purposeful activities provide an opportunity to develop skills in sensory, neuromotor, cognitive, psychological, and social components. Through feedback from the human and nonhuman environments, the individual learns about assets, limitations, potential, and the environment itself. Mosey suggests that routine purposeful activities are so much a part of daily life that they often go unnoticed until or unless something unusual happens such as a change in performance or behavior. For example, if one tries to use the nondominant hand to perform actions usually done with the dominant, the routine and simple becomes unusual and difficult, for example, signing a check. Changes in behavior such as habits are also noticed as when a person who is known for remembering numbers suddenly cannot remember a local telephone number. A third instance occurs when the purpose is clear to the person but not to others. For example, a person throws his or her handbag or wallet in the trash although the exterior appears to be in good condition. The logic may be difficult to understand until the owner explains that the interior is ripped and the stitches are coming apart.

DiJoseph suggests that purposeful activity requires the triad of mind–body–environment to be successful (9). She hyphenated the three to stress the interconnectedness. Thus, higher-level purposeful activity (not instinctual behavior) is based on the triad of mind–body–environment and purposeful activity is the core of occupational therapy.

Kielhofner and Nelson say there are two different perspectives on the profession's view of activity (10). The first viewpoint sees activity as a generic philosophy without any specific theoretical base. The second viewpoint sees activity as part of the theoretical ideas of moral treatment and humanistic theory. The first viewpoint is illustrated by the practice of diversional occupational therapy, which operated on the common sense principle that it was good for patients to be busy. The second viewpoint was based on three assumptions. First, the individual "maintains and balances itself in the world of reality by being in active life and active use" (11). Second, the loss of occupation resulted in psychological deterioration that undermined physical recovery and psychological morale (12). Third, mental illness was viewed as the result of a flood of pathological thoughts entering the consciousness. Activity could replace those thoughts with healthy thoughts that occurred in context with performing normal, routine life activity. Because the mind could only attend to one thought at a time, the healthy thoughts of activity would crowd out the pathological ones (13).

In the position paper, Hinojosa, Sabari, and Rosenfeld defined purposeful activity as "tasks or experiences in which the person actively participates" in their daily life routine (14). They stated that the "engagement in purposeful activity requires and elicits coordination between one's physical, emotional, and cognitive systems." An individual who is involved in purposeful activity directs attention to the task itself, rather than to the internal processes required for achievement of the task.

Breines (15) believed that the concept of purposeful activity is based on the work of Dewey who proposed that "occupation is conceptually allied with purposive action inherent in play and work . . . (and) that the elements of personal choice and self-direction are enabled by (purposive) active occupation" (16). Breines felt that the occupational therapy founders adopted and adapted the concept of purposive action to their ideas of health care. She stated that the lack of agreement about what is a purposeful activity may stem from occupational therapists tendency to "define their practice by the tools they use rather than by the process in which patients engage." Thus, the lack of agreement with the profession of a definition of purposeful activity "may reflect therapist role identity conflicts rather than conceptual foundation criteria." Unfortunately, reliance on the tools as definers of purposeful action or purposeful activity misses the point of therapy. Occupational therapy is the application of a process to health and health problems not the application of any given tool or tools. A tool defines a technician such as a perfusionist who operates a heart lung machine. The tool defines the job. Tools do not define the job of occupational therapy because the use of tools is part of the process and not the end product itself. Thus, as Breines stated, "purpose or purposeful action cannot be defined in terms of the tools with which, or the activity in which, therapists engage their patients. Purposeful activity must be defined in terms of the unique directions of individual patients and the enabling of patients toward enhanced (health and wellness)." According to Breines, the criteria for a purposeful action or activity is whether it elicits personal choice by the client and/or provokes individual development within the client.

Mosey, in 1986, redefined purposeful activity from her previous definition as "doing processes that require the use of thought and energy and are directed toward an intended or desired end result" (17). She contrasted purposeful activity with random activity, stating that the random activities are "undirected and without a predetermined goal." In addition she contrasted purposeful activity with "busy work" or mindless repetitive tasks, which are "designed primarily to keep one physically occupied and out of mischief."

Purposeful activity occurs when there is a reason for engaging in the activity that is apparent to the doer. Purposeful activity may be related to the process or to the end result (purpose). An example of process is the use of purposeful activity to decrease the impact of depression. An example of end result is the use of purposeful activity to teach a person to prepare a meal with one hand. However, the end result does not have to be a tangible product. The end result could be knowledge, such as knowing the difference between hot and cold water. Even when there is a product, the product may be less important than the process.

Also in 1986, purposeful activity was defined in relation to young children in a position paper as "the interaction of the child with the environment in a goal-directed task that promotes development, neurological organization, and a sense of mastery" (18). The purpose of the position paper was to clarify the role of occupational therapy in early childhood development and to promote the use of occupational therapists in service programs for early childhood intervention.

In 1991, Henderson and colleagues stated that the "use of purposeful activity, including occupation, is the core of occupational therapy, that is, the therapeutic kernel of what makes change in patients" (19). They suggested, however, there are three provisos: "First, that the definitions of purposeful activity must be multidimensional; second, that purposefulness and meaningfulness are attributes of persons and not of activities; and third, that it be recognized that legitimate occupational therapy services include techniques other than purposeful activity." Nonpurposeful activities include interpersonal interaction, orthotics, physical agents, family counseling, biofeedback, and the shaping of behavior. The meaningfulness of these techniques is supposedly "in their power to enhance the effectiveness of an activity or to facilitate performance."

According to the position paper adopted by the Representative Assembly in 1993, purposeful activity "refers to goal-directed behaviors or tasks that comprise occupations" (20). An activity is purposeful if the individual is an active, voluntary participant and if the activity is directed toward a goal the individual considers meaningful. The purposefulness of an activity lies with the individual performing the activity and with the context in which it is done.

Johnson stated that "purposeful activity is a concept central to occupational therapy theories, the implication being that activity (doing), when purposeful, lead to change" (21). She also stated that purposeful activity "motivates a person to participate because it has meaning and is related to his goals, regardless of its actual or perceived unpleasantness, difficulty or pleasure."

Trombly stated that "purposeful activity is circumscribed; it demands particular responses and is used to facilitate change in impairments and functional limitations" (22, p. 237).

Creek said in relation to purposeful activities that the "purpose and meaning are located in the client, not in the activity. An activity has no purpose independent of the person who is carrying it out, or who wishes it to be carried out. The occupational therapist uses her skills in analysis and reflection to select activities which will both meet therapeutic goals and have purpose and meaning for the client" (23).

Mocellin made two comments concerning purposeful activities (24). First, studies have found that some choices are fairly obvious but in other cases it is often difficult to determine why people choose as they do. The answers may depend on subtle variables that are not immediately obvious—even to the person doing the choosing. People are not always aware what causes their actions or reactions.

Second, voluntary participation requires that the person understand the situation: namely the person has free choice to select by free will or impulse what occupation or activity in which to engage, and is legally able to consent to the program as outline by the therapist. If a person has been judged incompetent by the court, clearly such consent is impossible. Such consent is also improbable with persons who have advanced dementia, are comatose, are taking heavy doses of medication, or are too young to understand the explanation.

Possible Historical Links to Purposeful Activity

Because the history of the term and concept of purposeful activity is unclear, an exact description of the historical tracing cannot be stated. Breines suggested the link to the philosopher, John Dewey (15, 16). In addition to philosophic ties are those from psychology. At the time the professional organization was being formed, several psychological ideas about the concept of purpose were being discussed. Among the leaders were William McDougall and Edward C. Tolman, who are collectively known for their support of purposive psychology (25). McDougall believed that all behavior was purposive; that is, purpose is the mainspring of action (26). According to McDougall, purpose rather than pleasure was the primary energy that directed a person to a goal-seeking future event. He believed that practical objectives such as food, shelter, and rest, as well as abstract objectives such as honor and virtue, are ends in and of themselves because they are worthwhile, not just because they give us pleasure (27). He even named this theory hormic energy. Hormic is derived from a Greek word meaning "directed toward a goal." McDougall, however, used the concept of purposiveness both as an internal and external mechanism.

Tolman accepted McDougall's assumptions with one major modification. He discarded the internal mechanism of purpose. Accord to Tolman, purposeful behavior is the readiness to persist through trial and error toward a goal. In other words, the behavior had to be observable (25).

The phrase purposeful activity does not appear in the descriptions of purposive, but the concept of goal direction is similar. Quite possibly purposive and purposeful are synonyms.

Other Uses of the Term Purposeful

Purposeful Function

In 1958 Ayres stated that purposeful function is the essence of occupational therapy (4): "It is here proposed the essential and distinctive quality of occupational therapy in *purposeful function*. Man is designed and built to perform in terms of *purposeful function*. It therefore logically follows that *purposeful function* must be utilized for maximal rehabilitation" (italics added). She said the purposeful motor function is defined as "the use of the motor system as a means toward accomplishing a goal which is inherent in the nature of the activity demanding the function." In 1960 (28) the definition was rephrased as the "use of the motor system as a means of accomplishing a goal that is inherent within or autonomous to the nature of the activity required to function."

Purposeful Movement and Purposeful Tasks

In 1963, Ayres was writing about purposeful movement in neuromuscular training (29). Ayres quoted Curran's (30) definition of purposeful movement as "voluntary movement with conscious focused on the end result." Specifically, Curran said that purposeful movement refers to the fact that the conscious effort is primarily directed toward an end object and not focused on the movement itself. Ayres asserted that goal-directed activity may be considered synonymous. She later stated the following:

> Thus a *purposeful task* has an implicit goal—one of its own. This purpose exists in addition to the therapeutic one. Reaching for a ball has the implicit purpose of grasping the ball; the therapeutic purpose is more likely to be neuromuscular integration. . . . Usually, the principle of *purposeful function* is employed along with the other principles, to a lesser extent in the less well integrated nervous systems and to a greater extent when the development of skill is desired. (Italics added)

In the same chapter she continued: "Willed movement, with attention focused on movement, is not natural—it is not the reason for which the neuromuscular system evolved. It evolved to fulfill *purposeful tasks.*"

Purposeful Action and Doing

Fidler and Fidler spoke of purposeful action as doing (31). The word doing was chosen "to convey the sense of performing, producing, or causing." In contrast to random activity, purposeful action is directed toward developing or testing skills, clarifying relationships or creating an end product. "*Doing* is viewed as enabling the development and integration of the sensory, motor, cognitive and psychological systems; serving as a socializing agency, and verifying on's efficacy as a competent, contributing member of one's society."

Purposeful Way

Curran stated that "Rood advocates utilizing a movement pattern in a purposeful way as soon as feasible" (30).

Summary

Occupational therapists did not create the term "purposeful activity." The term probably is derived from the psychology literature. Ayres, with the help of Curran and Rood, made the first serious use of the term in relation to occupational therapy although only two authors—Brienes (15) and Cynkin (32)—in current discussions about purposeful activity reference her work. Occupational therapists have difficulty keeping track of the origins of their concepts; thus, the original definitions and meanings attached to them may be lost.

Clearly, purposeful activity must be considered a goal toward which to work. With some consumers, the goal is quickly reached and the person is able and willing to actively participate in the criteria for and selection of activities and occupations in which to engage. However, there are also a large group of consumers for whom the goal is considered but seldom reached. There is, however, a second use of the term purposeful activity that is more concerned with process than goal. The ideas of meaning and doing are processes. Perhaps the concept of purposeful activity is really more a philosophical statement than a concrete reality. Occupational therapists strive to empower consumers to make their own choices concerning activities. Some achieve the goal, and some gain from the process even if the goal is not attained. The goal is not invalidated because it is not achieved 100 percent of time. Sometimes the journey, not the destination, is the real goal.

A summary of the assumptions about purposeful activity is provided in Appendix A to this chapter. The summary is from the works of Mosey, Nelson and Peterson, and Pedretti.

ROUTINE

Webster's New Universal Unabridged Dictionary defines routine as related to persons as the following:

1. A customary or regular course of procedure;
2. Common place tasks, chores, or duties that must be done regularly or at specified intervals; typical or everyday activity:
3. Regular, unvarying, habitual, unimaginative, or rote procedure;
4. An unvarying and constantly repeated formula, as of speech or action; convenient or predictable response;
5. An individual act, performance, or part of a performance, as a song or dance, given regularly by an entertainer;
6. Of the nature of, proceeding by, or adhering to routine; routine duties; and
7. Dull or uninteresting; commonplace. (1)

The word routine has not been widely used as a concept in occupational therapy. However, aspects inherent in the concept of routine have been discussed. Those aspects include a time or temporal dimension; doing or performing; task or procedure; and orderly, regular, rote, or ritualistic quality.

Christiansen and Baum define routines as "occupations with established sequences, such as the morning ritual surrounding showering and dress for the day"(2). They quote Bond and Feather who wrote that "a routine has a stability about it that extends over time and pertains to a particular set of activities within a defined situation" (3).

Daily routines also seem to take place at particular times of the day. ADLs tend to cluster in the morning (4).

Hagedorn defines routines as "chains of tasks with fixed sequence which become automated and habitual" (5). She suggests that effective routines may help to reduce the amount of sensorimotor effort and energy as well as the need for cognitive aspects of attention and planning. Routines may contribute to the successful production of an activity or effect outcome. Also, some routines have a sequence or order inherent in the way the tasks are accomplished such as taking a shower before putting on one's clothes. Doing the reverse—that is, getting dressed and then taking a shower—cleans the clothes but not necessarily the body. Other routines develop for some convenience such brushing teeth, putting on makeup, or shaving and then brushing and combing the hair. The tasks do not inherently need to be done in that order but the order has evolved as a comfortable pattern to ensure that an important aspect of "getting dressed for the day" is not overlooked.

Routines can become counterproductive if the sequence, order, or pattern becomes overly rigid and cannot be changed even when the circumstances change. For example, on a camping trip, putting on makeup or shaving may not be necessary or expected. Inability to adapt or change the routine becomes a problem in and of itself and may discourage creativity or problem solving.

Allen does not describe the concept of routine per se but rather links routine to task (6). She then defines routine tasks as the "activities that a person does on a daily basis." Routine tasks usually involve "food, clothing, shelter, transportation, general health precautions and money management." Routine tasks are commonly referred to as activities of daily living. Actually the concept of routine tasks includes both basic ADLs and instrumental ADLs.

Cynkin and Robinson use the word routine but do not define it (7). For example, consider the following: "each individual has . . . a distinctive set of routines and a specific repertoire of activities." The authors are talking about patterns and configurations. Patterns are defined as "combinations of qualities, acts, tendencies, etc., forming a consistent or characteristic arrangement" (8). An idiosyncratic activities pattern is "a graphic representation of the daily use of time by one individual at one specific period of the life span." A configuration is "a picture of the distinctive life-style of one person at one particular point in the life span." Routines may be present in these graphic representations, but they are not identified as such.

Summary

The concept of routine is fairly new to model building in occupational therapy. Whether it is actually a useful concept remains to be seen. Other terms that may appear as synonyms are pattern and configuration.

TASK

The dictionary defines task in three ways and provides three synonyms: a) a definite piece of work assigned to, falling to, or expected of a person; duty; b) any piece of work; and c) a matter of considerable labor of difficulty (1). The three synonyms are job, assignment, and chore.

Miller defines task as "any set of activities, occurring at the same time, sharing some common purpose that is recognized by the task performer" (2). Christiansen shortens the definition to "a set of activities sharing some purpose recognized by the task performer" (3). He continues by suggesting that a task has dimensions related to complexity, degree of structure, and purpose. *Complexity* refers to the number and characteristics of the steps, sequences, or patterns in the task. *Degree of structure* refers to the specific methods or flexibility and creativity permitted by the task itself or by the criteria for performing the task imposed by others. The *purpose* may be for self-maintenance, productivity, or leisure. Also important is whether the task requires cooperation or competition and whether it is performed in public or private.

As Reber points out in defining task, the term task "has enormous latitude in usage; it is used for simple physical movements as well as for life-goals, it covers personal tasks set by an individual or external demands established by others" (4). However, in general task is "something that needs to be done, or an act that one must accomplish."

"Tasks are pervasive in everyday life, representing the context and focus of much of human behavior" (5). Fleishman and Quaintance suggest two categories of definitions of task. The first explores the breadth of the tasks while the second explores whether the task is external or internal in relation to the performer. Each can be divided into two parts so there are four types of definitions. The first describes *task as the totality of the situation* imposed upon the performer. Thus all aspects of the physical, social, and personal environment are relevant. The second type of definition treats a *task as a specific performance.* Such performances can be described as steps or instructions to follow in performing the task. The third type of definition is based on the assumption that the a *task is external* to the person and thus is defined in terms of what has been imposed upon the performer. A fourth type of definition occurs by assuming the *task is intrinsic* to the person. Such definitions consider the propensity of some people to redefine any task in terms of personal needs, values, or experiences. Thus, the task becomes whatever the individual perceives it to be. All tasks are defined by the person idiosyncratically and subjectively. Occupational therapy practitioners appear to use all four of the definitions of task described by Fleishman and Quaintance. The reader of occupational therapy literature must keep in mind the wide spectrum of the word definition and concept of task.

Christiansen and Baum incorporate the concept of task in the model of person–environment–occupational performance (6). They define tasks, plural form, as "combinations of actions sharing a common purpose recognized by the performer." The definition suggests an intrinsic view; that is, a task is whatever the person says it is. On the other hand, Dunn, Brown, and McGuigan use the concept of task in relation to the environmental context and demands for performance (7). This use of the concept of task appears to illustrate the first type of definition in which all aspects of the physical, social, and personal aspects of the task are considered relevant to the performance of the task. Such a definition and use of the concept of task is quite broad in its application. This broad approach to applying the concept of task appears to apply to the contemporary task-oriented approach suggested by Mathiowetz and Bass Haugen (8). However, the emphasis appears to be on the external demand for task performance because of the emphasis on functional tasks that are required to be performed by the person.

In summary, the concept of task in occupational therapy literature is quite broad, having at least four variations. Thus, in reading or studying occupational therapy models in which the concept of task appears, the reader must discern the meaning attributed to the concept of task to fully understand the model. In research studies, the concept of task must be clearly defined because the four different means may require different methods of research to determine their construct validity.

FUNCTION

The word function appears frequently in the occupational therapy literature. It may appear by itself or in combination with another word, such as in the phrases functional assessment and evaluation, functional ability, functional capacity, functional independence, functional limitation, functional performance, and functional status. In addition, one can speak of functional electrical stimulation, functional range of motion, functional skills, functional strength, and functional tasks. Finally, according the Position Paper of the American Occupational Therapy Association, the word function can be used interchangeably with the word performance (1).

The word function is derived from the Latin word *functionem* meaning *of action,* formed of *fungi* meaning *to perform.* The Oxford English Dictionary lists six major definitions for the word function (2). They are as follows:

1. *In etymological sense:* The action of performing; discharge or performance of (something);
2. Activity; action in general whether physical or mental;
3. The special kind of activity proper to anything; the mode of action by which it fulfills its purpose. Also in generalized application, especially physics, as contrasted with structure;
4. The kind of action proper to a person as belonging to a particular class, especially to the holder of any office; hence the office itself, an employment, profession, calling, trade;
5. A religious ceremony; originally in the Roman Catholic Church; and
6. *Mathematics.* A variable quantity regarded in its relation to one or more other variable in terms of which it may be expressed, or on the value of which its own value depends.

   The first three definitions all relate to use of the word function in occupational therapy literature. Many therapists have defined function for themselves. Mosey defines function as "the ability to engage comfortably at an age-appropriate level in performance components and the areas of occupational performance with the context of one's cultural, social and non-human environment" (3). Fisher defines function as "ability (of the individual) to perform the daily life tasks related to ADLs and IADLs, work, and play and leisure . . . that he or she wants and needs to perform" (4). However, she also points out that each profession views the word function from a slightly different perspective as illustrated in Table 9.1. Jette, a physical therapist, points out that the word function has been used to define "the characteristic action of *body parts* (the 'function of the shoulder'); the performance of *bodily organs* ('kidney function') as well as the performance of an *individual* (to function in 'activities of daily living')" (5). The indiscriminate and ambiguous use of the word, he points out, leads to considerable conceptual and semantic confusion. Mixing descriptions of the attributes of body parts, body organs, and whole

Table 9.1.   Professional Views of Function

Profession	Frame	Methods	Goal
Occupational therapy	Occupational tasks, skills, and processes	Purposeful and meaningful tasks, skills, and processes	Occupational role performance
Physical therapy	Motion and movement	Therapeutic exercise and physical agents	Physical mobility and capacity
Medicine	Disease and illness	Drugs and surgery	Symptom reduction and elimination
Nursing	Health	Helping and caring	Healthiness and sense of well-being
Social work	Social and community organizations	Social change and helping process	Social interaction and relationships
Recreational therapy	Recreation and leisure	Recreational and leisure activities for fun and amusement	Counterbalance work and obligation activities

Adapted from: Fisher AG. Functional assessment and occupation: critical issues for occupational therapy. New Zealand Journal of Occupational Therapy 1994;45(2):13–19.

individuals leads to unclear thinking and even less clear action. Ultimately, it becomes difficult to determine what is functioning let alone how well "it" functions.

Dysfunction

Mosey defines dysfunction as

the inability to engage comfortably at an age-appropriate level in performance components or the areas of occupational performance within the context of one's cultural, social, and nonhuman environment. Dysfunction may be due to sequelae arising from disease, injury or deficit . . . or . . . may be the loss of a particular skill or the lack of development of a particular skill in the usual course of maturation.

Functional Assessment

One of the oldest definitions of functional assessment is given by Lawton (6). He defined functional assessment as meaning

any systematic attempt to measure objectively the level at which a person is functioning in any of a variety of areas such as physical health, quality of self-maintenance, quality of role activity, intellectual status, social activity, attitude toward the world and toward self, and emotional status.

Functional Limitation

Nagi defines functional limitation as a "limitation in performance at the level of whole organism or person" (7). The Institute of Medicine says functional limitation is a "restriction or lack of ability to perform an action or activity in the manner or within range considered normal that results from impairment" (8). The National Center for Medical Rehabilitation Research defines functional limitation as a "restriction or lack of ability to perform an action in the manner of range consistent with the purpose of an organ or organ system" (9). Granger defines functional limitation as "a consequence of a health problem and represents an inability to meet a standard of an anatomical, physiological, psychological, or mental nature (impairment)" (10).

Functional Performance

Kielhofner defines functional performance as the "ability to complete tasks and functions needed for daily living" (11).

Summary

The word and concept function has been used extensively in occupational therapy models. While some model developers think the word should be banned from conceptual models others find the word useful. There are many words and concepts in occupational therapy with multiple meanings which provides as many opportunities to love the word and hate the meaning or vice versa.

HABIT

The word habit is from the Latin word *habitus* meaning condition, appearance, attire, character, or disposition. Other synonyms are habitude, practice, usage, custom, use, and wont. Habit is a word with many meanings. Samples of the multiple meanings from two unabridged dictionaries are given in Table 9.2.

Habit first appears in occupational therapy in Tracy's book *Studies in Invalid Occupation*. In the preface written by Fuller, he says the following

> for many nervous invalids who have gradually shut themselves away from all association with others and whose self-seclusion has become a bit—the result of morbid fear—the occupation room offers a most effective opportunity for annihilating this fear and establish the patient again in normal habits and natural relations with his fellow beings. (1)

Thus, the use of occupation to facilitate normal habits of living and interpersonal relations is suggested.

Adolf Meyer used the word habit in his explanation of schizophrenic behavior. His concept of habit became the basis of the first practice model in occupational therapy called habit training developed by Eleanor Clarke Slagle. In Meyer's textbook *Psychobiology,* habit is explained as "the essential fabric of the reactive resources of the organism" (2). The doing of things forms the basic structure of the mental life, and habit formation is a process that applies to every item of human behavior. When Meyer speaks of the disorganization of habits in the parergasia processes, it is the deterioration of the learned but fundamental ways of meeting life to which he is drawing our attention—a withdrawing into dreamlike states in which the prophylactic corrective of action is not permitted. Habits of action and bringing things to completion are the basic conative resources of the organism.

In his paper on habit disorganization, Meyer suggests that one cause of mental disorders is the "disharmony of habits, disharmony of those regulations which shape a well-balance economy: the intestinal and circulatory functions, the sexual life, and above all the trend of interests depending in its integrity and efficiency on a certain equilibration" (3). Meyer credits William James, a psychologist, for recognizing that habits can be observed and be related to certain bodily functions. James proposed "the phenomena of habit in living beings are due to the plasticity of the organic materials of which their bodies are composed" (4). He states that

> plasticity means the possession of a structure weak enough to yield to an influence, but strong enough not to yield all at once. Each relative stable phase of equilibrium in such a structure is marked by what we may call a new set of habits . . . and habit diminishes the conscious attention with which our acts are performed.

Table 9.2. Current Definitions of the Word "Habit"

Webster's Third New International Dictionary defines habit as:	*Webster's New Universal Unabridged Dictionary* defines habit as:
1. a) clothing, apparel, mode of dress; b) a garment or a suit of clothes: outfit 2. a) a costume indicative or characteristic of a calling, rank, or function; b) riding habit 3. bearing, conduct, behavior; 4. a) bodily appearance or makeup; physical type; physique; b) the body as a physiological organism; the system of bodily processes; c) the body's surface 5. The prevaling disposition or character of a person's thoughts and feelings; mental makeup 6. a) a settled tendency of behavior or normal manner of procedures; custom, practice, way; b) of a thing; a usual manner of occurenace or behavior; tendency 7. a) a behavior pattern acquired by frequent repetition or developed as a physiologic function and showing itself in regularity; b) an acuired or developed mode of behavior of function that has become nearly or completely involuntary 8. Characteristic mode of growth or occurrence 9. The characterisitic crystalline size and form of a substance 10. Close acquainstance; familiarity. 11. A generic entiry occurring as an external or supermantural reality or force constitutive of or acting on an individual 12. Addition	1. An acquired behavior pattern regularly followed until it has become almost involuntary 2. Customary practice or use 3. A particular practice, custom, or usage 4. A dominant or regular disposition or tendency; prevailing character or quality 5. Addiction, especially to narcotics 6. Mental character or disposition. 7. Characteristic bodily or physical condition 8. The characteristic form aspect, mode of growth, etc., of an organism 9. The characteristic crystalline form of a mineral 10. Garb of a particular rank profession, religious order, etc. 11. The attire worn by a rider of a saddle horse 12. To clothe; array

Meyer suggests that by studying the habits of patients various types of habit disorganization, then can be identified. Once a habit disorder is identified, it can be treated by habit training.

The primary objective of habit training is the reorganization or reestablishment of habit reactions. Occupation is used to overcome habits, to modify others and construct new ones with the purpose of restoring and maintaining health (5). The primary objective is to require the patient's attention and to build on the habit of attention. To accomplish the objective a 24-hour schedule is arranged with physician, nurses, attendants, and occupational therapist.

Slagle actually divided patients into three groups. The first were those who resided in the so-called "backwards" of the hospitals who were the most backward or regressed in their behavior. Most of these patients were not expected to leave the hospital although occasionally one did make the transition to community life. The second group was expected to return to community life, and the third group was thought to benefit or profit from participation in a work clinic or occupational center with the idea that such patients could learn to prevent subsequent hospitalizations.

The term "habit training" is most associated with the first group where following a fixed schedule 24 hours a day was the primary objective. In reality, however, all three groups became part of the habit-training program. Naturally enough, the first treatment group is called "habit training." The second treatment group was called the "kindergarten group," and the third might be placed in either the "occupational center" or the "preindustrial group."

Habit training continued until Slagle died in 1942. Thereafter, the new ideas about psychoanalytic, projective, and expressive therapy became primary influences in the practice of occupational therapy in mental health, and the concepts of habit training diminished. Also the nursing staff took over the idea of 24-hour scheduling because they were on the wards at all times and the occupational therapist was not.

Habit Dysfunction

Kielhofner, Barris, and Watts proposed a concept of habit dysfunction based on the idea of functional habit patterns (6).

> A person with functional habit patterns is able to organize everyday behavior into routines that are both personally satisfying and environmental adaptive . . . Habit dysfunction is characterized by behavior output that is either overly rigid, . . . or conversely, by the absence of an automatic patterned response.

They propose that habits are governed by rules that are information in the system operating to put constraints or boundaries on action. An individual with adaptive habit patterns is balancing demands with the internal system and the external environment in a wide variety of situations. Habit dysfunction occurs, on the other hand, when the person is unable to balance the internal and external demands because the habits are incongruent with the demands.

References

PURPOSEFUL ACTIVITY

1. Bowman E. Psychology of occupational therapy. Arch Occup Ther 1922;1(3):172.
2. Alessandrini NA. Play: a child's world. Am J Occup Ther 1949;3(1):9.
3. Bunnell S. Occupational therapy of hands. Am J Occup Ther 1950;4(4):148.
4. Ayres AJ. Basic concept of clinical practice in physical disabilities. Am J Occup Ther 1958;12(6):300–302,311.
5. Representative Assembly Minutes. The philosophical base of occupational therapy. Am J Occup Ther 1979;33(11):785.
6. Clark PN. Human development through occupation: A philosophy and conceptual model for practice, Part 2. Am J Occup Ther 1979;33(9):577–585.
7. Gilfoyle EM, Grady AP, Moore JC. Children Adapt. Thorofare, NJ: Slack Inc., 1981.
8. Mosey AC. Occupational Therapy: Configuration of a Profession. New York: Raven Press, 1981:99–107.
9. DiJoseph LM. Independence through activity: mind, body, and environment interaction in therapy. Am J Occup Ther 1982;36(11):740–744.
10. Kielhofner G, Nelson C. A study of patient motivation and cooperation/participation in occupational therapy. Occup Ther J Res 1983;3(1):35–45.
11. Meyer A. The philosophy of occupation therapy. Arch Occup Ther 1922;1(1):1–10.
12. Tracy SE. The Study of Invalid Occupations: A Manual for Nurses and Attendants. Boston: Whitcomb & Barrows, 1910.
13. Dunton WR. Reconstruction Therapy. Philadelphia: Saunders, 1919.
14. Hinojosa J, Sabari J, Rosenfeld MS. Purposeful activities. Am J Occup Ther 1983;37:805–806.
15. Breines E. The issue is: an attempt to define purposeful activity. Am J Occup Ther 1984;38(8):543–544.
16. Dewey J. Democracy and Education. New York: Free Press, 1916.
17. Mosey AC. Purposeful activities. In: Mosey AC. Psychosocial Components of Occupational Therapy. New York: Raven Press, 1986:227–241.
18. Morroni K, Hickman L. Early childhood intervention: position paper. Am J Occup Ther 1986;40(12):834.
19. Henderson A, Cermak S, Coster W, et al. Occupational science is multidimensional. Am J Occup Ther 1991;45(4):370–371.
20. Hinojosa J, Sabari J, Pedretti L. Position paper: purposeful activity. Am J Occup Ther 1993;47(12):1081–1082.
21. Johnson SE. Activity analysis. In: Turner A, Foster M, Johnson SE. Occupational Therapy and Physical Dysfunction: Principles, Skills, and Practice. 4th ed. New York: Churchill Livingstone, 1996:101–124.
22. Trombly CA. Purposeful activities. In: Trombly CA. Occupational Therapy for Physical Dysfunction. 4th ed. Baltimore: Williams & Wilkins, 1996:237–253.
23. Creek J. Approaches to practice. In: Creek J. Occupational Therapy and Mental Health. 2nd ed. New York: Churchill Livingstone, 1997:73.
24. Mocellin G. Occupational therapy: a critical overview. Part 1. Br J Occup Ther 1995;58(12):502–506.

25. Peters RS. Brett's History of Psychology. London: George Allen & Unwin Ltd., 1953:669–676.
26. Roback AA. William McDougall and hormis psychology. In: Roback AA. History of American Psychology. New York: Library Publishers, 1952:253–263.
27. Guilford JP. Fields of Psychology. New York: Van Nostrand, 1940:642–645.
28. Ayres AJ. Occupational therapy for motor disorders resulting from impairment of the central nervous system. Rehab Lit 1960;21(10): 302–310.
29. Ayres AJ. Occupational therapy directed toward neuromuscular integration. In: Willard HS, Spackman CS. Occupational Therapy. 3rd ed. Philadelphia: Lippincott, 1963: 443,445.
30. Curran PA. A study toward a theory of neuromuscular education through occupational therapy. Am J Occup Ther 1960;14(2):80–87.
31. Fidler GS, Fidler JW. Doing and becoming: purposeful action and self-actualization. Am J Occup Ther 1978;32(5):305–310.
32. Cynkin S. Activities. In: Royeen C. The Practice of the Future: Putting Occupation Back into Practice. Number 7. Rockville, MD: American Occupational Therapy Association, 1994.

ROUTINE
1. Webster's New Universal Unabridged Dictionary. New York: Barnes & Noble, 1996.
2. Christiansen C, Baum C. Understanding occupation: Definitions and concepts. In: Christiansen C, Baum C. Occupational Therapy: Enabled Function and Well-Being. Thorofare, NJ: Slack Inc., 1998:16.
3. Bond MJ, Feather NT. Some correlates of structure and purpose in the use of time. J Pers Soc Psychol 1988;55(2):321–329.
4. Baltes MM, Wahl HW, Schmid-Furstoss U. The daily life of elderly Germans: activity patterns, person control, and functional health. J Geronol 1990;45(4):173–179.
5. Hagedorn R. Occupational Therapy: Perspectives and Processes. Edinburgh: Churchill Livingstone, 1996:81–82.
6. Allen CK. Independence through activity: the practice of occupational therapy (psychiatry). Am J Occup Ther 1982;36:734.
7. Cynkin S, Robinson AM. Occupational Therapy and Activities Health: Toward Health Through Activities. Boston: Little Brown & Co., 1990:16–17.
8. Random House Dictionary of the English Language. New York: Random House Publishing, 1987.

TASK
1. Webster's New Universal Unabridged Dictionary. New York: Barnes & Noble, 1996.
2. Miller RB. Task taxonomy: science or technology? In: Singleton WT, Easterly RS, Whitfied DC. The Human Operator in Complex System. London: Taylor & Francis, 1967.
3. Christiansen C. Occupational therapy: Intervention for life performance. In: Christiansen C, Baum C. Occupational Therapy: Overcoming Human Performance Deficits. Thorofare, NJ: Slack Inc., 1991:29.
4. Reber AS. Dictionary of Psychology. London: Penguin Books, 1985:759.
5. Fleishman EA, Quaintance MK. Taxonomies of Human Performance: The Description of Human Tasks. New York: Academic Press, 1984.

6. Christiansen C, Baum C. Occupational Therapy: Enabling Function and Well-Being. Thorofare, NJ: Slack Inc., 1997:55.
7. Dunn W, Brown C, McGuigan A. The ecology of human performance: a framework for considering the effect of context. Am J Occup Ther 1994;48:595–607.
8. Mathiowetz V, Bass Haugen JB. Motor behavior research: implications for therapeutic approaches to central nervous system dysfunction. Am J Occup Ther 1994;48: 733–745.

FUNCTION
1. American Occupational Therapy Association. Position paper. Occupational performance: occupational therapy's definition of function. Am J Occup Ther 1995;49(10): 1019–1020.
2. The Oxford English Dictionary. Oxford, England: Clarendon Press, 1933.
3. Mosey AC. Occupational Therapy: Configuration of a Profession. New York: Raven Press, 1981:82.
4. Fisher AG. Functional measures, part 1: What is function, what should we measure, and how should we measure it? Am J Occup Ther 1992;46(2):183–185.
5. Jette AM. Concepts of health and methodological issues in functional assessment. In: Granger CV, Gresham GE. Functional Assessment in Rehabilitation Medicine. Baltimore: Williams & Wilkins, 1984:46–64.
6. Lawton MP. The function assessment of elderly people. J Am Geriatr Soc 1971;19: 465–481.
7. Nagi SZ. Some conceptual issues in disability and rehabilitation. In: Sussman MB. Sociology and Rehabilitation. Washington, DC: American Sociological Association, 1965:100–113.
8. Pope AM, Tarlow AR. Disability in America: Toward a National Agenda for Prevention. Division of Health Promotion and Disease Prevention, Institute of Medicine. Washington, DC: National Academy Press, 1991.
9. National Advisory Board on Medical Rehabilitation Research. Draft V. Report and Plan for Medical Rehabilitation Research. Bethesda, MD: National Institute of Health. National Center for Medical Rehabilitation and Research, 1992.
10. Granger CV. A conceptual model for functional assessment. In: Granger CV, Gresham GE. Functional Assessment in Rehabilitation Medicine. Baltimore: Williams & Wilkins, 1984:14–25.
11. Kielhofner G. Conceptual functions of occupational therapy. 2nd ed. Philadelphia: FA Davis, 1997:344.

HABIT
1. Fuller DH. The need of instruction for nurses in occupations for the sick. In: Tracy SE. Studies in Invalid Occupations: A Manual for Nurses and Attendants. Boston: Whitcomb & Barrows, 1910.
2. Meyer A. Psychobiology. Springfield, IL: Charles C Thomas, 1957.
3. Meyer A. Remarks on habit disorganization in the essential deteriorations, and relation of deterioration of the psychasthenic, neurasthenic, hysterical and other constitutions. In: Winters E. The Collected Papers of Adolf Meyer. V. II. Psychiatry. Baltimore: John Hopkins Press, 1951. (Originally a speech delivered in 1905.)

4. James W. Habit. In: James W. The Principles of Psychology. Vol. 1. (104–127). New York: Dover Publications, 1887. (Originally published in Popular Science Monthly in February, 1887.)
5. Slagle EC. Training aides for mental patients. Arch of Occup Ther 1922;1(1):11–17.
6. Kielhofner G, Barris R, Watts JH. Habits and habit dysfunction: a clinical perspective for psychosocial occupational therapy. Occup Ther Mental Health 1982;2(2):1–21.

Purposeful Activities

Mosey and others have described several characteristics of purposeful activities that may be viewed as assumptions which support the concept of purposeful activities.

I. Purposeful activities are universal. They exist and prevail in all times, places, and cultures.

   A.   There is an endless variety of purposeful activities, but all are directed toward a planned or anticipated end result.

   B.   Everyday or routine purposeful activities are part of the fabric of life. Thus, they often are given minimal attention and often go unnoticed.

   C.   Everyday or routine purposeful activities catch one's attention when they must be performed with considerable thought and effort.

   D.   The purpose in a purposeful activity may not be apparent to the observer but is known to the individual although the individual may have difficulty articulating this purpose.

   E.   The therapeutic value of everyday or routine purposeful activities may be questioned because some societies and cultures expect therapy to be magical and to "work" in mysterious ways.

   F.   The acceptance of purposeful activities as therapeutic tools may be hastened because the tasks and tools are already known to the client.

II. Purposeful activities are fundamental to optimal growth and development.

   A.   Purposeful activities facilitate the acquisition, maintenance, and elaboration of sensorimotor, cognitive, and psychosocial components or skills. They are acquired through active goal-directed interaction with the environment.

   B.   Purposeful activities constitute occupational performance because social roles are comprised of an integrated cluster or group of purposeful activities.

   C.   Most purposeful activities require the performance of several performance components. The exceptions are cognitive thought, thinking, daydreaming, or contemplation.

   D.   Purposeful activities provide the means through which the individual gains knowledge about the human and nonhuman environment and about him or herself.

III. Purposeful activities are comprised of tasks and performance components.
    A. Tasks and performance components can be identified and analyzed individually or as elements within the purposeful activity.
    B. Tasks and performance components can be facilitated or taught individually or as elements within the purposeful activity.
    C. Analysis and instruction can include examination of the motions used; the procedure and process; material and equipment; the result of the process, the interpersonal relations that influence the process or are influenced by the process, the context in which the activity occurs; the cultural meanings; the influence of age and gender; and relationship of the performance components to the occupational performance and adaptive potential

IV. Purposeful activities are holistic.
    A. The whole activity (occupation) must be understood as an entity because the whole activity is different from the sum of the tasks and performance components.
    B. Tasks and performance components may be viewed as changed by the totality of the whole. (A boring task may be tolerated because the whole is viewed as pleasing or useful.)
    C. The whole process and the whole product must be considered in relation to the individual's sense of competency, mastery, and satisfaction, and to the impact on the environment.

V. The tasks and performance components (elements) of a purposeful activity may be arranged or manipulated in a variety of combinations to suit the needs of or be made useful to an individual person.
    A. Such arrangement and manipulation of a purposeful activity is an asset to therapeutic intervention because the therapist can change the activity or task to the manner most beneficial to the client.
    B. The same characteristics of arrangement and manipulation can be limitations because anyone, including the client, can change the purpose of the activity, which may negate the beneficial aspects designed by the occupational therapy personnel.
    C. Such changes may include substitution of materials or equipment, failure to follow instructions as given, getting help from others instead of performing the tasks individually, taking more or less time, quitting the task or project, etc.

VI. Purposeful activities can be changed so as to elicit or promote different responses from different individuals.
    A. Level of mastery required to complete the activity can be changed.
    B. Environmental location and factors can be changed (indoors or outdoors, ward or clinic, lighting, temperature, ventilation, noise).

C. Number of people and their relationship to the individual can be changed.
D. Characteristics of the activity may be changed such as need for fine or gross motor movements.
E. The inherent characteristic of the activity, such as messy or neat, clean or dirty, simple or complex, quickly done or long-term project, can be matched to the characteristics of the individual's temperament or personality type.
VII. Purposeful activities can be graded along a continuum or dimension. Examples include degree or amount of complexity, structure, stimulation, creativity, variety of procedures, number of steps required to completion, or social interaction required.
A. An activity can be varied several dimensions or just one dimension.
B. This gradually allows the occupational therapy personnel to select activities that best meet the needs of the client at any given point in the intervention process and to meet the desired goal.
VIII. Purposeful activities enhance communication.
A. The enhanced communication may be verbal or nonverbal.
B. The verbal and nonverbal communication may be congruent (in agreement) or incongruent (one communication says one thing, and another communication says something different).
IX. Purposeful activities have a focusing and organizing effect on human action and behavior.
A. Performing (doing) a purposeful activity has a converging effect that allows feelings and ideas to be integrated into words, action, or product.
B. Performing (doing) a purposeful activity has an organizing effect that can facilitate the integration or gestalt of a single task or activity (microscopic organizing effect).
C. Performing (doing) a purposeful activity can have an organizing effect that can facilitate the integration or gestalt of many tasks or activities into a larger gestalt such as a schedule or routine for a day, week, month, or year (macroscopic organizing effect).
D. Performing (doing) a purposeful activity in the context of a group may provide a degree of structure and organization that is not possible individually and that may benefit several groups members.
E. Performing (doing) a purposeful activity may provide a framework that allows expression of ideas and feelings within known or agreed upon limits.
F. Performing (doing) a purposeful activity provides a tangible means of measuring progress. Purposeful activity is often inherent in setting measurable objectives and outcomes.

X. Purposeful activity emphasizes action and doing.
   A. Action and doing are important because they cannot be taken back or denied as words can.
   B. Purposeful activity proves concrete evidence (through action and doing) of skills in actual situations not just abstract knowledge and verbal skills.
   C. Performance of purposeful activity provides opportunity to understand the consequence of action and doing.
   D. Performance of purposeful activity provides a storehouse of action and doing experiences important and necessary to human function.
   E. Purposeful activity facilitates collaboration in identifying difficulties in action and doing.
   F. Participation in purposeful activity minimizes denial, rationalization, or evasion of responsibility relative to actual proficiency in performance.
XI. Purposeful activity involves (engages) the nonhuman environment.
   A. There is considerable variation in the amount of nonhuman environment involved in the performance of various purposeful activities.
   B. Not all interactions with the nonhuman environment are necessarily purposeful.
XII. Awareness of purposeful activity varies on a continuum from conscious to not conscious/unconscious.
   A. One continuum is the variation between subcortical and cortical levels of function. Depending on the task or skill some learning may occur at the subcortical level while other learning is acquired at the cortical level. An example is learning to ride a bicycle. Balance is learned subcortically whereas direction of travel requires cortical learning to know what is safe or dangerous and to get to a specific destination.
   B. A second continuum is the variation in the amount of conscious or unconscious focus of attention used or required. When a task or skill is being learned, the focus of attention is greater than when a task or skill is very familiar and repetitive. An example is tying one's shoe laces. Learning requires attention. After several repetitions, the task and skill become automatic.
   C. Purposeful activity can "tap" the unconscious by permitting a focus on maladaptive behavior or intrapsychic conflict (psychoanalytic model).
XIII. Purposeful activity can vary on a continuum from real to symbolic.
   A. Purposeful activity can be real, symbolic, or a combination of both.
   B. Tasks that are unstructured, ambiguous, nonverbal, and allow for creativity and self-expression tend to promote expression and production of symbols.

C.   Tasks may be similar to a symbolic object or interaction that occurs in normal development or is part of daily life such as expression of feelings through painting or knitting a sweater to give as a gift.

D.   Tasks may be symbolic of real environmental interactions such as a therapist providing a nurturing (parenting) relationship with a client.

XIV. Purposeful activity can vary on a continuum from simulated to natural.

    A.   Simulation often occurs in the clinic such as preparing a meal.

    B.   For simulation to be successful, the tasks or activity must be relevant to the development of skills the individual will need for successful participation in the community, arouse and sustain the individual's interest in the learning process, and be designed to resemble as closely as possible the activity patterns the individual is likely to encounter in the community.

    C.   A natural purposeful activity is one that takes place in the community. Such activities may occur in the company of the occupational therapy personnel, or with fellow clients, or the client may act independently.

    D.   Prescribed purposeful activities are those natural activities in which the therapist is not involved. Such activities are agreed on by the client and therapist for the purpose of testing and practicing new skills. The occupational therapy personnel may serve as a resource person providing support and guidance in problem solving and reinforcement.

XV. Purposeful activities can add purpose to exercise (Nelson and Peterson, 1989).

    A.   There are three types of added purposes to exercise.

        1.   Naturalistic activities are those that occur spontaneously as a result of everyday work and play. *Example:* A construction worker or farmer may get exercise through the activities inherent in the occupation. An office worker may get exercise by playing a game of racquetball or swimming.

        2.   Simulated activities are those in which the environmental context is more or less contributed by the therapist so as to resemble naturalistic activities. *Example:* The therapeutic kitchen may support simulated cooking activities.

        3.   Imagery-based activities are those based or verbal or pictorial stimuli to elicit imaged or "visualized" activity even though physical support may not be present in the immediate environment. *Example:* Directions such as "reach for the stars" or "fly like an airplane" invoke imagery.

XVI. Purposeful activity can divert attention away from pain or discomfort.

XVII. Purposeful activity can have negative consequences (Nelson and Peterson, 1989).

    A.   The added stimuli may distract an individual when conscious attention is desirable.

B.   The additional motives may be distracting and make focusing atten-
     tion on the goal difficult.
C.   Purposeful activities may be difficult to grade in accordance with the
     goal or need of the client.
D.   Involvement in a favorite activity or occupation during rehabilitation may
     have undesirable consequences when the person discovers how difficult
     it is to perform an activity or occupation which was once easy to do.
E.   Some easy-to-use activities for therapeutic purposes may be culturally
     out of favor or be gender-bound.
F.   Some purposeful activities can be easily confused by client families
     and administrators as "camp crafts" or "busy work."

XVIII.   Purposeful activity can be organized into a continuum of treatment for
         physical disabilities (Pedretti, 1996).
A.   The treatment continuum has four stages.
     1.   Adjunctive methods are procedures that prepare the patient for
          occupational performance but are preliminary to the use of pur-
          poseful activity. Examples include rote exercise, facilitation and
          inhibition techniques, positioning, sensory simulation, selected
          physical agent modalities, and devices such as braces and splints.
     2.   Enabling activities are those created to simulate purposeful activ-
          ities such as sanding boards, riding a skateboard, stacking cones
          or blocks, using practice boards for mastery of clothing, using fas-
          teners and hardware, using diving simulators, using work simu-
          lators, and doing table-top activities such as working with peg-
          boards for training perceptual-motor skills. Others include special
          equipment such as wheelchairs, ambulatory aids, special clothing,
          communication devices, and environmental control systems.
     3.   Purposeful activity includes activities having an inherent or au-
          tonomous goal and are relevant and meaningful to the client.
          Usually, they are part of the daily life routine or occur in the con-
          text of occupational performance. Examples are feeding, com-
          pleting personal hygiene tasks, dressing, getting around (mo-
          bility), communicating, doing arts and crafts, playing games or
          sports, working, and participating in educational activities.
     4.   Occupational performance and occupational roles are those the
          client resumes or assumes in his or her living environment and
          in the community.

Adapted from: Mosey AC. Purposeful activities. In: Mosey AC. Psychosocial components of occupational therapy.
1986:227–241; Nelson DL, Peterson CQ. Enhancing therapeutic exercise through purposeful activity. A theoretic
analysis. Topics in Geriatric Rehabilitation 1989;4(4):12–22; Pedretti LW. Occupational performance: a model for
practice in physical dysfunction. In: Pedretti LW. Occupational Therapy: Practice Skills for Physical Dysfunction. 4th
ed. St. Louis: Mosby, 1996:3–12.

CHAPTER 10

Tools

The term tools is used in this chapter to convey both the internal and external approaches practitioners have to encourage clients to participate in their intervention program. Occupation is the large one but occupation often requires interest or some other type of motivation to attract the client's attention and energy. Furthermore, occupation can be subdivided into occupations related to daily activities, leisure, play, and work. Activity is discussed because of its frequency in the occupational therapy literature and its controversial role therein.

OCCUPATION

Occupation has been described by occupational therapy personnel in many ways. First there is the question of reviewing the dictionary definitions of the verb form "to occupy" because it is unclear whether the founders were using the verb or noun definitions when the term "occupation" became accepted. Because language usage changes over the years, a comparison was made between a dictionary based on language usage during the time of the founder's writings and a dictionary that more closely reflects language usage today. These comparisons are shown in Tables 10.1 through 10.4.

The earliest definition of occupation in the occupational therapy literature appears in Tracy's book *Studies in Invalid Occupation* (1). She quotes Dewey from his book *The School and Society* (incorrectly cited as The School and the Child) originally published in 1900:

> By occupation is not meant any kind of "busy work" or exercise that may be given to the child to keep him out of mischief or idleness when seated at his desk. By occupation I mean a mode of activity on the part of the child which reproduces or runs parallel to some form of work carried on in the social life. The fundamental point in the psychology of an occupation is that it maintains a balance between the intellectual and the practical phases of experience. (2, p. 132)

Tracy felt it was important that occupations maintain the connection with the social or real life of the individual whenever possible. She was concerned the individual would have "feelings of being interrupted in his legitimate work, of being relegated to the physical repair shop" (1, p. 13).

Table 10.1. Definitions of the Word "Occupy" 100 Years Apart

1897 Definition	1997 Definition
In 1897 The *American Encylopaedic Dictionary* defined to occupy as:	In 1997 the *Webster's New Universal Unabridged Dictionary* defined to occupy as:
1. To seize; to take possession of and hold	1. To take or fill up (space, time, etc.)
2. To hold in possession; to possess, to fill	2. To engage or employ the mind, energy, or attention of
3. To fill, to cover; to take up the room or space of	3. To be a resident or tenant of
4. To possess, to enjoy (with an obscene quibble)	4. To take possession and control of (a place) as by military invasion
5. To use in business; to make use of; to employ in traffic	5. To hold (a position, office, etc.)
6. To use; to make use of	6. To take or hold possession
7. To employ, to engage, to busy (often used reflexively)	
8. To give employment to; to employ, to maintain	
9. To attend to, to follow, as a business, profession, or employment	

Words in common: space, engage, employ, hold, possession, take or take up, fill or fill up, Words not in common: seize, cover, room, business, employ, busy, maintain, profession, employment, mind, energy, attention, resident, tenant, control, military, invasion, position, office

Hall, who started using occupation as therapy in 1906, said the following:

The therapeutics of occupation is a curiously complex thing. No one claims that prescribed occupation can, as a rule, of itself, cure anything. But it is beyond controversy that the patient pleasantly and usefully occupied is a better subject for medical treatment of any kind that one who is discouraged, introspective, and idle. In many people and in many disabilities, the fatigue point, the breaking-down point, is so easily reached that life is hopelessly ineffective. By means of manual work carefully prescribed, it is often possible to push this point along, to build up a degree of resistance which is in itself worthwhile. Such gains may tip the scale toward recovery, may develop a morale, a courage, which is of more value than medicine. (3)

The importance of Hall's statement is that early practitioners of occupational therapy did not claim there was direct benefit from applying occupation to the acute stages of the disease or disorder. Rather, occupational therapy was used during convalescence to assist with the return to productive or normal life. It was not

Table 10.2. Comparison in the Usage of the Word "Occupy" From 1933 to 1986

1933 Definition	1986 Definition
In the 1933 *Oxford English Dictionary* the verb "occupy" is defined as:	The 1986 *Webster's Third New International Dictionary* defined occupy as:

1933 Definition:

1. a) To take possession of, take for one's own use, seize
   b) specifically to take possession of (a place) by settling in it, or by military conquest, etc.; to enter upon the possession and holding of
2. a) To hold possession of; to have in one's possession or power; to hold (a position or office)
   b) To reside in and use (a place) as its tenant or regular inhabitant; to tenant
   c) To hold possession or office; to dwell, reside; to stay, abide
3. To take up, use up, fill (space or time); also in weakened sense, to be situated or stationed in, to be in or at (a place or position)
*4. To employ, busy, engage (a person, or the mind, attention, etc.)
5. To make use of, use (a thing)
*6. a) To employ oneself in, engage in, practice, perform, carry on; to follow or ply as one's business or occupation
   b) To be busy or employed (in some capacity); to exercise one's craft or function; to practice; to do business, to work
7. To employ (money or capital) in trading; to lay out, invest, put out to interest, trade with; to deal in
8. To deal with or have to do with sexually; to cohabit

1986 Definition:

1. To engage the attention or energies of; busy, employ
2. a) To fill up (a place of extent)
   b) To take (a specified time)
3. a) To take possession of by conquest; seize
   b) To take up residence in; settle in
   c) To maintain possession or control by military occupation
4. a) To hold possession of
   b) To fill and perform the functions of
5. To reside in as an owner or tenant

Words in common: possession, take, military, hold or holding, reside or residence, tenant, fill or fill up, place, engage, attention, employ, busy, function, occupation.

Table 10.3. Definitions of Occupation 100 Years Apart	
1897 Definition	**1997 Definition**
In 1897 *The American Encylopaedic Dictionary* defined occupation as:	In 1997 *Webster's New Universal Unabridged Dictionary* defined occupation as:
1. The act of occupying or taking possession of and holding; a seizing and holding; as, the occupation of a town by an enemy 2. The act or state of occupying or holding; the time during which one is an occupier; occupancy, tenure, holding; as during his occupation of the farm 3. The state of being occupied or employed in any way; that which engages one's time or attention; work, employment 4. The business of one's life; profession, business, trade, calling, vocation	1. A person's usual or principle work or business 2. Any activity in which a person is engaged 3. Possession, settlement, or use of land or property 4. The act of occupying 5. The state of being occupied 6. The seizure and control of an area by military forces 7. The term of control of a territory by foreign military forces 8. Tenure or the holding of an office or official function

Words in common: occupying or occupied, possession, holding, seizing or seizure, tenure, engages or engaged, work, business.

Words not in common: time, occupancy, employed, attention, employment, trade, calling, vocation, activity, settlement, property, control, military forces, territory, office, official function.

until the 1950s that the word "occupation" was applied to self-care or activities of daily living (4).

In 1983, the project to identify the philosophy of occupational therapy operationally defined occupation as "volitional, goal-directed behavior aimed at the development of play, work and life skills for optimal time management . . . the essence of the occupational process, and an optimally healthy person will be seen as one whose occupation (how one occupies time) reflects a balance of play, work and rest proportional to the needs of the individual" (5).

Nelson has taken the word occupation a step further and created new phrases (6, 7). Occupation as defined by Nelson is the relationship between an occupational form and an occupational performance. Occupation is something (the form) that is done (the performance). Occupational form is the objective set of circumstances, external to the person, that elicits, guides, or structures the person's occupational performance. An occupational form typically has a physical dimension as well as a sociocultural dimension. Occupational forms are usually nouns and

Table 10.4.	Comparison in the Usage of the Word "Occupation" From 1933 to 1986
1933 Definition	**1986 Definition**
In 1933 the *Oxford English Dictionary* gave the definition of occupy as:	In 1986 the *Webster's Third New International Dictionary* gives the definition of occupy as:

1. The action of taking possession, especially of a place or of land; seize, as by military conquest, etc.; entrance upon possession
2. a) Actual holding or possession, especially of a place or of land; rarely, also, of an office or position; tenure; occupancy
   b) A piece of land occupied by a tenant; a holding
3. The taking up of space or time (*rare*)
4. a) The being occupied or employed with, or engaged in something; that in which one is engaged; employment, business
   b) With plural. A particular action or course of action in which one is engaged, especially habitually or studiedly; an employment, business, calling
5. Use, employment (*of* a thing) *Obsolete*
6. The exercising (*of* any business or office); exercise, discharge *Obsolete*
7. Attribution, as occupation franchise, the right to vote at parliamentary elections as a tenant or occupier; occupational bridge, a bridge for the use of the occupiers of the land, e.g., one connecting parts of a farm, etc., separated by a canal or railway; occupation road, a private road for the use of the occupiers of the land
	1. a) An activity in which one engages; a way of passing the time
	   b) The principal business of one's life: a craft, trade, profession or other means of earning a living: employment, vocation
	2. The function or use of something.
	3. a) The actual possession and use of real estate (as by lease); occupancy, tenancy
	   b) The possession or settlement of a place or area: tenure
	4. The act or process of occupying or taking possession of a place or area: seizure
	5. a) The usual temporary holding and control of a country or a part of a country by a foreign military force
	   b) The military force occupying a country or the policies carried out by such a force

adjectives as apposed to verbs and adverbs. The physical dimension of an occu-pational form can include shapes, sizes, distances, weights, textures, and lighting, as expressed by temporal aspects or human aspects. The sociocultural dimension can include symbols, norms, sanctions, roles, and typical uses or variations as ex-pressed by levels of society or language. Occupational performance is the volun-tary doing by the person in the context of the occupational form. Occupational performance is usually described by verbs or adverbs. It requires complex se-quences or chains of movement and postural control. It depends both on the oc-cupational form and on the unique abilities, or structure, that the individual brings to the situation. Potentially, an occupation might never be performed exactly as it was before because of the variations in the abilities and structure that the individ-ual brings to the occupational performance.

Breines has suggested another approach to expanding the view of occupation (8, 9). She suggests that occupation be described according to three interrelated con-cepts: egocentric, exocentric, and consensual. Egocentric is represented by the phase "to be occupied." Breines states that "[w]hen one is occupied, one is engaged both in mind and in body, sometimes simultaneously, sometimes alternatively. When performing a task, mind and body integrate. When the mind is occupied, the body performs. When the body is occupied, the mind is distracted or engaged."

The exocentric is represented by the phrase "to occupy." Breines explains that "[w]hen engaged in tasks, one occupies space and occupies time; one is interact-ing with these elements of the environment, while these elements themselves in-teract. That is, the individual learns to adapt to the world and/or the environment is adapted to the individual."

Finally the consensual aspect is represented by "occupation." Occupation in-cludes "vocation or work, but also represents interactive play or other endeavors in which one collaborates, competes or otherwise engages with or for others in so-cially responsible behaviors."

Yet another view of occupation is expressed by Levine and Brayley (10). They define occupation as the "engagement in activities, tasks, and roles for the purpose of meeting the requirements of living." Thus, a hierarchical relationship is estab-lished between activities, tasks, and roles. Activities are viewed as the "foundation of the doing process" and are defined as any specific action or pursuit. Tasks form the next level, which are more complex units of doing and are goal-directed. The components of tasks that create the complexity include temporal boundaries, rules or structures, and social–emotional dimensions. The highest level consists of roles that define or govern the tasks and activities necessary for performance that is both competent and meets sociocultural expectations. In addition to this activ-ity, task or role is influenced by some aspect or aspects of the human or nonhuman environment.

Finally, Christiansen and colleagues define occupation(s) as "the ordinary and familiar things that people do every day" (11). Occupations are viewed as "having both performance and contextual dimensions because they involve acts with defined setting." They also may have a temporal dimension if they extend over time. In addition, occupation may be "driven by an intrinsic need for mastery, competence, self-identity, and group acceptance," which gives them a psychological dimension. Furthermore, occupation(s) often have a social or occupational role that is identified with a specific culture, thus giving occupation a social and symbolic dimension. Finally, individuals endow or infuse occupation with meaning in relation to the their individual lives, thus giving occupation a spiritual dimension. Spiritual is used to refer to the nonphysical and nonmaterial aspects of occupation. Therefore, occupation(s) has a multidimensional view.

Occupation Versus Activity

There also has been an ongoing discussion regarding the differences, if any, between the word *activity* and the word *occupation*. Part of problem may be explained by the increased use of the word *activity* in the English language. Whereas the number of definitions for occupation have decreased from 1933 to 1986 (12, 13), the number of definitions for the word activity increased from four to seven. In 1933, activity was defined as shown in Table 10.5.

The key words appear to be occupied, employed, or engaged in employment, action, business, or calling in 1933 whereas the 1986 definition includes passing of time or engaging in a craft, business, trade, profession, or vocation.

Although the dictionary and thesaurus view activity and occupation as synonyms, several occupational therapists have suggested that the two words as concepts to describe occupational therapy are quite different. Darnell and Heater state that describing *occupation* as "purposeful activity" is not adequate because reflex activity, cardiovascular activity, and molecular activity both have a purpose but are not "purposeful activity" in the sense that an occupation is considered "purposeful activity" (14). They point out that the word *occupation* could not be substituted for the word *activity* in either reflex activity or cardiovascular activity. The phrases "reflex occupation," "cardiovascular occupation," and "molecular occupation" do not convey the same meaning as activity. *Activity* includes the actions or functions of body organs, cells, and molecular structures, but the word *occupation* does not. At the level of body organs, cells, and molecular structures, the words *activity* and *occupation* are not and cannot be synonyms and thus are not interchangeable. Occupation is used to describe what humans do, or "human doing." It does not describe what is going on inside the bodily organs, cells, and molecular structures.

Another way in which activity and occupation are different is in reference to the amount of action. Activity is usually confined to a specific type of action such as *physiological activity, business activity,* or *radioactivity.* Occupation, on the other

Table 10.5. Comparison in the Usage of the "Activity" From 1933 to 1986

1933 Definition

In 1933 the *Oxford English Dictionary* defined activity as:

1. The state of being active; the exertion of energy, action
2. The state or quality of being abundantly active; brisk or vigorous action; energy, diligence, nimbleness, liveliness
3. Physical exercise, gymnastics, athletics
4. Anything activity; an active force or operation

1986 Definition

In 1986 the *Webster's Third New International Dictionary* definitions for the word activity as:

1. The quality or state of being active (the sphere of his activity, solar activity)
2. Physical motion or exercise of force as
   a) Vigorous or energetic action: liveliness, (to restrict his liveliness),
   b) Adroit or skillful physical action: agility (an athlete's agility)
3. Natural or normal function or operation as

a) A process (as moving or digesting) that an organism carries on or participates in by virtue of being alive,
b) Any similar process (as searching, desiring, learning, or writing) that actually or potentially involves mental function: specifically and educational procedure designed to stimulate learning by first hand experience or observation, experiment, injury, and discussion
4. a) An actuating force,
   b) A creative agency or process.
5. a) An occupation, pursuit, or recreation in which a person is active— often used in plural, (business activities, social activities)
   b) A form of organized, supervised and often extracurricular recreation (as athletic games, dramatics, or dancing)
6. a) The characteristic of acting rapidly or of promoting a rapid reaction,
   b) The apparent or effective concentration of a substance (chemistry)
7. An organizational unit for performing a specific function; also its duties or functions

hand, can be much broader in encompass and express human purpose or action throughout the life span. West said the following:

> Let us consistently use and more imaginatively implement the concept as well as them occupation as the common core of occupational therapy. It is infinitely more expressive and encompassing than "purposeful activity" and will continue to broadly describe of our particular mode of intervention. (15)

Hagedorn suggests there are several differences between the words "occupation" and "activity" as they apply to occupation (16). She states that:

> A person *possesses* occupations and owns occupational and social roles as part of the individual's personal identity of "who I am."

Table 10.6. Classification of Occupations

I. Locality
  A. Bed
  B. Ward
  C. Shop
  D. Outdoor—sawing fire wood
  E. Unlimited—knitting
II. Interest
  A. Plain or drab—sawing fir wood, sweeping, dusting, folding paper, hemming towels or napkins.
  B. Occupations which are somewhat stereotyped, but require some effort of attention to perform them properly—sawing or planing wood; nailing wood to form boxes or other objects, the material being prepared by others; knitting and crocheting in some forms; sorting materials as to size or color, although with some patients the handling of colors may give such aesthetic gratification as to warrant placing such occupation under group V.
  C. Occupations which are stereotyped, which require fairly constant attention, but permit frequent rest periods. Examples: Painting; polishing or sawing metal; ploughing; wood work in some forms; type setting; leather punching or tooling; basket weaving in plain pattern, as the borders and fancy weavers will remove this to group IV.
  D. Occupations requiring quiet constant attention, which may be discontinued at the option of the worker, but in which variety or development create interest. Examples: Clay modeling, paper mache, leather carving, embroidery.
  E. Occupations which require constant attention. These should be sub-divided into stereotyped and varied.
    1. Stereotyped: feeding a printing press, corn cutter, or similar machine; doing many things in groups, such as pulling a wagon or lawn roller, pulling on a rope.
    2. Varied: Developing photographic prints or negatives; dyeing; making a plaster cast.
  F. Occupations in which the surprise element does much to promote interest. Rest periods not an option of workers. Examples: Group games, tennis, baseball, group singing, orchestra playing.

From Dunton WR: Prescribing Occupational Therapy. Springfield Ill, Charles C Thomas, 1928, p 20–21 and Dunton WR: Some problems in occupational therapy. Maryland Psychiatr Quart 9:37, 1919.

A person *performs* activities and task but does think of the activities as describing the self.

Example: I am a business man (occupation). I perform business activities.

An occupation *defines and organizes* a particular sphere of action over an extended period of time.

An activity is the *means* whereby a specific purpose is achieved on a particular occasion.

Example: I have been in business for 25 years (occupation). Last month my company sold 101 new cars (activity).

An occupation *is an organized form* of human endeavor.

An activity *may form part of* a human occupational endeavor, or be non-occupational.

Example: Orchard farming (occupation) can be a risky business. Sometimes the fruit freezes (activity of freezing), drops off the trees, or is eaten by worms, beetles or birds.

An occupation *has a name and* associated social or occupational *role title*.

An activity *may or may not have a specific name* and may or may not bring with it a specific social or occupational role.

Example: Farming (occupation) requires many things. Among them is the right conditions to ripen (activity) the fruit or grow (activity) the wheat.

An occupation is described as a sociocultural phenomenon with attributes which can be defined and observed.

An activity is identified by a short description of active and objective.

Example: A good musician must practice many long hours. The sound activity of a violin occurs as a string vibrates and causes the wood to resonate.

SUMMARY

The founders of occupational therapy stated in the original constitution for the National Society for the Promotion of Occupational Therapy that "[t]he object of our society shall be the advancement of occupation as a therapeutic measure; the study of the effects of occupation upon the human being; and the dissemination of scientific knowledge of the subject." Clearly, the founders wanted occupation, not activity, to be the principle focus of the profession. Unfortunately, they did not attempt to elaborate of the meaning of the word "occupation." Perhaps they were wise enough to know that any definition would be short-sighted and out of date as the society, culture, and language changed over the years.

Mocellin has been critical of the wide spectrum of what can be included under the word occupation according to occupational therapists (17). He questions whether all "human goal-oriented behaviors, tasks and roles, including bathing toileting and dressing, eating, work, watching television, making love, and recreational, creative, relaxation, social and spirtual activities" are really occupations (17, p. 505). Have occupational therapists gone too far in expanding the concept of occupation to include so many human activities as occupation?

ACTIVITY

Thus, occupational therapy has had an uneasy relationship with the word *activity*. There have been three distinct uses of the word in the occupational therapy literature. In one, the word is used as a synonym for the word occupation. In another, the word is considered *not* occupation. And in the third, the word is considered to be a part of a hierarchy of occupation. Some discussion about the concept of occupational therapy was covered in the discussion of occupation, especially regarding the differences between activity and occupation. That issue is included in this discussion but also included are the meaning of term activity and the historical trends.

Webster's New Universal Unabridged Dictionary provides nine definitions of which seven are general definitions for the word activity (1). The general definitions are: a) the state or quality of being active; b) a specific deed, action, function or sphere of action: social activities; c) work, especially in elementary grades at school, that involves direct experience by the student, rather than textbook study; d) energetic activity; animation; liveliness; e) a use of energy or force; an active movement or operation; f) normal mental or bodily power, function, or process; and g) an organization unit or the function it performs.

The word activity may be expanding its usage in the English language. In 1933 only four definitions are provided: a) the state of being active; the exertion of energy, action; b) the state or quality of being abundantly active; brisk or vigorous action; energy, diligence, nimbleness, liveliness; c) physical exercise, gymnastics, athletics, and d) anything active; an active force or operation (2).

The first definition of activity appearing in the occupational therapy literature appears to be in 1980. Reed and Sanderson defined activity as "a specific action, function, or sphere of action that involves learning or doing by direct experience"(3). This definition is based on the definitions in the *American Heritage Dictionary of the English Language* (4).

The word activity has been used in occupational therapy literature since its formal beginning, but until recently the term was used primarily as a synonym for occupation. In 1920 Dr. Pattison used the word, but did not define it, as part of his definition of occupational therapy, which was as follows: " My notion of occupational therapy is mental or physical *activity* definitely prescribed and guided for the distinct purpose of contributing to and hastening recovery from the effects of disease or injury. Unless prescribed to promote recovery the *activity* is not therapy" (italics added) (5).

Dr. Pattison was presumably trying to convey the idea that the use of arts and crafts, recreation, amusements, occupations, and other media was not simply a case of suggesting that patients or clients do something but rather that occupational therapy required a prescription or purpose and a plan of action. The specific plan should be directed at assisting the person to recover from the impact of a disease or injury.

In 1928 Dr. Dunton continued the use of activity and occupation as synonyms by stating the following:

A great variety of activities of normal life; amusements, study, and occupation of various kinds, have been, and are being used under direction to promote recovery from physical or mental disability. When so used *they are occupations* used therapeutically, or occupational treatment. (6, italics added)

He uses the words *activity* and *occupation* together throughout his book. In fact, he quotes Dr. Pattison's definition on the first page and also quotes the definition attributed to the Boston School of Occupational Therapy which begins by stating that "[o]ccupational therapy aims to furnish a scheme of scientifically arranged activities."

The intermixing of activity and occupation continues to occur in definitions of occupational therapy. In 1977, the definition recommended for state licensure was as follows: "Occupational therapy is the application of occupation, any activity in which one engages" (7). In 1981, the definition read as follows: "Occupational therapy is the use of purposeful activity" (8). In 1987, Evans proposed that occupation be defined as the "process of a person engaged in goal directed, intrinsically gratifying and culturally appropriate activity"(9).

In 1966, Reilly stated that the word activity "requires no . . . commitment to knowledge or purpose and permits one to deny that man's economic nature exists" (10). In contrast, she used the term occupational to acknowledge that "man, in addition to having a social and sexual nature, has an economic nature as well." Thus, Reilly opposed the use of the word activity.

In 1984, Nelson suggested that the word activity was used in two different ways (11). One way involved "activity as form" whereas the other way involved "activity as action." Activity as form is evident in such activities as dining, playing a game, or working—according to Nelson. Activity as action, in other words, the specific operation being carried out, is evident by stating I eat, play, or work. In summary, one can discuss or talk about activities in terms of general procedures that anyone would do to complete the activity (form) or one can talk about the specific procedures a given individual does to accomplish an activity (action). In 1988, Nelson suggested there is too much ambiguity in the use of the word activity, among others, and suggested there are better terms such as occupational form for "activity as form" and occupational performance as "activity in action" (12). In 1996 Nelson continued his work in further defining and describing occupation and therapeutic occupation (13). He again stated that the word *activity* is overly broad and includes meanings such as volcanic activity and intestinal activity. Instead he recommended the words occupation or occupational be substituted to avoid confusion in meanings not intended. West also suggested that occupation was "infinitely more expressive and encompassing" than the term activity (14). In 1998, Christiansen and Baum chose the word *actions* rather than activity as the most basic unit in their model of person–environment–occupational performance (15).

Hagedorn continued the theme that activity is not occupation (16). She made two distinctions. One is that the person *possesses* occupations whereas the person *performs* activities. The other distinction is related to the time perspective. Occupation occurs over an extended period of time whereas an activity is performed on a particular occasion. Thus she described activity as follows:

> An activity is identified by a short description of action and objective. An activity takes place on a specific occasion, during a finite period, for a particular purpose, and has both stable and situational elements. A completed activity results in a change in the previous state of objective reality or subjective experience.

In contrast, she defined an occupation as "an organized form of human endeavor, having a name and associated role title. A participant engages in an occupation over an extended period of time." In summary, Hagedorn felt that activity is not a synonym for occupation and vice versa. Foster concisely stated that "activity is *doing,* whereas occupation is a state of *being*" (17) .

Finally, Polatajko suggested that activity is too narrow a concept because activity is only one of many tools available to occupational therapists (18). Others include technology, assistive devices, environmental adaptation, attitudinal shift, family education, social education, and policy change. She suggested the word activity be replaced by the phrase occupational perspective. Thus, it is apparent that occupational therapists have both an attraction for and an avoidance of the word *activity.* At the present time, the reader cannot be sure of the intended meaning unless a definition is provided or the author can be questioned.

One significant addition is the concept of an organization unit that seems to be the definition being used in current literature. Activity is viewed as the initial step or stage in a sequence or hierarchy of terms. The sequence continues with task, occupation, and role. Beginning in 1991, Levine and Brayley used the sequential approach is discussing occupation (18). They wrote that engagement in activities, tasks, and roles are used for the purpose of meeting the requirements of living. The idea is that activity forms the basic level of the occupational therapy process. The task and role levels are assumed to be constrained by the activity level but the higher levels rule the activity level. Thus, activity is defined as "any specific action or pursuit" (p. 600). They then proposed a hierarchy of three terms, activity, tasks and roles, of which activity is the basis or foundation of the hierarchy. Tasks are "a set of activities sharing some common purpose recognized by the task performer" (p. 618). Role relates to "expectations or requirements for the performance of specific activities and tasks necessary to fulfill positions in society" (p. 621).

Examples of activities given in the text include brushing teeth, cooking hot dogs, weaving a mat, swinging in a net, or riding a scooter board. Categories of activities include, functional activities, diversional activities, development activities, activities related to gender, and culturally influenced activities. Activities can also be discussed in relationship to characteristics such as physical, sensory, perceptual, cognitive, psychological, or social.

In summary, the concept of activity has been used with three different focuses within occupational therapy literature. Historically, the term was a synonym for occupation. Next, the term was considered *not* a synonym for occupation. Currently, the term is being used as a basic componenet or substage within a hierarchy. Thus the concept of activity has had an uneasy relationship with occupational therapy. The concept may have come full circle from acceptance as a synonym, to nonacceptance as not the same as occupation, to acceptance in a different perspective within a hierarchy of terms.

ACTIVITIES OF DAILY LIVING

Although daily living activities has been a concern of the occupational therapist for many years, the systematic assessment of such activities did not begin until 18 years after the founding of the occupational therapy national organization. In 1935, Sheldon, a teacher of orthopedic physical education who later became a physical therapist, published a list of daily living activities for children (1). In 1945, Deaver and Brown, a physician and physical therapist, published a rating scale of 37 items called Physical Demands of Daily Living, based in part on Sheldon's work (2). Deaver is credited with coining the term activities of daily living (3, p. 20) although a written account of him using the term has not been located.

The first scale printed in the occupational therapy literature appeared in the first edition of Willard and Spackman (4). This scale was based on the one developed by Deaver and Brown. The first scale developed and published by an occupational therapist appears in the *American Journal of Occupational Therapy* in 1950 (5). Livingston developed a form to assess the skills of children with cerebral palsy and record their achievements. Since that time, numerous scales have been published by occupational therapists alone or in combination with other professionals. However, many, many scales designed to measure activities of daily living have been created by persons without any input from occupational therapists. It should be very clear that occupational therapy does not own and never did own the exclusive rights to assess persons regarding performance of activities of daily living.

Definitions for the concept of activities of daily living did not appear in occupational therapy literature when the scales first appeared. Spackman did not define activities of daily living in 1947 (3). Edgerton did not define activities of daily living, but he did define self-help activities as "those activities aimed at training or retraining the patient to be able to care for his personal needs in self-toileting, dressing and grooming, and self-reliance at the dining table, the telephone and in travel by public conveyance" (6, p. 54).

The term activities of daily living first appeared in an article written by an occupational therapist in 1950. Connell began the article using the term "daily living activities," but at the end of the first paragraph the phrase "activities of daily living" is used (7, p. 219). No definition was included, only a description about knowing the limitations, abilities, and potentialities of the individual. Just a few pages before the Connell article was one by Brown—the physical therapist who worked with Deaver—which provided a short history of the development and included the scale she developed (8). Although she also occasionally used the term activities of daily living, she only described but did not define it.

The first extensive coverage of activities of daily living by an occupational therapist was in 1963. Zimmerman wrote a 37-page chapter in the third edition of Willard and Spackman (9). Once again, however, no definition was provided. In 1971, Zimmerman described the concept of activities of daily living by saying that "[o]riginally the emphasis was upon self-care, but now it includes any activity necessary or desirable for each individual. Communications and travel . . . , various hand skills . . . , homemaking and clothing . . . , and specialized equipment or self-help devices" are also included (10).

The first definition found occurred in 1978. The Standards of Practice glossary defines activities of daily living as "the components of everyday activity including self-care, work and play/leisure activities" (11). In 1980, Reed and Sanderson defined activities of daily living in their glossary as follows: "The tasks which a person must be able to perform in order to care for the self independently, including self-care, communication and travel" (12). The following year, Pedretti's definition was as follows: "Activities of daily living (ADL) are tasks of self-maintenance, mobility, communication, and home management that enable an individual to achieve personal independence in his environment" (13, p. 109). In 1983, Trombly suggested that "activities of daily living (ADL) are those occupational performance tasks that a person does each day to prepare for, or as an adjunct to, role tasks" (14, p. 458). It should be apparent that occupational therapists do not have a single, unified concept of activities of daily living.

In recent years, the concept of activities of daily living has been divided into two or more parts. Trombly divides the concept into two parts. She defines self-care activities as those "activities or tasks done routinely to maintain the client's health and well-being, considering the environment and social factors" (15, p. 352). Instrumental activities of daily living are "[m]ore complex activities of tasks a person does to maintain independence in the home and community" (15, p. 44). Foti and Pedretti adopt a similar division: "ADL tasks include mobility, self-care, communication, management of environmental hardware and devices, and sexual expression. I-ADL include home management and community living skills, health management, and safety preparedness" (16, p. 463). Christiansen and Baum also concur with the division (17, p. 12). Activities of daily living are referred to as "personal care tasks including toileting, bathing, dressing, eating, and grooming (including oral hygiene)." Instrumental activities of daily living are listed as "telephone, food preparation, housekeeping, laundry, shopping, money management, use of transportation, and medication management." The list of IADLs is based on Lawton who first proposed the term instrumental activities of daily living (18).

The division into two major groups has reached general agreement with the profession of occupational therapy. Outside the profession, the debate continues. Cammack and Eisenberg suggest three parts: physical activities of daily living or PADL, instrumental activities of daily living (IADL), and mobility (19, p. 4). PADL "refers to the most basic of personal care tasks," IADL "is concerned with the more complex activities needed for independent living," and mobility is the "ability to negotiate one's environment which may also encompass components of the first two categories." Vreede also suggests a triad division to include ODL, ADL, and IDL (20). ODL are the "physical, mental or functional *operations* needed for daily living, for example sight or movement of one's hands." ADL are "the actual *activities* of daily living which make use of basic mental or physical functions, including more complex intentional activities such as kneeling or washing." IDL are the *ideas* about daily pursuits that have a shared value or common social purpose such as cooking a meal or playing marbles. The triad is considered hierarchical because "an ADL cannot be performed unless all the required ODLs are available. Nor will an ADL be performed unless it is part of an IDL." Vreede compares the triad to the WHO classification of impairment, disability, and handicap by suggesting the "impairment is the equivalent of a disturbed ODL, disability is the equivalent of a disturbed ADL, and handicap is the equivalent of a disturbed IDL."

To further illustrate the complexity of the term activities of daily living, consider the working definitions of activities of daily living and self-care on the MED-LINE database. On MEDLINE, activities of daily living is defined as the performance of the basic activities of self-care, such as dressing, ambulation, eating, etc., in rehabilitation. Implied is the idea that health professionals are assisting in the performance of the self-care tasks. Self-care is the performance of activities and tasks traditionally performed by professional health care providers. Thus, activities of daily living is the term used when assistance is required. Self-care is the term used when no assistance is necessary.

This discussion of activities of daily living should serve as a reminder to anyone discussing ADLs with another therapist or professional. There is very little shared meaning within the profession of occupational therapy and practically none at all outside the profession. Assuming a shared meaning is a high-risk behavior. Either define the term or assume no one really understands the context in which the term activities of daily living is being used.

INTEREST

Of the 20 definitions of the word interest in *Webster's New Universal Unabridged Dictionary*, the first four seem most relevant (1). They are as follows: a) the feeling of a person whose attention, concern, or curiosity is particularly engaged by something; b) something that concerns, involves, draws the attention of, or arouses the curiosity of a person; c) power of exciting such concern, involvement, etc.; quality of being interesting; and d) concern or importance.

Dunton defined interest in 1928 as meaning "the state of consciousness in which the attention is attracted to a task, accompanied by a more or less pleasurable emotional state. That is to say, an emotion is produced by the performance of a task, motor action, or by a sensory stimulus" (2). In his article on interest published in 1951, Dunton defined interest as follows:

> A. Excitement of feeling, whether pleasant or painful, accompanying special attention to some object, concern. *Interest* expresses mental excitement, which may be intellectual, or sympathetic or emotional, or merely personal, as interest in philosophical research, in human suffering, in money getting. B. A propensity to attend to and be stirred by a certain class of objects. C. That which causes such excitement or attention, has interesting quality, as a book of interest or scholarly interest.

In 1969, Matsasuyu developed the NPI Interest Check List, an assessment of five categories of interests—manual skills, physical sports, social, recreation, adl, and cultural/education and three levels of expressed strength of interest—casual, strong, and no interest (3). She did not cite any of Dunton's writings. Her citations were primarily to works on vocational interests and to the study of interest by psychologists. She did quote the *Psychiatric Dictionary*, which says "to interest is to attract and hold the attention, to occupy and engage a patient's concern to the extent of employing his time . . . This is one of the basic principles upon which occupational therapy is applied." Matsasuya stated six propositions (assumptions) regarding interest which were as follows:

1. Interests are family influenced. Interests are determined by early developmental contingencies that are primarily localized in the family unit where early intra-familial experience influences direction.
2. Interests evoke affective response. Interest can evoke affective response with persons, things, and ideas and can be expressed as likes, dislikes, indifferences or as preferences.
3. Interest are choice states. The capacity to make interesting choices serves the process of commitment to life roles for work, through occupational choice, and for play, through recreation and leisure.
4. Interest can be manifest in effective action. Interest in a subjective experience can lead the individual to engage in pertinent activities that can be satisfying and have adaptive value

5. Interest can sustain action. Degree of strength of interests varies according to the level and type of interaction with the event and can serve to sustain action during the learning stages or to maintain functional achievement.
6. Interests reflect self-perception. Expressed interests are subjective statements which reflect self-perception.

Matsasuya credited William James as identifying attention as the main criteria of interest (5). In his chapter on reasoning, he stated:

> But what determines which element we shall attend to first? There are two immediate and obvious answers: first our practical or instinctive and interests; and, second, our aesthetic interest.
>
> Interest alone gives accent and emphasis, light and shade, background and foreground—intelligible perspective, in a word. (6)

She also credited Dewey (7). Dewey proposed that a child has four types of interest: "the interest in conversation, or communication; in inquiry, or finding out things; in making things, or construction; and in artistic expression."

Matsasuya continued by suggesting that interest had been studied in two major directions (4). One looks at interest "as a task, an activity or description of an event." Interest is thus measured in terms of interest inventories, often in relation to vocational choice. The other approach looks at interest in relation to the development of personality. As such, interests may be described as "feelings, drives or reactions which are interest states and related to attitudes, values and other motivational indices such as attention, direction and sentiments." She suggested that the greater yield for occupational therapy is in the study of interest in relation to personality. Specific theorists mentioned are Allport, Roe and Seligman, and Murphy (8, 9, 10).

She quoted Allport as stating that the mature personality possesses "sophisticated and stable interest." Allport used the concept of interest in two ways: "1) a cognitive relationship of the person to the environment, and 2) a subjective relationship to his ego values."

Roe and Seligman were credited with suggesting that personality is subject to the same principles of development as other aspects of development. Interest is defined as "any activity (action, thought, observation) to which one gives effortless and automatic attention."

Murphy was credited with defining interest as "the attitude with which one attends to anything; the feeling accompanying attention; . . . interests are dispositions defined in terms of objects which one easily and freely attends to or which one regards as making a difference to oneself."

Matsasuya continued by suggesting that the concept of interest should be viewed within the context of White's concept of competence or the organism's capacity to interact effectively with its environment (11). More specifically, she suggested that interest is related to the effectance, the motivational aspect of competence.

Kielhofner has incorporated the concept of interest, specifically interests, into his model of human occupation (12). The concept of interests is one of three traits comprising the volition subsystem. Interests are defined as "disposition to find pleasure and satisfaction in occupations and the self-knowledge of our enjoyment of occupations." Interests involve attraction to and preference for occupation. Attraction is "a proclivity to enjoy certain occupations or certain aspects of performance." Preference is "the propensity to enjoy particular ways of performing or particular activities over others." Thus, a person comes to learn about the potentials for enjoyment and satisfaction in occupations through interests.

LEISURE

Webster provides three definitions for the word leisure, three for the phrase *at leisure* and one for *at one's leisure*. For leisure, the definitions are as follows: a) freedom from the demands of work or duty; b) time free from the demands of work or duty, when one can rest, enjoy hobbies or sports, etc.; and 3) unhurried ease.

For the phrase *at leisure*, the definitions are as follows: 1) with free or unrestricted time; 2) without haste; slowly; and 3) out of work; unemployed. For the phrase *at one's leisure,* the definition is "when one has free time; at one's convenience."

The concept of leisure has been in occupational therapy literature since the early years of the organized profession. Hall, in 1923, describes leisure as "well-earned repose, in every way desirable" (2). He contrasts leisure with idleness, especially idleness continued too long, as "deadening to the spirit as it is disabling to the body . . . and in the end, increased suffering." Such enforced idleness, or enforced rest, occurs in long illness or in delayed convalescence.

The first edition of the Uniform Terminology defined play/leisure as referring to "skills and performance in choosing, performing, and engaging in activities for amusement, relaxation, spontaneous enjoyment, and/or self-expression" (3). These activities include play or leisure exploration and play or leisure performance according to the second edition (4). In the third edition (5), play or leisure exploration includes "identifying interest, skills, opportunities, and appropriate play or leisure activities." Performance includes "planning and participating in play or leisure activities, maintaining a balance of play or leisure activities with work and productive activities and activities of daily living as, and obtaining, utilizing, and maintaining equipment and supplies." Leisure is not defined separately in any of the editions.

Mosey stated that, within the context of leisure, a person "seeks physical and emotional health, a degree of freedom, self-knowledge, to be wanted by and useful to others, and to find one's place in the universe" (6). Leisure is usually defined as a "time when one is free from family and other social responsibilities, activities of daily living, and work. It is characterized by a feeling of comparative freedom and self-determination." Mosey suggested that the choice and involvement in leisure activities are motivated primarily by personal satisfaction and enjoyment. She also believed that leisure should not just be considered a balance mechanism for work, self-care, and family responsibilities but that leisure should be considered on its own merits. She rejected the Greek concept of leisure in which work was the means toward achieving leisure. Finally, Mosey outlined that leisure pursuits are influenced by age, gender, occupation, marital status, and education. They may be solitary or group situations.

In 1991, Davidson stated that leisure is "characterized by relative choice and is usually shared by people of like interests" (7). Leisure is a "time away from work and responsibilities, a time to restore oneself and find meaning in life."

Primeau summarized the issues in the leisure literature (8). There are three viewpoints as to what constitutes leisure: 1) leisure as time, 2) leisure as activity, and 3) leisure as an experience or state of mind. The amount of time available for leisure continues to be a cited as a negative item for many people. For persons without disability, the more frequent complaint is that there is not enough time for leisure activities. For person with disabilities, there may be too much time for leisure activities. According to literature cited by Primeau, some ideas regarding leisure as time suggest that technology, especially computers, has changed the perception of time to the expectation of a faster pace. People want to get through everything faster supposedly to have more leisure time. Time to do what? Another idea is that there are rising aspirations about the use of time. More people want to do more things. They want to take advantage of the increasing choices and goals available to them. Thus, there is not enough time to do everything they want to do. Time to do what? A third idea is that time is being perceived by more people as a precious commodity. As work, self-care, and family take more time, there is less time to call their own. Time to do what? The major problem with measuring leisure as time is that there is no agreement about what leisure time really is. There has never been a satisfactory definition of leisure in relation to time. Is leisure time that which remains after everything else is done? Is leisure time "free time," discretionary time, residual time, or unobligated time? Is leisure time the time in which the individual gets to choice how it will be spent? Is there a magic formula for figuring how much leisure time each person is entitled to have? Does society owe each citizen a guarantee that time will be divided into equal intervals of 8 hours of work, 8 hours of self-care and family responsibilities, and 8 hours of leisure time? What happens if some person wants 9 hours or 7 hours of leisure time? Who determines the entitlement to leisure time in the first place? Is leisure time a birthright? Is leisure time earned according to the number of work hours a person does? Do employers owe their employees so much leisure time? How does a person with a job, a home to maintain, and a family to raise figure the amount of leisure time he or she is owed? Is leisure time owed by the minute, day, week, month, year, or age? Can leisure time be stored or put in a leisure time bank to be used at some later time? Who is in charge of the leisure time bank? How does a person collect or get paid for the leisure time that is owed? How does a person make a withdrawal from the leisure time bank? Should the leisure time bank be required to send monthly statements on the amount of leisure time accumulated? It should be clear that measuring leisure in relation to some number unit of time is not realistic. The assumptions can be too quickly challenged by those who feel another viewpoint regarding leisure as time are more useful or more valid.

The second issue is time as activity. Activities (or occupations) depending on the definition are divided into categories. One of the categories is called leisure activities. The other categories might be called work activities, self-care activities, obligatory activities, family responsibilities, subsistence activities, or any other label deemed important. Most studies using the leisure as activity approach are records of how many people did what leisure activity, the frequency in which specific leisure activities are engaged, and preferences for some leisure activities as opposed to others. Immediately, the problem is apparent. What constitutes a leisure activity? Must everyone agree on what is a leisure activity. What happens to people who play sports for a living? Is basketball a leisure activity for persons who play professional basketball? What happens to activities that some people consider leisure activities but others do not? Can a leisure activity be a leisure activity in some situations and not in others? For example, is shopping always a leisure activity or does it sometimes belong in another category? Does the definition of leisure activity change over the lifespan? What about social and cultural variations?

The third issue is leisure as experience or state of mind. Key descriptors are focused on meaning and quality of life. In other words, what is the meaning of leisure to the individual? Does leisure contribute positively or negatively to the person's quality of life. Is leisure satisfying or not satisfying to the person? Primeau summarized the qualities expressed in definitions as including freedom of choice, intrinsic motivation, enjoyment, low work-relation and role constraint, aesthetic appreciation, relaxation, novelty, self-expression, companionship, intimacy, and lack of evaluation. Such qualities suggest that people use leisure to experience a variety of qualities in their lives. The real question is whether these same qualities can be used to express experiences in work, self-care, family, or other categories? In other words, is leisure a distinct and separate category of life experience that is measured in meanings or qualities which are different than any other category of human experience? Is it possible for work and leisure to occur together, for example? Do some people enjoy their work and thus find the same quality of satisfaction in their work that they might find in leisure? Do some professional basketball players enjoy their work on the basketball court or is basketball just a way to earn a good living? Do some occupational therapy personnel enjoy their work enough to volunteer hours not required of the employer, or is work always work and leisure always preferred over work? Primeau quoted Csikszentmihalyi who suggested consideration of what is both important and enjoyable is that a person act with the fullness of his or her abilities in a setting where the challenges stimulate growth of new abilities and whether the setting is work or play, productive or recreational, does not matter (9).

However, in studies that attempted to explore optimal experiences in work and leisure, Csikszentmihalyi and LeFevre found that participants still claimed to have increased motivation and relaxation when engaged in leisure rather that work (10). The increased enjoyment in leisure was reported even though the individuals had more optimal experiences at work. At least in the North American culture, people seem to feel a social obligation not to report enjoyable experiences at work regardless of how they actually felt.

Primeau concluded that occupational therapists must find ways of studying leisure that do not juxtapose leisure with work. Socially defined categories and expectations are not necessarily good descriptors of the individual human experience. Such techniques as participant observation, in-depth interviewing, life histories, and narrative inquiry may help occupational therapy personnel to understand the meaning and purpose of leisure to the individual without being bound by social or cultural rules. Affective experience may be quite different without the culturally bound expectations.

Occupational therapy practitioners may want to consider placing less emphasis on the categories of leisure and other subdivisions of occupations and put more emphasis on the total occupational experience in a person's life. Perhaps occupational therapy personnel need to help persons with disability or other lifestyle changing events to see their occupations as a whole or gestalt and avoid reinforcing the sociocultural divisions of leisure versus some other division of occupation into categories. If all occupation is important to individuals, why are certain types of occupation preordained as more important than others? Should not occupational therapy promote occupation as a whole or gestalt and deemphasize the divisions that do not seem to work well anyway?

PLAY

The word play is even harder to define than the word leisure. *Webster's* lists 94 definitions. Under synonyms, the explanation includes: "Play, fame or sport refers to forms of diverting activity. Play is the general word for any such form of activity, often undirected, spontaneous, or random."

The concept of play has been part of occupational therapy literature from the beginning. In 1922, Meyer made a statement in his lecture about big four rhythms or cycles of "work and play and rest and sleep" (2). Play is neither defined or described beyond the relationship within the phrase. In the article that followed, Slagle talked about the play spirit which must be created or recreated because there is "little opportunity for spontaneous play at any time in their lives" (3). Slagle credited Jane Addams with saying that the play spirit needs to be continued to avoid "the fatal passivity that leads to social deviation." Slagle suggested folk dancing, gymnastics, playground activities, competitive games, and others within the model of habit training.

In the same issue of the journal, Brush stated that for children with cardiac disease *"the play-cure meets these requirements better than any other"* (italics in the original) (4). He refered to the need to inculcate the ways of life that will facilitate the "main pursuits" of happiness and service. Play is not defined but rather described in terms of games, dances, and tournaments. He also added that "work-therapy meets with a great deal of resistance; play mellows and reaches all, builds happily upon itself, and gives the more nearly adequate all-round physical and mental exercise." In his summary, however, the word recreation, not play, was used.

These initial references do not make a distinction between play as occupation for children as opposed to play as an occupation for adults. The next references specify one or other.

Hall, in 1923, discussed play in relation to adults:

> To the adult American, play means out-of-door sports, baseball, tennis, basket ball, medicine. Ball. These games are, of course, for the most part impossible for the hospital convalescent . . . Success here is not only fun, but the play may be so encouraging and developing as to take rank with the medical agents . . . I wonder if a great deal of the O.T. work may not be fulfilling the requirements of play. (5)

The fluid relation of work and play has been recognized in the field for many years. Wade in 1947 stated:

> In some activities it is impossible to distinguish between those that are work and play, or occupation and recreation. The difference may be determined only by the patient's reaction and acceptance of a given activity . . . Work and play possess common elements, particularly in relation to their values as vehicles of resocialization. (6)

In 1950, Davis provided a list of 12 aspects of play which considers part of recreation for persons with mental disorders (7). The aspects are listed as the psychodynamics of play.

1. Play is above all natural and therefore allows the individual to express his or her own personality without the inhibitions that frequently distort behavior in the mentally sick.
2. Play is free and expressive. There is a sheer physical abandon in play activity that is not present in other types of active behavior.
3. Play is extroverting, serving to free the patient from him or herself into the interests and activities of others.

4. Play is modifiable, with its many forms and gradations providing activity suited to the capacity and interests of many types.
5. Play may be competitive, awakening, and expressing the aggressive traits.
6. Play may be cooperative, developing team organization and group feeling.
7. Play may be redirective, pointing the patient's interest toward more social behavior.
8. Play may be sublimating, serving as an outlet to blocked impulses, urges, or desires, leading to a more acceptable level of behavior.
9. Play is interpretative, unfolding the patients' nature and showing his or her attitude toward the his or herself, the environment, and life in general.
10. Play may be progressive, enabling the patient to attain high steps of social and physical advancement.
11. Play is integrative, enabling the patient to focus attention and to organize motor and mental fields into a constructive pattern.
12. Play is inherently satisfying, attracting many patients who are unable to do other things into pleasurable and constructive activities.

In 1954, Driver stated that the significance of play in healthy development is important for therapists to understand because "play provides the child with opportunities for practice and exploration of all his skills and interest" (8). In the hospital, play links the child to the normal environment and provides an area of familiarity and security. Because the child invests so much interest in play, it could be said that "play is his business." This idea taken from Alessandrini (9) who introduced the concept of play in 1949 as the work of children. She said that in play the child engages the self "with the same attitude and energy that we engage ourselves in our regular work." Through play the child experiments, investigates, and learns. She suggested that play should include physical, dramatic, creative, and constructive activities to promote development.

In 1966, Reilly spoke about adults being allowed to "play" with the doing of the performance first (10). The play stage is the first of three stages she proposed in the learning process for teaching skills in the occupational behavior model. The second stage is to provide a "clear-cut teaching-learning experience," and the third is to encourage performance "for real." By 1969, Reilly had clarified the concept of play as part of a development continuum with work (11). She said the following:

> Play, in a chronological or a longitudinal sense, we believe, is the antecedent preparation area for work . . . The entire development continuum of play and work we designate as occupational behavior.

Reilly never really defined play although she did describe play as a cobweb (12). Shannon, one of Reilly's students, stated that play includes all forms of playful, recreative, leisure time activities. Instead of defining play, Reilly described three stages of play development: exploratory behavior, competency behavior, and achievement behavior (13). Exploratory behavior occurs as a result of intrinsic motivation of pleasure in exploring the environment to test reality and search the imagination for rules. Competency behavior is dominated by the efficiency or competency drive to deal with the environment, to influence it actively, and to be influenced by it through feedback mechanisms. Through practice, various tasks are mastered, and self-confidence or self-reliance is gained. Achievement behavior is linked to expectancies, particularly the standards of winning or losing. Achievement is based on competition and a known standard of excellence.

In 1971, Florey, another of Reilly's students, created a classification scheme for the development of play behavior, which she believed was based on intrinsic motivation (14). She defined play as action on human and nonhuman objects. Human objects include parents, peers, and self. Nonhuman objects are also divided into three subgroups. Type I objects are creative or unstructured media that change shape or form intrinsically when manipulated, e.g., paints, clay, sand, or water. Type II objects change shape or form when combined with another similar object or many dissimilar objects, e.g., beads, blocks, tinker toys, craft materials, or constructional media. Type III objects do not change shape or form when manipulated, e.g., rattles, balls, dolls, or play equipment.

Takata, also a student of Reilly, provides six principles regarding play based on her analysis of existing theories of play (15):

1. Play is a complex set of behaviors that is characteristically "fun," pleasurable, and spontaneously initiated.
2. Play may be sensory, neuromuscular, mental, or a combination of all three.
3. Play involves exploration, experimentation, repetition of experience, and imitation of one's surroundings.
4. Play proceeds with its own time and space boundaries.
5. Play serves to function as integrator of the children's internal world to the social world.

Play follows a sequential, developmental progression.

She then suggested that there are four salient elements derived from the principles: human, nonhuman, qualitative aspect, and quantitative aspect. The first two are self-explanatory. Qualitative refers to what is available, who is available, and how the child interacts with or uses them in play. Quantitative refers to time spent at play and the amount of time needed for learning through play to occur.

Bundy, one of the more recent model developers in the area of play, created the model of playfulness, which is discussed in the section on models (16).

Assessments

Several assessment instruments on play have been developed. Among these are the Play History by Takata (17), Preschool Play Scale by Knox (18), Play Skills Inventory by Hurff (19), Inventory of Occupational Choice Skills by Shannon (20), and Test of Playfulness by Bundy (21).

WORK

Webster's New Universal Unabridged Dictionary lists 54 definitions for the term work. Perhaps because occupational therapy deals with everyday aspects of human life, the use of everyday words is appropriate. However, the multiple meanings of these words do little to clarify the concepts applied to occupational therapy practice.

Work has been a central concept of occupational therapy since its beginning. However, the meaning of work has been changed many times, which makes the contribution of occupational therapy practice difficult to follow. McKeever identified seven themes of work which are as follows: religion and morality, self-confidence, prevention and cure, knowledge, skills and habits, economic benefit, good citizenship, and quality of life (2).

The first theme is religious morality. In 1915 Hall and Buck wrote a book on handicrafts (3). One of the major concerns was that "thousands of men and women . . . are . . . doomed to idleness and dependence because of injury or some illness that makes ordinary work out of the question." The concern that idleness was the devil's workshop was apparent in several articles. Bowers, in a paper presented at the founding meeting in 1917, quotes a Teuton proverb as saying that "idleness is the parent of all vice and evil" and continues by quoting an unnamed churchman as saying that the "devil seeks the unemployed first of all" (4). Bowers continues saying that "[w]ork dispels all this trouble which idleness produces." Clearly, work was the road to salvation for those with physical and mental disabilities.

The recognition that work could improve a person's self-confidence is shown in Hall's sentence: "The one great end to be obtained is self-forgetfulness and a pride and satisfaction in work and in life" (5, p. 32). Faulkes discussed the value of the curative workshop by stating the "patient may pass a judgment upon his own progress and become interested in some form of vocational work" (6). Barton discussed a man who seemed to have no energy or interests but the idea of constructing a good hen-house got the man started by investigating nearby hen-houses, which required him to walk (7). As he walked, he regained strength, and as he drew drawings of what he saw, he learned to draw. Construction of the hen-house developed carpentry skills. Kidner continued the theme of self-confidence by suggesting that training in an occupation reestablished a person's "belief in himself" that may have been weakened by a prolonged illness. (8)

The third theme is prevention and cure. Hall says, "It is conceivable that . . . work . . . might . . . do much toward preventing the unfortunate mental states which come from unrelieved complications of social and business life" (5, p. 31). In other words, work can be used to relieve psychological stress. Dunton emphasized that the "primary purpose of occupational therapy is *cure*" (9, p. 317). Hall simply titled his report on the therapeutic application of manual work the "Work-Cure" (10). Hall and Dunton were physicians so their perspective was the prevention and cure of disease. Kidner, a manual arts instructor and architect, had a different point of view (8, p. 446). He stated that the "purpose of the pre-industrial shop is to assist the patient in his readjustment to normal living" regardless of whether the person will continue to live in an institution or can return to the community. Kidner was more concerned with results of impairment, usually called disability, than with the particular disease itself. Thus, the word "cure" refers to both a direct meaning by reducing the effects of the disease or injury and indirect meaning by reducing the consequences of disease or injury such as disuse or loss of skills. Faulkes continued the disability theme by stating that the value of the curative workshop is in removing or minimizing the "factors which prolong . . . disability" (6). In other words, curative workshops did not cure disease but rather "cured" disability.

A fourth theme is work as a means to improve knowledge, skills, and work habits. Hall observed that manual work could increase the accuracy and precision of the person's movement (5). Barton felt that if a person could not return to previous employment, the new trade should incorporate "the greatest amount of his old knowledge and ability" (11, p. 64). Dunton did not entirely agree with Barton on the value of old or previously learned knowledge (9, p. 320). Dunton believed the work should lead to an increase in the patient's knowledge. Kidner stressed the use of the preindustrial shop to "development of habits of industry that have been impaired by disease or accident" (8, p. 446). Kidner understood that work habits might have to be established or reestablished after prolonged periods of unemployment.

The fifth theme is work and the economic benefit to the individual and society. Hall argued that patients were capable of "turning out excellent work of considerable commercial value" that could be sold in a shop (5). Furthermore, knowledge of a trade might provide "comfortable support in later years," which was important in 1905 because the social security retirement program was not passed until 1933. Brown named his pottery business the Arequipa Sanatorium for Tuberculous Wage-Earning Girls (12). As evidenced by the name, the purpose of the business was to have females with tuberculosis make, or assist in making, ceramic pottery that would be sold. Thus, women with a chronic disability, tuberculosis, were provided a source of economic return. In justifying the start of a work program run by the Illinois Society for Mental Hygiene, Thomson stated that "work was needed, from both a therapeutic and an economic standpoint" if the Society was to be of any real help to its clients because work was "an important element in restoration" (13).

The economic value to society is stressed by Johnson, who stated that one of the industries used by patients has been established on a commercial basis to manufacture tennis nets (14). Faulkes continued the theme of social benefit by stating that the role of curative workshops is to cut down compensation awards and re-turn the worker to the job within a shorter time (6). Evans supported the curative workshop role saying that "insurance companies and industrial plants are finding it profitable to send the disabled employee to us because it saves them dollars and cents" (15, p. 50). The same could be said for work-hardening programs today. The theme of work and economics was a major factor in the development of oc-cupational therapy and continues to exert an influence today.

The sixth theme is that work promotes socially accepted values such as good citizenship. Thomson concluded that workshops for the disabled would make useful "many who otherwise would be a burden to their friends, the state, or them-selves" (13, p. 398). The concept of burden seems to imply that the person should feel guilty about being a burden and embrace the opportunity to gain the more so-cially acceptable role of self-sufficiency. In the introduction to Hall and Buck's book, the authors quote a newspaper editorial stating that men who are incapac-itated should be "grateful to pick up sufficient knowledge [of work skills] to make them partially or entirely self-supporting for the rest of their shattered lives" (3, p. vii). One of the goals stated for the American Occupational Therapy Association is to reestablish the capacity for social usefulness (16).

The seventh theme is that work can increase the quality of life through happi-ness. Hall observed that "if we give to each a fair share of the blessing of self-forgetfulness and consequent happiness we have done well . . . " (5, p. 32). Thom-son suggested that school and workshops for the disabled could make the clients happy (13). Newton says that Consolation House, founded by George Barton, rep-resented a movement away from institutional life toward one in which the indi-vidual can "be happy, get well . . . and do the same for others" (17).

Thus, the concept of work is well-established in occupational therapy litera-ture. The question is one of focus. Should the focus of work be on the therapeu-tic contributions, the wage earning potential, or the relationship of temporal and economic productivity to self-care and more discretionary pursuits in leisure and play? Should the moral aspect of work continue to be stressed, or should the spir-itual value of work be emphasized? Does work still promote self-confidence, self-work, and self-identify? Can work contribute to prevention and cure of disorders, or is work a primary contributor to disorder and injury? What knowledge, skills, and habits are necessary for work and can occupational therapy practitioners pro-vide the learning experiences necessary to clients to gain such knowledge, skills, and habits? Does participation in work settings make clients better citizens, how-ever good citizenship may be defined? How does work contribute to quality of life and life satisfaction? What is the relationship in today's environment between vo-cational rehabilitation and occupational therapy?

The answers to these questions and others related to work in the practice of oc-cupational therapy would clarify the role of occupational therapy in health care delivery specifically and society in general.

THE ENVIRONMENT

Wester's New Universal Unabridged Dictionary (1) lists four meanings for the term environment: a) the aggregate of surrounding things, conditions, or influences; surroundings; milieu; b) *Ecology.* The air, water, minerals, organisms, and all other external factors surrounding and affecting a given organism at any time; c) the social and cultural forces that shape the life of a person or a population; d) an indoor or outdoor setting that is characterized by the presence of environmental art that is itself designed to be site-specific; and e) *Computers.* The hardware or software configuration, or the mode of operation of a computer system. Synonyms include local and environs. Environment, milieu, ambiance, setting, and surroundings all refer to what comprises the atmosphere or background against which someone or something is seen. Environment may refer either to actual physical surroundings or to social or cultural background factors. Milieu refers to intangible aspects of the environment. Ambiance applies to the atmosphere of the surroundings, their mood, or tone. Setting suggests a background that sets something apart from another. Surroundings alludes specifically to the physical aspects of the environment.

In addition to the aspects of environment identified in the dictionary definition, other terms and aspects have been used in occupational therapy to describe environment. Context is another term encountered in occupational therapy literature. Context refers to the set of circumstances or facts that surround a particular event or situation (1). Context emphasizes the historical events or situations that might be influencing the current situation such as a person's response to occupational therapy intervention.

Another aspect is the internal environment of the individual meaning mind–body aspects that influence or shape a person's actions and responses. Furthermore, one can discuss the natural or nature environment, the physical or inorganic environment, the economic environment, the health care environment, the political environment, the family environment, the institutional environment, the hospital environment, and others. In other words, the concept of environment can be examined from a micro or macro perspective.

Origins

The role of the environment as a therapeutic medium has been recognized since occupational therapy began. In 1845, Earle stated the following:

> It is the intention of the Committee and the offices to make the (Bloomingdale) Asylum a comfortable home for the patients . . . and that . . . various auxiliaries to moral treatment are abundantly supplied to the patients. Among these are manual labor, various games and other amusements, a good library, and horses and carriage for riding. (3)

A chaplain was also employed. Earle has synthesized the ideas of moral treatment which stressed that the physical environment should be home-like, not a prison, and that normal daily activities such as laboring, playing games, reading, and riding should be provided. Going to church on Sunday was also encouraged as part of regular routine. Allison, in 1886, also stressed the importance of comfortable and attractive surroundings, books for diversion, recreation and amusements, and pleasant companionship to facilitate recovery (3).

Hall made three references to the environment (4, p. 48). He suggested that the "patient's whole personality is at war with its environment . . . and . . . that the environment of the neurasthenic is almost invariably bad." Especially concerned about the daily life of an average neurasthenic, he continued by stating concern with two things: "the attitude of the patient toward his environment and also with that environment." Furthermore, he contended that the improvement is at least in part dependent on being able to secure an improved environment. Thus, the dual concern for the environment is stated: the significance of changing the person's response to the environment and the potential of changing the environment to better "respond to" or fit the needs of the individual.

Current Studies

One of first occupational therapy practitioners to focus on environment as a concept was Dunning (5). She suggested that occupational therapy practitioners should consider three aspects of the environment: space, people, and task. Analysis of the three aspects should be evaluated by considering the givens (what exists), the possibility for change (those givens that could be altered), and preference (what was most acceptable to the client). The result is an environmental grid containing three columns subdivided into three aspects.

Dunning stated several important assumptions about the environment from the view of occupational therapy. The first is that there is only the total environment of which human beings are simply one kind of component. In other words, no dichotomy exists between the person and the environment. Analysis by components such as physical, social, economic, political, or cultural is for the convenience of study, but the components operate as one environment in real life. Second, human psychological functioning is more frequently an indication of the demands made on the person than a reflection of the inherent nature of the person. Thus, to better understand the individual, the occupational therapy practitioner must understand the environment in which the person lives and analyze the environmental demands. Third, although human goals are many and varied, their sum and substance depends on learning, which occurs through socialization. Fourth, the environment can be viewed as a system with many subsystems to which the individual responds and which shape those responses. The system is dynamic and changed. Occupational therapy practitioners can be change agents who facilitate the change process.

Kannegieter suggested five inferences that could be drawn regarding behavior on a hospital ward (6). Although the study concerns psychiatric wards, the inferences are not limited to mental health clients. Therefore, the five inferences will be stated in generic terms. The first is that variations in the structure and organizational management of the therapeutic environment can be measured through client and staff perceptions. An example is the Ward Atmosphere Scale, which measures relationships such as involvement, support, and spontaneity; personal development such as autonomy, personal problem orientation, practical orientation, and anger and aggression; and system maintenance and change such as order and organization (7). Second, client behavior is affected by individual differences, setting differences, and interactions between individuals and setting. There are two behavioral responses that can be observed: those responses owing to individual differences, called response-specific behaviors, and those owing to setting differences, called situation-specific behavior. An early study by occupational therapists Pishkin, Mackenthum, and Stump demonstrated that therapist's attitude such as friendliness or firmness affected the behavior of clients (8). Third, client perceptions of themselves, others, and the therapeutic environment are related to elements in the therapeutic environment. The results of research studies suggests that clients' behavior varies with what the staff emphasizes (9). Fourth, therapeutic environments are persistent over time and clients unless active intervention procedures are implemented. The status quo is very entrenched unless deliberate attempts are made to change the environment. Resistance to change will be strong. Fifth, therapeutic environments are differentially related to treatment outcomes. The research results have been mixed regarding the relations of the therapeutic environment and client outcome (9). However, a high correlation occurs if clients' expected outcomes are matched to the type of therapeutic environment designed to support such outcomes. In summary, the interface between and client and occupational therapy practitioner can have a significant influence on the outcome for that client.

Barris continued the exploration of the environment in relation to occupational therapy practice (10). In particular, she discussed the concept of press or environmental demands in relation to the ways the environment communicates expectations for the person to perform and the impact of that performance on the developments of skills, habits, and roles. She also discussed how different environment settings affect performance over the life span. For example, an infant is not expected to participate in formal education, but as a child, the role of student becomes an expectation. The expectation may increase in adolescence. In adulthood, the student role is decreased, and in old age, the student role is probably not a significant expectation.

Llorens concentrated her discussion on using the environment to tip the balance from dysfunction to function through the use of purposeful activity as a change agent (11). She strongly encouraged studying the occupational therapy process to verify the concept of the environment as a positive change agent toward function.

Multiple Terms

The concept that a link exists between the humans and their environment has been expressed several ways in occupational therapy literature. Llorens (11) speaks of the individual and the environment, DiJoseph (12) uses the phrase mind–body–environment link, Dunn and colleagues (13) prefer the term ecology, and Barris (10) writes about the person–environment interactions. Although person-environment seems to be the preferred term in current literature, the older terms appear to be synonyms (14, 15). All are concerned with the relationship of humans to their environment and the use of the right amount and right kind of environment as a therapeutic tool in occupational therapy to facilitate better function, health, and sense of well-being. Right amount and right kind of environment requires further study to more fully understanding the role of the environment as a therapeutic tool in occupational therapy practice.

Low-stimulus Environment

Parent explored the oppose problem of too little environment called low-stimulus environment (16). She noted that psychology literature has shown that low-stimulus and meaningless environments can lead to behavioral deficits. Low-stimulus environments include sensory and perceptual deprivation, immobilization, and isolation. All three can occur in intensive care units (ICU). The walls, ceiling, equipment, and bed linens are often white with no pattern or variation, the person is usually confined to the room to facilitate nursing care, and usually only one person is assigned to a room with visiting hours limited to 15 minutes twice a day. The ICU is a nearly perfect example of a low-stimulus environment. How many behavioral problems occurring in such units result from the low-stimulus environment rather than the health problem for which the person was assigned to the ICU in the first place? Although the problem behaviors occurring in low-stimulus environments have been identified in the literature for more than 20 years, ICUs continue the same patterns of care today. The only exception is the addition of a television set.

Environment in Conceptual Models of Occupational Therapy

Specific reference to the environment in conceptual models began in 1980 and soon several other models followed. Again, however, it must be stressed that environment has always been a part of occupational therapy practice. The question is one of recognition and extent of use. Kielhofner and Burke proposed a model of human occupation in which man is viewed as a system that interacts with the environment (17, p. 573): "The environment is the physical, social, and cultural setting in which the system operates." In the same year, Reed and Sanderson proposed a conceptual model of occupational therapy called personal adaptation through occupation. In the model, the environment is subdivided into the physical, psychobiological, and sociocultural components. The physical environment involves the inorganic or nonhuman world, the psychobiological environment involves the organic or individual aspects, and the sociocultural environment includes the superorganic or collective being aspects. Major assumptions are that all occupations are determined by the environment, that occupations are developed and exist because of the environment, and that occupations which no longer fulfill environmental needs or demands are phased out. Thus, the job opportunities for playing piano music in silent movie theaters, making horse-drawn buggies, or being a conductor on a train's caboose are infrequent in today's job market.

SUMMARY

Occupational therapy is only one field of study interested in the environment. The wide interest is evident in the reviews of environmental assessments by occupational therapy authors (14, 19, 20). Psychology, social work, and nursing have been particularly active in publishing. Occupational therapy practitioners must show how the use of environment as a therapeutic medium can be achieved through conceptual and practice models of occupational therapy in ways that are unique to the vision of occupational therapy.

References

OCCUPATION
  1. Tracy SE. Studies in Invalid Occupation: A Manual for Nurses and Attendants. Boston: Whitcomb & Barrows, 1980:13.
  2. Dewey J. The School and Society. Chicago: University of Chicago Press, 1900. (Reprinted 1990.)
  3. Hall HJ. OT: A new profession. Concord, MA: Rumford Press, 1923:48.
  4. Edgerton WM. Activities in occupational therapy. In: Willard HS, Spackman CS. Principles of Occupational Therapy. Philadelphia: Lippincott, 1954:54.
  5. Shannon PE. Project to identify the philosophy of occupational therapy. (Report to the Representative Assembly.) Rockville, MD: American Occupational Therapy Association, 1983.
  6. Nelson DL. Occupation: form and performance. Am J Occup Ther 1988;42:633–641.
  7. Nelson DL. Occupational form, occupational performance, and therapeutic occupation. In: Royeen CB. The Practice of the Future: Putting Occupational Back into Therapy, Part 2. Bethesda, MD: American Occupational Therapy Association, 1994.
  8. Breines EB. Occupational Therapy Activities from Clay to Computers: Theory and Practice. Philadelphia: FA Davis, 1995.
  9. Breines EB. Understanding "occupation" as the founders did. Br J Occup Ther 1995;58(11):458–460.
 10. Levine RE, Brayley CR. Occupation as a therapeutic medium. In: Christiansen C, Baum

C. Occupational Therapy: Overcoming Human Performance Deficits. Thorofare, NJ: Slack Inc., 1991:591–631.
11. Christiansen C, Clark F, Kielhofner G, Rogers J. Position paper: Occupation. Am J Occup Ther 1995;49(10):1025–1018.
12. Murray JAH, Bradley H, Graigie WA, Onions CT. The Oxford English Dictionary. Oxford, England: Clarendon Press, 1933.
13. Gove PB. Webster's Third New International Dictionary of the English Language Unabridged. Springfield, MA: Merriam-Webster Inc, 1986.
14. Darnell JL, Heater SL Occupation therapist or activity therapist: which do you choose to be? Am J Occup Ther 1994;48(5):467–468.
15. West WL. A reaffirmed philosophy and practice of occupational therapy for the 1980s. American Journal of Occupational Therapy 1984;38(1):15–23. Quote from p. 22.
16. Hagedorn R. Occupational Therapy Perspectives and Processes. Edinburgh: Churchill Livingstone, 1995.
17. Mocellin G. Occupational therapy: a critical overview, part 1. Br J Occup Ther 1995; 58(12):502–506.
18. Hunter R. The American Encyclopedic Dictionary. Chicago: R.S. Peale & JA Hill, 1897.

ACTIVITY

1. Webster's New Universal Unabridged Dictionary. New York: Barnes & Noble, 1996.
2. Murray JAH, Bradley H, Craigie WA, Onions CT. The Oxford English Dictionary. Oxford, England: Clarendon Press, 1933.
3. Reed KL, Sanderson SR. Concepts of Occupational Therapy. Baltimore: Williams & Wilkins, 1980:233.
4. Morris W. American Heritage Dictionary of the English Language. Boston: Houghton Mifflin, 1985.
5. Pattison HA. [Address]. National Society for the Promotion of Occupational Therapy, Proceedings of the Third Annual Meeting. Towson, MD: The Society, 1919:55
6. Dunton WR. Prescribing Occupational Therapy. Springfield, IL: Charles C Thomas, 1928:1–2.
7. AOTA Representative Assembly. Minutes. Am J Occup Ther 1977;31:599.
8. AOTA Representative Assembly. Minutes. Am J Occup Ther 1981;35:792.
9. Evans AK. Nationally speaking: definition of occupation as the core concept of occupational therapy. Am J Occup Ther 1987;41:627.
10. Reilly M. A psychiatric occupational therapy program as a teaching model. Am J Occup Ther 1966;20(2):66.
11. Nelson DL. Children with Autism and other Pervasive Disorders of Development and Behavior: Therapy through Activities. Thorofare, NJ: Slack Inc., 1984:34.
12. Nelson DL. Occupation: form and performance. Am J Occup Ther 1988;42(10): 633–641.
13. Nelson DL. Therapeutic occupation: A definition. Am J Occup Ther 1996;50(10):778.
14. West WL. A reaffirmed philosophy and practice of occupational therapy for the 1980s. Am J Occup Ther 1984;38(1):22.
15. Christiansen C, Baum C. Person-environment occupational performance: a conceptual model for practice. In: Christiansen C, Baum C. Occupational Therapy: Enabling Function and Well-Being. Thorofare, NJ: Slack Inc., 1998:50.

16. Hagedorn R. Occupational Therapy: Perspectives and Processes. Edinburgh, Churchill Livingstone, 1995:79.
17. Foster M. Theoretical frameworks. In: Turner A, Foster M, Johnson SE. Occupational Therapy and Physical Dysfunction: Principles, Skills and Practice. 4th ed. New York: Churchill Livingstone, 1996:39.
18. Polatajko HJ. Dreams, dilemmas, and decision for occupational therapy practice in a new millennium: a Canadian perspective. Am J Occup Ther 1994;48(7): 593–594.
19. Levine RE, Brayley CR. Occupation as a therapeutic media. In: Christiansen C, Baum C: Occupational Therapy: Overcoming Human Performance Deficits. Thorofare, NJ: Slack Inc., 1991.

ACTIVITIES OF DAILY LIVING

1. Sheldon MP. A physical achievement record. J Health Phys Ed 1935;6:30–31,60.
2. Deaver GG, Brown ME. Physical Demands of Daily Life. New York: Institute for the Crippled and Disabled, 1945.
3. Frey WD. Functional assessment in the '80s: a conceptual enigma, a technical challenge. In: Halpern AS, Fuhrer MJ. Functional Assessment in Rehabilitation. Baltimore: Paul H. Brookes Publishing Co., 1984:11–43.
4. Spackman CS. Occupational therapy for patients with physical injuries. In: Willard HS, Spackman CS. Principles of Occupational Therapy. Philadelphia: Lippincott, 1947:231–233.
5. Livingston DM. Achievement recording for the cerebral palsied. Am J Occup Ther 1950;4:66–67,74.
6. Edgerton WM. Activities in occupational therapy. In: Willard HS, Spackman CS. Principles of Occupational Therapy. 2nd ed. Philadelphia: Lippincott, 1954:43–60.
7. Connell KA. An occupational therapist's approach to the vocational problems of the cerebral palsied. Am J Occup Ther 1950;4(5):214–223,238.
8. Brown ME. Daily Activity Inventory and Process Record for those with atypical movement. Am J Occup Ther 1950;4(5):195–204; 1950;4(6):261–272; 1951;5(1):23–29,38.
9. Zimmerman ME. Occupational therapy in the A.D.L. program. In: Willard HS, Spackman CS. Occupational Therapy. 3rd ed. Philadelphia: Lippincott, 1963:320–357.
10. Zimmerman ME. Activities of daily living. In: Willard HS, Spackman CS. Occupational Therapy. 4th ed. Philadelphia: Lippincott, 1971:217–256.
11. Representative Assembly. Glossary of terms used in the occupational therapy standards of practice. In: American Occupational Therapy Association: Manual on Administration. Rockville, MD: The Association, 1978:73–75.
12. Reed KL, Sanderson SR. Glossary of terms. In: Reed KL, Sanderson SR. Concepts of Occupational Therapy. Baltimore: Williams & Wilkins, 1980:233–249.
13. Pedretti LW. Treatment methods for physical dysfunction: Activities of daily living. In: Pedretti LW. Occupational Therapy: Practice Skills for Physical Dysfunction. St. Louis: Mosby, 1981:109–162.
14. Trombly CA. Activities or daily living. In: Trombly CA. Occupational Therapy for Physical Dysfunction. 2nd ed. Baltimore: Williams & Wilkins, 1983:458–479.
15. Trombly CA. Occupational Therapy for Physical Dysfunction. 4th ed. Baltimore: Williams & Wilkins, 1995.
16. Foti A, Pedretti LW. Activities of daily living. In: Pedretti LW. Occupational Therapy: Practice Skills for Physical Dysfunction, 4th ed. St. Louis: Mosby, 1996:463–506.

17. Christiansen C. Understanding occupation: definitions and concepts. In: Christiansen C, Baum C. Occupational Therapy: Enabling Function and Well-Being. Thorofare, NJ: Slack Inc., 1998:3–25.
18. Lawton MP. The functional assessment of elderly people. J Am Geriatr Soc 1971;19(6):465–481.
19. Cammack S, Eisenberg MG. Key Words in Physical Rehabilitation: A Guide to Contemporary Usage. San Diego: Springer Publishing Co., 1995.
20. Vreede CF. The need for a better definition of ADL. Int J Rehab Research 1988; 11(1):29–35.

INTEREST

1. Webster's New Universal Unabridged Dictionary. New York: Barnes & Noble, 1996.
2. Dunton WR. Prescribing Occupational Therapy. Springfield, IL: Charles C Thomas, 1928:6.
3. Matsasuya JS. The Interest Check List. Am J Occup Ther 1969;12(4):323–328.
4. Hinsie LE, Campbell RJ. Psychiatric Dictionary. 3rd ed. New York: Oxford University Press, 1960:400.
5. James W. Reasoning. In: James W. The Principles of Psychology. v. 2. New York: Dover Press, 1950:344. (Original article appeared in J Speculative Phil 1978;7:236.)
6. James W. Attention. In: James W. The Principles of Psychology. v. 1. New York: Dover press, 1950:402.
7. Dewey J. School and the life of the child. In: Dewey J. School and Society. Chicago: University of Chicago Press, 1990. (Original publication 1900, revised 1915.)
8. Allport GW. Personality and Social Encounter. Boston: Beacon Press, 1960.
9. Roe A, Seligman M. The Origin of Interests. Washington, D.C.: American Personnel and Guidance Association, 1964.
10. Murphy G. [no chapter cited]. In: Hahn ME, MacLean MS. Counseling Psychology. New York: McGraw-Hill, 1955.
11. White RW. Motivation reconsidered: The concept of competence. Psychol Rev 1959; 66:297–333.
12. Kielhofner G. A Model of Human Occupation: Theory and Application. Baltimore: Williams & Wilkins, 1995:47–48.

LEISURE

1. Webster's New Universal Unabridged Dictionary. New York: Barnes & Noble, 1996.
2. Hall HJ. OT: A New Profession. Concord, MA: Rumford Press, 1923:2.
3. American Occupational Therapy Association. Uniform Terminology System for Reporting Occupational Therapy Services. Rockville, MD: Author.
4. American Occupational Therapy Association. Uniform Terminology for Occupational Therapy. 2nd edition. Am J Occup Ther 1989;43:808–815.
5. American Occupational Therapy Association. Uniform Terminology for Occupational Therapy. 3rd Edition. Am J Occup Ther 1994;48:1047–1054.
6. Mosey AC. Psychosocial Components of Occupational Therapy. New York: Raven Press, 1986:85.
7. Davidson HS. Performance and the social environment. In: Christiansen C, Baum C. Occupational Therapy: Overcoming Human Performance Deficits. Thorofare, NJ: Slack, Inc.:162–163.

8. Primeau LA. Work and leisure: Transcending the dichotomy. Am J Occup Ther 1996; 50(7):569–577.
9. Csikszentmihalyi M. Beyond Boredom and Anxiety. San Francisco: Jossey-Bass, 1975.
10. Csikszentmihalyi M, Le Fevre J. Optimal experience in work and leisure. J Person Soc Psych 1989;56:815–822.

PLAY

1. Webster's New Universal Unabridged Dictionary. New York: Barnes & Noble, 1996.
2. Meyer A. Theory of occupation therapy. Arch Occup Ther 1922;1(1):1–10.
3. Slagle EC. Training aides for mental patients. Arch Occup Ther 1922;1(1): 11–17.
4. Brush F. Recreational therapy for heart disease. Arch Occup Ther 1922;1(1):25–32.
5. Hall HJ. Work and plan. In: Hall HJ. OT: A New Profession. Concord: Rumford Press, 1923:30–35.
6. Wade BD. Occupational therapy for patients with mental disease. In: Willard HS, Spackman CS. Principles of Occupational Therapy. Philadelphia: Lippincott, 1947: 87–88.
7. Davis JE. Recreational Therapy. In: Dunton WR, Licht S. Occupational Therapy: Principles and Practice. Springfield, IL: Charles C Thomas, 1950:320–231.
8. Driver M. Occupational therapy in pediatrics. In: Dunton WR, Licht S. Occupational Therapy: Principles and Practice. Springfield, IL: Charles C Thomas, 1954:198.
9. Alessandrini NA. Play—a child's world. Am J Occup Ther 1949;3(1):9.
10. Reilly M. A psychiatric occupational therapy program as a teaching model. Am J Occup Ther 1966;20(2):64.
11. Reilly M. The educational process. Am J Occup Ther 1969;23(4):302.
12. Reilly M. An explanation of play. In: Reilly M. Play as Exploratory Learning. Beverly Hills: Sage Publications, 1974:146–148
13 Shannon RD. The work-play model: a basis for occupational therapy programming in psychiatry. Am J Occup Ther 1970;24:215.
14. Florey L. An approach to play and play development. Am J Occup Ther 1971;26 (6):275–280.
15. Takata N. The play milieu—a preliminary appraisal. Am J Occup Ther 1971; 25(6):281–284.
16. Bundy A. Play theory and sensory integration. In: Fisher AG, Murray EA, Bundy AC. Sensory Integration: Theory and Practice. Philadelphia: FA Davis, 1991:48–68.
17. Takata N. Play as prescription. In: Reilly M. Play as Exploratory Learning. Beverly Hills: Sage Publication, 1974:209–246.
18. Knox SH. A play scale. In: Reilly M. Play as Exploratory Learning. Beverly Hills: Sage Publication, 1974:247–266.
19. Hurff J. Play skills inventory. In: Reilly M. Play as Exploratory Learning. Beverly Hills: Sage Publication, 1974:267–283.
20. Shannon PD. Occupational choice: decision-making play. In: Reilly M. Play as Exploratory Learning. Beverly Hills: Sage Publication, 1974:285–314.
21. Bundy AC. Play and playfulness: what to look for. In: Parham LD, Fazio LS. Play in Occupational Therapy for Children. St Louis: Mosby, 1997:52–66.

WORK

1. Webster's New Universal Unabridged Dictionary. New York: Barnes & Noble, 1996.

2. McKeever G. The Role of Work for Occupational Therapy in Mental Health. [Unpublished master's thesis] Houston: Texas Woman's University, 1997.
3. Hall HJ, Buck MMC. The Work of Our Hands. New York: Moffat, Yard & Co., 1915:viii.
4. Bowers PE. Work in the treatment of insane criminals. Modern Hosp 1917;8:406–408.
5. Hall HJ. The systematic use of work as a remedy in neurasthenia and allied conditions. Boston Med Surg J 1905;CLII (2):29–32.
6. Faulkes WF. The curative workshop from the viewpoint of industrial accident compensation. Occup Ther Rehabil 6(4):253–264.
7. Barton GE. Inoculation of the bacillus of work. Modern Hosp 1917;8:399–403.
8. Kidner TB. The hospital pre-industrial shop. State Hosp Q 1924/25;10:447–453.
9. Dunton WR. The principles of occupational therapy. Pub Health Nurse 1918; 10:316–321.
10. Hall HJ. Work-cure. J Am Med Assoc 1910;LIV(1): 12–14.
11. Barton GE. Teaching the Sick. Philadelphia: Saunders, 1919.
12. Brown PK. The potteries of Arequipa Sanatorium. Modern Hosp 1917;8:394–396.
13. Thomson EE. Occupation and its relation to mental hygiene. Modern Hosp 1917;8:397–398.
14. Johnson SC. Occupational therapy in New York City institutions. Modern Hosp 1917;8:414–416.
15. Evans EV. The organization of a curative workshop. Occup Ther Rehabil 1929; 8(1):49–62.
16. American Occupational Therapy Association. Principles of Occupational Therapy (Bulletin No. 4). New York: The Association, 1923.

THE ENVIRONMENT

1. Webster's New Universal Unabridged Dictionary. New York: Barnes & Noble, 1996.
2. Earle P. Historical and descriptive account of the Bloomingdale Asylum for the insane. Am J Insanity 1845;2:1–13.
3. Allison HE. The moral and industrial management of the insane. Alienist and Neurologist 1886;7:286–297.
4. Hall HJ. Neurasthenia. A study of etiology. Treatment by occupation. Boston Med Surg J 1905;CLIII(2):47–49.
5. Dunning H. Environmental occupational therapy. Am J Occup Ther 1972;26(6): 292–298.
6. Kannegieter RB. Environmental interactions in psychiatric occupational therapy-some inferences. Am J Occup Ther 1980;34(11):715–720.
7. Moos RH. Evaluating Treatment Environments. New York: John Wiley, 1974.
8. Pishkin V, Mackenthum DH, Stump BE. Experimental attitudes affecting behavioral changes in neuropsychiatric patients. Am J Occup Ther 1961;15(2):57–60,81.
9. Moos RH, Houts PS. Differential effects of the social atmosphere of psychiatric wards. Human Relations 1970;23:47–69.
10. Barris R. Environmental interactions: an extension of the model of occupation. Am J Occup Ther 1982;36(10):637–644.
11. Llorens LA. Changing balance: environment and individual. Am J Occup Ther 1984;38(1):29–34.

12. DiJoseph LM. Independence through activity: mind, body, and environment interaction in therapy. Am J Occup Ther 1982;36(11):740–744.

13. Dunn W, Brown C, McGuigan A. The ecology of human performance: a framework for considering the effect of context. Am J Occup Ther 1994;48:595–607.

14. Letts L, Law M, Rigby P, et al. Person-environment assessment in occupational therapy. Am J Occup Ther 1994;48(7):608–618.

15. Christiansen C, Baum C. Person-environment occupational performance: a conceptual model for practice. In: Christiansen C, Baum C. Occupational Therapy: Enabling Function and Well-Being. Thorofare, NJ: Slack Inc., 1990:47–70.

16. Parent LH. Effects of a low-stimulus environment on behavior. Am J Occup Ther 1978;32(1):19–25.

17. Kielhofner G, Burke JP. A model of human occupation, part 1. Conceptual framework and content. Am J Occup Ther 1980;34(9):572–581.

18. Reed KL, Sanderson SR. Towards a theory of occupational therapy. In: Reed KL, Sanderson SR. Concepts of Occupational Therapy. Baltimore: Williams & Wilkins, 1980:225–231.

19. Spencer JC. Environmental assessment strategies. Topics in Geriatric Rehabil 1987;3(1):35–41.

20. Davidson H. Assessing environmental factors. In: Christiansen C, Baum C. Occupational Therapy: Overcoming Human Performance Deficits. Thorofare NJ, Slack Inc., 1991:427–452.

The Consumer
Domain Base

CHAPTER 11

Disability

Over the years the definition of disability has been focused on the individual. *Webster's New Universal Unabridged Dictionary* defines disability as the following:

1. Lack of adequate power, strength, or physical or mental ability; incapacity.
2. A physical or mental handicap, esp. one that prevents a person from living a full, normal life or from holding a gainful job.
3. Anything that disables or puts one at a disadvantage.
4. The state or condition of being disabled.
5. Legal incapacity; legal disqualification. (1)

The International Classification of Impairments, Disabilities, and Handicaps (ICIDH) also has focused on the individual as the source of the disability (2). As Table 11.1 illustrates, the definitions of disability describe what the person cannot do. The phrases used are "lack of ability to perform an activity," "reduction of a person's activity," and "inability to engage in any substantial gainful activity." Such definitions are based on the belief that it is the person who cannot do or perform. Consideration for environmental obstacles such as architectural barriers or social stigma is not acknowledged. This social attitude seems to be based on the "able-bodied sailor" concept. If a person is "able-bodied," he or she can work and do other things. If a person is not "able-bodied," he or she cannot perform.

In contrast, the definition by Hulst describes disability as the "disadvantage or restriction in the organization of society, which prevent[s] an individual . . . from fully participating" (3). Finkelstein takes a similar position by stating that disability is a "disadvantage or restriction of activity *caused by a social organization* which takes no or little account of the people who have physical impairments" (italics added) (4). Because the social organization does not consider or pay attention to the needs of people with physical impairments, these people are excluded from the "mainstream of social activities." In other words, the environment, especially the social environment, is largely responsibility for disability. Disability, therefore, occurs because people in society do not acknowledge or take the time necessary to reduce the barriers to full participation by all citizens. Instead, citizenship is reserved as a privilege for those without disability. Individuals must overcome their disability if they are be considered real citizens. Those who view the source of dis-

Table 11.1.   Definitions of Disability

- A disability is any restriction or lack (resulting from an impairment) of ability to perform an activity in the manner or within the range considered normal for a human being. (ICIDH, WHO, 1980)
- Any temporary or long-term reduction of a person's activity as a result of an acute or chronic condition. (ICIDH, 1987)
- The inability to engage in any substantial gainful activity by reason of a medically determinable physical or mental impairments which can be expected to result in death or has lasted or can be expected to last for a continuous period of not less than 12 months. (ICIDH, 1989)
- The inability or limitation in performing social roles and activities such as in relation to work, to family, or to independent living. There are two dimensions of organismic performance (physical and emotional) and two dimensions of disability (work and independent living). (Nagi S. An epidemiology of disability among adults in the USA. MMFQ/Health and Society 1996:439–467)
- Disability is the disadvantage or restriction in the organization of society, which prevents an individual with a functional limitation or impairment from fully participating. (Hulst R. Vox Nostra. Magazine of Disabled People International 4. December, 1992)
- Disadvantage or restriction of activity caused by a social organization which takes no or little account of people who have physical impairments and thus excludes them from the mainstream of social activities. (Finklestein V. Planning services together with disabled people. World Health Statistics Quarterly 42:177–179, 1989)
- Disability manifests itself as a degree of modification, in excess or default of the ability to accomplish a physical or mental activity, as a result of a deficiency or deficience. There is, therefore, a need to classify abilities and define a severity scale. (Bergeron H, Michel G St, Cloutier R. Proposed Nomenclature of Abilities Working Document, Societe Canadienne de la CIDIH, Comite Quebecois sur la CIDIH, October, 1990)
- Inability or limitation in performing tasks, activities, and roles to levels expected with physical and social contexts. (American Society of Hand Therapists. Clinical Assessment Recommendations. 1992)

From: Brandsma JW, Lakerveld-Heyl K, Van Ravensberg CD, Heerkens YF. Reflection on the definition of impairment and disability as defined by the World Health Organization. Disability and Rehabilitation 1995;17(3/4):119–127.

ability to be certain social organizations strongly protest the view that those with disability are the problem or the source of the problem.

To summarize, there has been a social stigma attached to people with physical, cognitive, and mental impairments. Therefore, the two different types of definitions of disability are differentiated by where they attribute the stigma or problem: to the individual or to physical and social environments. The result is similar; people with disabilities are frequently denied the opportunity to perform and participate fully in occupational and social roles.

BRIEF HISTORY OF DISABILITY

The stigma associated with disability has been a part of the social history of western culture and civilization. In the 18th century, disability was explained in terms of religion or the supernatural. Either the disability occurred because of sin in the family or it was a curse or spell by some demonic spirit. For relief, one petitioned God to forgive the sin or petitioned the demons to lift the curse or undo the spell. Medical care or rehabilitation were not even considered.

In the 19th century, disability was defined legally. Persons with some disabilities such as blindness were legally entitled to educational programs and employment. Persons with other disabilities such as mental retardation or mental illness were to be sent to institutions for custodial care because these people lacked the moral values necessary to participate in society. Mentally ill persons were also exempted from crimes they committed because they were "morally insane." Some progress was made through scientific fields such as medicine to begin diagnosing disease and disability. The results have been called the "medicalization of disability." For relief, the disabled person or his or her family petitions the physician to change the diagnosis. For example, if a person who was diagnosed as mentally retarded is rediagnosed as mentally competent (normal), the stigma of mental retardation may be lifted.

In the 20th century, the three professions of religion, law, and medicine began to join forces to define disability. Using such themes as "the ravages of war" and "social good" as justifications, several entitlement programs were enacted that defined who is disabled (legal), who will diagnose disability (medicine), and who will provide comfort (religion). The concept of rehabilitation began with the Soldiers and Sailors Rehabilitation Act (PL 65–178), which was passed in 1918 to provide rehabilitation to service men injured during the war (5). In 1920, civilians were provided with similar entitlements through the passage of the Industrial (Vocational) Rehabilitation Act (PL 66–236) although the actual services provided by the states varied. Insurance of service personnel was first passed in 1914 (PL 65–90, War Risk Insurance). Civilians had to wait until the Social Security Act was passed in 1933 for Social Security Insurance (SSI) as part of the Social Security Act (PL 74–271) and for the Social Security Amendments that created medicare and medicaid in 1965 (PL 89–97).

People with disabilities started to demand their right to relief of their conditions in the 1960s. Many social movements concerning person with disabilities were started. Names such as the disability movement, the disability rights movement, or the disability equality movement began to appear in the popular press and finally in the scientific literature. One outcome of the disability movement was the first Independent Living Center established in 1972 in Berkeley, California.

In the 1970s, several important laws were passed. The Rehabilitation Act of 1973 Amendments (PL 93–112) contained Section 504, which legislated that persons with disabilities had equal civil rights in any building or institution built with federal money. In 1975 the Education for all Handicapped Act was passed (PL 94–142). It stated that all children, regardless of disability, were entitled to a free and appropriate education in the public schools. The act is now called the Individuals With Disabilities Education Act (IDEA) to comply with the changing concepts about terminology. The term "handicap" has been relegated to the sports of golf and horse racing. In 1978 the Comprehensive Services and Developmental Disabilities Amendments (PL 95–602) were passed to provide better services to persons with mental retardation and multiple disorders starting at birth if the condition was identified at birth.

Finally, in 1990 the Americans With Disabilities Act (ADA) passed as Public Law 101–336. This act is designed to protect the civil rights of all persons with disabilities in the work place and public areas including stores and sports arenas. Separate acts for housing and transportation had been published earlier. A summary of the significant dates appears in Table 11.2.

MODELS OF SERVICE DELIVERY TO PERSONS WITH DISABILITY

The two models in Table 11.3 illustrate the differences in how people with disabilities should be viewed in delivery of service. In the traditional rehabilitation paradigm, the person with a disability is a patient or client with impairments, lack of work skills, functional limitation, lack of motivation and cooperation, and maladjustment. The role of the professional is to diagnosis, prescribe, manage, and control such persons. The solution is the intervention by rehabilitation professionals who can provide evaluation and training. Desired outcomes include maximum performance of activities of daily living, gainful employment, improved motivation, and completion of treatment. In contrast, the independent living paradigm describes the person with a disability as a consumer of services. The services should not make the person dependent on others, but rather should provide adequate social support and should address architectural and economic barriers. The role of the professional should be that of peer, consultant, helper, advocate, mentor, and role model. The solution is peer counseling, advocacy, and self-help. Desired outcomes are self-direction, living arrangements in the least restrictive environment possible, and social and economic productivity.

THE PROCESS OF DISABILITY

Disability, unlike acute illness, does not happen all of a sudden. The process leading to disability has four or five stages. This disability process or disablement process has been studied for more than 20 years. Figure 11.1 is a summary of the concepts used in the models to illustrate comparisons and contrasts. Nagi was the first to provide a model of the disability process as shown in Figure 11.2 (6). He suggested four stages in the disability process: active pathology, impairment, func-

Table 11.2. Short History of the Disability Movement

18th century	Disability was understood in religious and supernatural terms. For relief, one petitions God to forgive the sin, lift the curse, or undo the spell.
19th century	Disability was admitted to the category of "disabled" by early legal authorities who decided whom would have the entitlements. For relief, one petitions the courts concerning presence or absence of moral values.
19th century	Medicine through "science" began to diagnose and pronounce on disease and disability. Called the "medicalization of disability." For relief, one petitions physicians to change the diagnosis.
20th century	In this country, the three professions (religion, law, and medicine) joined forces using "rages of war" and "social good" as justifications to pass a number of "entitlement" laws for defining who is disabled (legal), who will diagnose disability (medicine), and who will provide comfort (religion). Insurance groups (governmental and private) decided who would be paid.
1916	War Risk Insurance Act passed.
1918	Soldiers and Sailors Rehabiltation Act passed.
1920	Civilian Industrial Rehabilitation Act passed. (First of the Vocational Rehabilitation Acts.)
1933	Social Security Act passed.
1960s	People with disabilities started to demand relief of their conditions as a right and initiated the social movement of persons with disabilities called variously, disability movement, disability rights movement, or disability equality movement.
1972	The first Independent Living Center was established in Berkeley, California.
1973	Rehabilitation Act of 1973 Amendments. Contained Section 504. Public Law 93–112.
1975	Education for All Handicapped. Public Law 94–142. Now Individuals with Disabilities Education Act.
1978	Comprehensive Services and Developmental Disabilities Amendments. Public Law 95–602.
1990	Americans With Disabilities Act (ADA) passed. Public Law 101–336. 42 U.S. C. Sec. 12101.

Table 11.3. Comparison of the Tradition Rehabilitation Model and Independent Living Model

ITEM	TRADITIONAL REHABILITATION MODEL	INDEPENDENT LIVING MODEL
Role of person with disability	Patient/client	Consumer
Role of service provider	Professional Prescriber and manager of treatment Controller of access to service Diagnostician	Peer Consultant and role provider model Helper and advocate Mentor
Definition of problem	Physical or mental impairment Lack of vocational skills Functional limitations Lack of motivation and cooperation Psychological maladjustment	Dependence on professionals, relatives, etc. Inadequate support services Architectural barriers Economic barriers
Locus of problem	In the individual with a disability	In the environment In the medical model In the rehabilitation process and the narrow "professional" attitudes they can promote
Solution to problem	Intervention by rehabilitation professional Evaluation and training Home and job site modification	Peer counseling Advocacy Self-help Consumer control Removal of community barriers and disincentives
Source of control	Professional	Consumer
Desired outcomes	Maximum activities of daily living (ADL) Gainful employment Improved motivation and psychological adjustment Completed treatment	Self-direction Least restrictive environment Productive (social and economic)

Adapted from: Schlaff C. From dependency to self-advocacy: redefining disability. Am J Occup Ther 1993;47(10):944.

Nagi

ACTIVE PATHOLOGY	IMPAIRMENT	FUNCTIONAL LIMITATION	DISABILITY	

Wood (ICIDH)

PATHOLOGY "DISEASE"	IMPAIRMENT	DISABILITY	HANDICAP	

NCMRR

PATHO- PHYSIOLOGY	IMPAIRMENT	FUNCTIONAL LIMITATION	DISABILITY	SOCIETAL LIMITATION

Institute of Medicine (Tarlov)

PATHOLOGY	IMPAIRMENT	FUNCTIONAL LIMITATION	DISABILITY	

Jette

PATHOLOGY	IMPAIRMENT	FUNCTIONAL (IN)CAPACITY	SOCIAL/ROLE (DIS)ABILITY	

Figure 11.1. Comparison of disablement concepts.

ACTIVE PATHOLOGY (interruption or interference with normal processes and efforts of the organism to regain normal state)	➡	IMPAIRMENT (anatomical physiological, mental, or emotional abnormalities or loss)	➡	FUNCTIONAL LIMITATION (limitation in performance at the level of the whole organism or person)	➡	DISABILITY (limitation in performance of socially defined roles and tasks within a socio-cultural and physical environment)

Figure 11.2. Model of disability process.

tional limitation, and disability. Active pathology involves the interruption or interference with normal processes and efforts by the organism to regain a normal state. Infection and injury are examples of such interruption or interference. Active pathology may lead to impairment. Impairment is an anatomical, physiological, mental, or emotional abnormality or loss. Fracture, atrophy, dementia, and loss of affect are examples. Impairment may lead to functional limitation. Functional limitation is a limitation in performance at the level of the whole organism or person. Loss of mobility, loss of strength, loss of memory, and "flat" or unemotional affect may result. Disability is a limitation in performance of socially defined roles and tasks within a sociocultural and physical environment. Loss of mobility

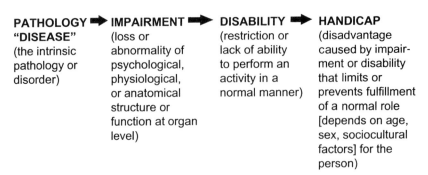

PATHOLOGY ➡ IMPAIRMENT ➡ DISABILITY ➡ HANDICAP
"DISEASE" (loss or (restriction or (disadvantage
(the intrinsic abnormality of lack of ability caused by impair-
pathology or psychological, to perform an ment or disability
disorder) physiological, activity in a that limits or
or anatomical normal manner) prevents fulfillment
structure or of a normal role
function at organ [depends on age,
level) sex, sociocultural
factors] for the
person)

Figure 11.3. Classification of disabilities. (From: World Health Organization. International Classification of Impairment, Disabilities, and Handicaps. Geneva: WHO, 1980.)

could mean the roofer could not climb a ladder to get to the roof. Loss of strength could mean the person who moves furniture no longer has the necessary strength to do so. Loss of memory could mean the person is unable to go to the grocery store without getting lost. Loss of emotion could mean that the person does not enjoy socializing with friends anymore. In 1980 the ICIDH, a part of the International Classification of Diseases (ICD), adopted a model similar to Nagi's, which is shown in Figure 11.3 and was proposed by Wood (2). The definitions remain similar in scope, but the term "disability" was substituted for "functional limitation" and the term "handicap" was substituted for "disability." The ICIDH model has been widely circulated and therefore is widely known.

For approximately 10 years, the ICIDH model remained unchallenged. Then two models were published almost concurrently. The National Center for Medical Rehabilitation and Research (NCMRR) changed the structure of the model by creating five stages instead of four as shown in Figure 11.4 (7). The first three are defined similarly to Nagi's model. The term "pathophysiology" is substituted for "active pathology." The difference is in the definitions of "disability" and "societal limitation." Disability in the NCMRR model is defined as a limitation or inability in performing tasks, activities, and roles to levels expected within physical and social contexts, and societal limitation is a restriction attributable to social policy or barriers that limit fulfillment of roles. Societal limitation is designed to identify those restrictions that are the direct or indirect result of social policy. An example is regulations that terminate health insurance covered by medicaid if a person with a disability makes more than a certain amount in wages. At first glance, there might not seem to be a problem because the person is earning money. However, the person with a disability may not be able to afford the larger-than-average premium that the insurance company may demand because the chronic disability is known to require ongoing medical management. As a result, the person with a disability is discouraged from working too much so as to avoid losing health insurance.

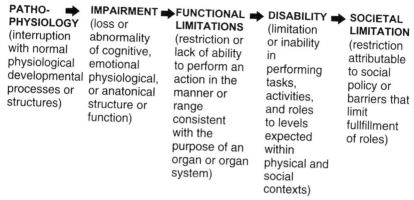

PATHO- ➡ PHYSIOLOGY (interruption with normal physiological developmental processes or structures)	IMPAIRMENT ➡ (loss or abnormality of cognitive, emotional physiological, or anatonical structure or function)	FUNCTIONAL ➡ LIMITATIONS (restriction or lack of ability to perform an action in the manner or range consistent with the purpose of an organ or organ system)	DISABILITY ➡ (limitation or inability in performing tasks, activities, and roles to levels expected within physical and social contexts)	SOCIETAL LIMITATION (restriction attributable to social policy or barriers that limit fullfillment of roles)

Figure 11.4. Revised classification. (From: National Advisory Board on Medical Rehabilitation Research. National Center Medical Rehabilitation Research. Bethesda, MD: National Institutes of Health, 1992.)

The second revised model shown in Figure 11.5 was proposed by the Institute of Medicine (8). This model did little to change the basic ideas proposed by Nagi. The major change is some clarification of the definition of "functional limitation" to explain that the criterion for performance of the action or activity is the manner it is done or within which range is considered normal. Nagi did not specify a criterion.

The fifth model shown in Figure 11.6, called the disablement model, was published by Jette, a physical therapist (9). He suggested the third and fourth categories should be called "functional (in)capacity" and "social/role (dis)ability." Functional incapacity is defined as restriction in basic physical and mental actions, such as ambulation, reaching, stooping, climbing stairs, producing intelligible speech, seeing standard print, etc. Social/role disability is defined a difficulty doing activities of daily living: working, managing one's household, doing personal care, engaging in hobbies, participating in leisure activities, socializing with friends and relatives, providing child care, running errands, sleeping, going on trips, etc.

HOW THE MODELS WORK

All five models are explained in similar terms. Figure 11.7 shows the process outlined by Nagi as diagrammed by Melvin (10). During the pathology stage, a medical diagnosis is made. Impairments identified during this stage such as signs, symptoms, and laboratory abnormalities are treated. Treatment is provided through medical care and/or rehabilitation. The response to treatment may be a cure, but residual impairment such as weakness, restricted joint motion, or pain may remain. Residual impairment is also treated through medical care and/or rehabilitation. If such treatment is successful, the person is cured. If treatment is not

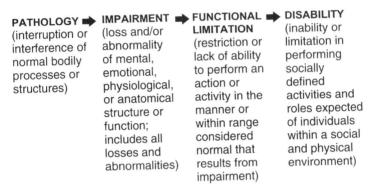

Figure 11.5. Second revised model of disability process. (From: Pope AM, Tarlov AR, eds. Disability in America: Toward a National Agenda for Prevention. Washington, DC: National Academy Press, 1991.)

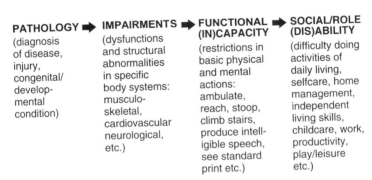

Figure 11.6. Disablement model. (Adapted from: Jette AM. Disablement outcomes in geriatric rehabilitation. Med Care 35(6 Suppl.):JS35.)

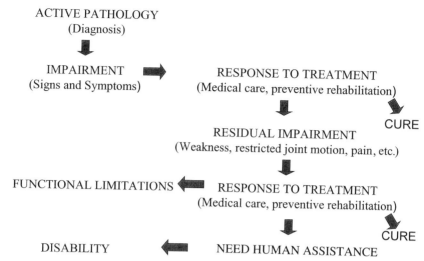

Figure 11.7. Pathway to disability. (Adapted from: Koshel JJ, Granger CB. Rehabilitation terminology: who is severely disabled? Rehabil Lit 1978;39(4):103.)

successful, then functional limitations may remain. The functional limitations may require human assistance and may, in turn, lead to the disability stage.

In Figure 11.8 the factors that influence the progression of the stages are identified. Three types of factors are discussed: risk factors, extraindividual factors, and intraindividual factors. *Risk factors* are see as having the most influence on the state of impairments. Risk factors, or predisposing factors, include demographics; lifestyle; and social, behavioral, psychological, environmental, and biological characteristics. *Extraindividual factors*, or those factors outside the individual, include medical care and rehabilitation; medications and other therapeutic regimens; external support available; and the built, physical, and social environments. *Intraindividual factors* include lifestyle and behavioral changes, psychosocial attributes and coping, and activity accommodations. Although occupational therapy is not specifically mentioned, occupational therapists can participate in each of the subcategories in dealing with extraindividual and intraindividual factors.

In Figure 11.9 Verbrugge and Jette suggest that disability is the result of a gap between capability and demand (11). In other words, the person does not have, for whatever reason, the capability to meet the demand imposed by the task environment. To decrease the gap, either the capability of the person must increase or the demand of the environment must decrease. In most cases, some of each probably occurs; that is, through intervention with the individual, the person's capability is improved. At the same time, intervention in the environment may reduce demands. For example, factors that might increase the capability of the individual

EXTRAINDIVIDUAL FACTORS: Medical care and rehabilitation; medications and other therapeutic regimens; external supports; and the built, physical, and social environment

THE MAIN PATHWAY

PATHOLOGY➡ IMPAIRMENTS ➡ FUNCTIONAL ➡ DISABILITY
                                                   LIMITATIONS

RISK FACTORS:
Predisposing characteristics, demographic, social, lifestyle, behavioral, psychological, environmental, and biological

INTRAINDIVIDUAL FACTORS:
Lifestyle and behavior changes, psychosocial attributes and coping, and activity accommodations

Figure 11.8. A model of the disablement process. (Adapted from: Verbrungge LM, Jette AM. The disablement process. Soc Sci Med 1994;38(1):1–14.)

INTRAINDIVIDUAL AND EXTRAINDIVIDUAL FACTORS AFFECTING *DEMAND*: Modifications of the built, physical, and social environment; activity accommodations; external supports; psychosocial attributes and coping

TASK ENVIRONMENT: DEMAND

PATHOLOGY➡ IMPAIRMENTS ➡ FUNCTIONAL ➡ DISABILITY
                                                  LIMITATIONS

PERSON: CAPABILITY

INTRAINDIVIDUAL AND EXTRAINDIVIDUAL FACTORS AFFECTING *CAPABILITY*: Medial care and rehabilitation, medications and other therapeutic regimens, lifestyle and behavior changes

Figure 11.9. Disability as a gap between capability and demand. (Adapted from: Verbrugge LM, Jette AM. The disablement process. Soc Sci Med 1994;38(1):1–14.)

are surgery, medications, rehabilitation services, and changes in lifestyle and behavior such as decreasing high-risk activities and ceasing smoking. Changes in the environment might include modification of the built or physical environment to reduce architectural and terrain barriers; activity accommodation through work simplification and energy conservation; development of external supports such as personal assistance and special equipment; and improvement of psychosocial skills such as increased self-esteem, competence, and coping.

Figure 11.10 illustrates how the process of intervention relates to the process of disability. Identification of pathology is the domain of the physician and laboratory personnel. Pathology is based on evaluating the signs, symptoms, and laboratory results against known diseases, disorders, or other conditions. Occupational therapy practitioners can contribute to the pathology stage especially if a team approach is used to evaluate the patients or clients. If the occupational therapy practitioner is working without a medical referral, it would be essential for the practitioner to determine if active pathology is present either by asking the person being evaluated or by direct assessment of the person. Impairments are usually identified by practitioners using clinical evaluation procedures. Examples include testing range of motion and flexibility, muscle strength, alertness, visual tracking, mood, and affect. The purpose is to determine how well the body systems are working. Such tests do not, however, indicate how well the systems function in the performance of tasks and activities.

Functional limitation is evaluated by using assessment instruments that measure the performance of basic activities of daily living (BADLs), instrumental activities of daily living (IADLs), and functional capacity evaluation (FCE) for job performance. The assessments may include those done by the occupational therapy practitioner and those completed by the patient or client—called self-reports. Self-reports should always be double-checked by the practitioner to ensure the accuracy of information. Functional limitations often correlate with impairments because difficulties with body system functions interferes with functional use. However, sometimes the functional limitations may continue after the body system regains capacity. The person may not realize that function is possible, or he or she may be afraid to try. Also, functional performance can be a "treatment" for impairment. In the process of doing or trying to do a functional activity, the person may improve the performance of the body system.

Disability can be evaluated by exploring the productivity responsibilities and social roles the person occupies. Assessment instruments for productivity and social roles must be selected based on the practitioner's knowledge of what the person's roles are. Standard protocols do not apply to evaluating the disability stage. Roles and the potential disabilities vary too much. The assessment must be developed from the roles and responsibilities the person actually performs.

SERVICE DOMAINS

Figure 11.11 shows the domain of rehabilitation in the disability models. The existence of pathology is not in itself an indicator of the need for rehabilitation services. Sickness also is not necessarily an indicator nor are most illnesses. For many pathologies, sicknesses, and illnesses, rehabilitation is not indicated or necessary. Even when the pathology is known to frequently cause impairment, the process toward disability may not always occur. However, when impairment does occur, a large percentage of cases are likely to need or benefit from rehabilitation services.

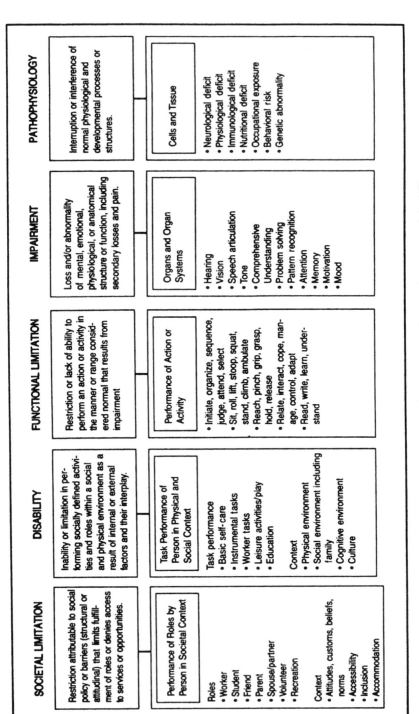

Figure 11.10. How the process of intervention relates to the process of disability.

SOCIETAL LIMITATION

Restriction attributable to social policy or barriers (structural or attitudinal) that limits fulfillment of roles or denies access to services or opportunities.

Performance of Roles by Person in Societal Context

Roles
- Worker
- Student
- Friend
- Parent
- Spouse/partner
- Volunteer
- Recreation

Context
- Attitudes, customs, beliefs, norms
- Accessibility
- Inclusion
- Accommodation

DISABILITY

Inability or limitation in performing socially defined activities and roles within a social and physical environment as a result of internal or external factors and their interplay.

Task Performance of Person in Physical and Social Context

Task performance
- Basic self-care
- Instrumental tasks
- Worker tasks
- Leisure activities/play
- Education

Context
- Physical environment
- Social environment including family
- Cognitive environment
- Culture

FUNCTIONAL LIMITATION

Restriction or lack of ability to perform an action or activity in the manner or range considered normal that results from impairment

Performance of Action or Activity

- Initiate, organize, sequence, judge, attend, select
- Sit, roll, lift, stoop, squat, stand, climb, ambulate
- Reach, pinch, grip, grasp, hold, release
- Relate, interact, cope, manage, control, adapt
- Read, write, learn, understand

IMPAIRMENT

Loss and/or abnormality of mental, emotional, physiological, or anatomical structure or function, including secondary losses and pain.

Organs and Organ Systems

- Hearing
- Vision
- Speech articulation
- Tone
- Comprehensive
- Understanding
- Problem solving
- Pattern recognition
- Attention
- Memory
- Motivation
- Mood

PATHOPHYSIOLOGY

Interruption or interference of normal physiological and developmental processes or structures.

Cells and Tissue

- Neurological deficit
- Physiological deficit
- Immunological deficit
- Nutritional deficit
- Occupational exposure
- Behavioral risk
- Genetic abnormality

Table 11.4.   Factors and Examples Related to the Disablement Process
Activity Accommodations: Changes in kinds of activities, procedures for doing them, frequency or length of time doing them. The what, how, how often, how long.
Built, Physical, and Social Environment: Structural modifications at job/home, access to buildings, and to public transportation, improvement of air quality, reduction of noise and glare, health insurance and access to medical care, laws and regulations, employment, discrimination, etc.
External Supports: Personal assistance, special equipment and devices, standby assistance/supervision, day care, respite care, Meals-on-Wheels, etc.
Lifestyle and Behavior Changes: Overt changes to alter disease activity and impact.
Medical Care and Rehabilitation: Surgery, physical and occupational therapy, speech therapy, counseling, health education, job retraining, etc.
Medications and Other Therapeutic Regimens: Drugs, recreation therapy/aquatic exercise, biofeedback/medication, rest/energy conservation, etc.
Psychosocial Attributes and Coping: Positive affect, emotional vigor, prayer, locus of control, cognitive adaptation to one's situation, confidant, peer support groups, etc.
Risk Factors: Predisposing characteristics: demographic, social, lifestyle, behavioral, psychological, environmental, biological.
Adapted from: Verbrugge LM, Jette AM: The disablement process. Soc Sci Med 1994:38(1):1–14.

When functional limitations and/or disability has occurred, all persons are candidates for rehabilitation services.

Guccione suggests that the domain of physical therapy is primarily in the areas of impairment and functional limitations (Fig. 11.11) (12). In particular, impairments in the cardiopulmonary, musculoskeletal, and neuromuscular body systems are seen as the domain of physical therapy practitioners. Functional limitations dealing with physical, psychological, and social aspects are likewise viewed as areas in which physical therapy practitioners can intervene with success. Guccione does not list anything for physical therapy in the areas of disability or handicap in social care.

Figure 11.12 is a suggested illustration of the domain of occupational therapy. Under impairment the body systems dealing with musculoskeletal, neuromuscular, cardiopulmonary, and cognitive and mental aspects are listed. Under function limitations, the components of sensorimotor, cognitive, and psychosocial aspects are listed. Under disability, the occupational areas dealing with self-maintenance, productivity, and leisure are listed. Occupational therapy practitioners are involved in social care, health care, and medical care.

Table 11.5.	Three Most Frequently Chosen Treatment Goals, at the Level of Impairments, Disabilities, or Handicaps					
Impairments		**%**	**Disabilities in**	**%**	**Handicaps in**	**%**
OT	motor impairments	48	personal care	48	mobility	26
PD	sensory impairments	15	locomotor skills	41	physical independence	24
	cognitive impairments	14	domestic skills	35	occupational role	19
OT	intrapersonal impairments	55	basic skills	72	occupational role	48
MH	cognitive impairments	34	leisure	51	social role	46
	motor impairments	6	relation	25	physical independence	19
PT	pain	66	normal tempo during work	27		
	restricted joint range of motion	46	walking	18		
	increased or decreased muscle tone	41	lifting	9		

Data from: Dekker J. Application of the ICIDH in survey research on rehabilitation; the emergence of the functional diagnosis. Disabil Rehabil 1995;17(3/4):200.

OUTCOME AS PROJECTED BY THE DISABILITY MODELS

Jette suggests that the outcome of disability models should be based on three interrelated factors: host, agent, and environment (9). Figure 11.13 shows the interaction of the three factors. Host factors are the attributes of the individual. They include preconditioning or risk factors as well as lifestyle and behavior changes, psychosocial attributes, coping skills, and accommodations made by the individual after the onset of the disability. Agent factors are the specific pathologies, diseases, or accidents that cause the disability. Environmental factors are the physical and social surroundings in which the social or role disability occurs. Rehabilitation may be included as an environmental factor that attempts to influence the outcome in a positive direction.

One outcome that has received much attention in the research literature is quality of life. Jette has suggested that quality of life for persons with disability depends on the individual's response to functional limitation and disability (13). Some factors that may influence the quality of life of a disabled person are shown in Figure 11.14. These include physical functioning, social interaction, and emotional status. Specific examples are emotional well-being, behavior competence, sleep and rest, energy and vitality, and overall life satisfaction. All of these occur at the personal and social system level rather than the body and organ system level.

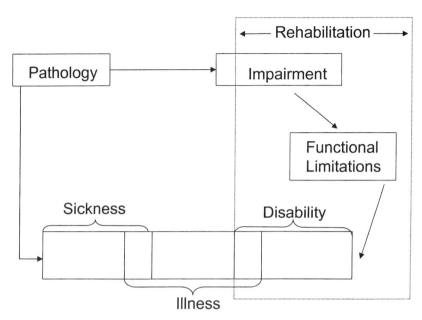

Figure 11.11. Concepts of concern to rehabilitation. (Adapted from: Granger CV, Greeshan GE. Functional Assessment in Rehabilitation Medicine. Baltimore: Williams & Wilkins, 1984:7.)

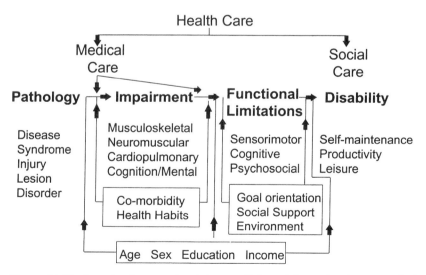

Figure 11.12. Domain of occupational therapy. (Adapted from: Guccione AA. Physical therapy diagnosis and the relationship between impairments and function. Phys Ther 1991;71(7):499–504.)

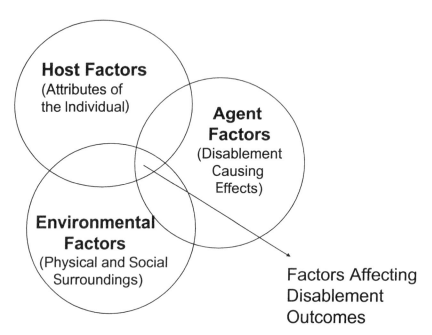

Figure 11.13. Variables affecting disablement outcome. (From: Jette AM. Disablement outcomes in geriatric rehabilitation. Med Care 1997;35(6 Suppl.):JS34.)

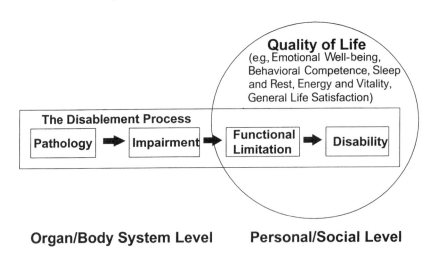

Figure 11.14. Relationship of quality of life to the disablement concepts. (Based on: Jette AM. Physical disablement concepts for physical therapy research and practice. Phys Ther 1994;74(5):384.)

OCCUPATIONAL THERAPY AND DISABILITY

Three studies have compared occupational therapy practice to other rehabilitation fields using the different models. Two used the ICIDH system. Dekker found that occupational therapists in the Netherlands practicing in both physical disabilities (PD) and mental health (MH) were able to reliability assess impairments, disabilities, and handicaps at an acceptable level or better (14). The best reliability occurred in identifying impairments (96% in PD and 93% in MH agreement), and the poorest occurred in identifying handicaps (82% in PD and 80% in MH agreement). In comparison, physical therapists in the Netherlands scored 78% agreement in assessing impairments and 88% in assessing disabilities. No figure was provided for assessing handicaps. Treatment goals of occupational therapy were highest for disabilities (56% PD, 48% MH). The remainder was approximately equally divided between impairments and handicaps. In physical therapy, slightly more than two-thirds of the goals are related to impairments, and the remaining one-third address disabilities. Thus, one difference between occupational therapy and physical therapy practice, based on the Dekker study, is the treatment focus for disabled persons. Occupational therapists focus primarily on disabilities but do address handicaps. Physical therapists focus primarily on impairments with less emphasis on disabilities.

Driessen and colleagues describe the assessment categories used in the Dekker study (15). The categories were derived from the models presented in Reed and Sanderson and the Canadian Association for Occupational Therapy (16, 17). The performance areas or components such as motor, sensory, cognitive, or spiritual, were considered impairments. The occupational areas such as self-care, leisure, and productivity were considered as disabilities. And the environmental areas were considered handicaps.

The third study explored the roles of members in rehabilitation teams in detecting certain disability (18). In the study, occupational therapists practicing in Ireland were best at detecting cognitive problems and dressing skills. Physical therapists were best at detecting balance and mobility problems. Nurses are best at detecting incontinence and pressure sores.

Cognition was measured using the Mini-Mental State Examination. No formal assessment was used in assessing dressing skills. Three levels of disability were measured for all disabilities: non, mild, and moderate/severe.

DISABILITY AND THE REAL WORLD

Occupational therapy practitioners must be aware that what appears to be disabling and what is actually disabling are not always the same thing. Furthermore, what really bothers persons with disabilities and what practitioners think bothers such persons do not always coincide.

Myers studied activities of daily living and instrumental activities of daily living in which the participants in England were ask to rank the degree of difficulty of 50 items (19). Eighty-five percent or greater of the participants reported no difficulty using the telephone, brushing their teeth or caring for dentures, preparing light meals, combing or brushing their hair, using an elevator, turning a faucet on and off, dressing or undressing, remembering to turn off appliances, or washing and drying dishes. The items with the highest mean difficulty include remembering shopping items, cleaning the bathtub, walking, vacuuming, remembering telephone numbers, getting on or off a bus or streetcar, remembering people's names, getting around outdoors in winter, cutting toenails, climbing and descending stairs, walking up and down hills, and caring for pets. Of note is the number of items related to memory and mobility. Unfortunately, the specific problems in caring for pets are not identified.

Suarez de Balcazar, Bradford, and Fawcett surveyed persons with disabilities to determine what concerned them most (20). Ranking included the percent of importance and percent of satisfaction for 18 items. The subjects were North Americans. Items ranked highest in importance were insurance for automobiles, life, and liability; utility bills; disability rights and advocacy; affordable and available health care; and social services. The lowest ranked item was affordable and available assistive devices. However, the range of the percentages was only nine points—from 80 to 89%. Items ranked highest in satisfaction were social services, health care, public access, accessibility of commercial services, and community support and responsiveness. Lowest rankings for satisfaction were utility bills; insurance for automobiles, life, and liability; availability of discounts for commercial services; and affordable, available, and accessible housing. The rankings ranged from 34 to 51%.

Occupational therapy practitioners need to be aware of what concerns the client has. A client concerned about obtaining insurance and paying utility bills may not be very concerned about accessing assistive technology even though the technology may improve functional performance.

SUMMARY

Disability is a multifaceted concept. Professionals and persons with disabilities differ on the meaning of disability and the problems associated with being disabled. The view of disability has also changed over the course of history. Especially in this century, many legislative initiatives have been passed that are related to the rehabilitation of persons with disabilities. Also, several models have been proposed to examine the process of becoming disabled and the process of rehabilitation. The World Health Organization is currently reviewing its model for disability, and substantial changes can be expected. Occupational therapy practitioners have demonstrated their ability to assess disability from various perspectives and to be able to plan intervention programs according to these differing perspectives. However, practitioners need to be aware that what is viewed by professionals as important may not be shared by the person with a disability. Serving individuals means keeping the client's view constantly in focus.

References

1. Webster's New Universal Unabridged Dictionary. New York: Barnes & Noble, 1996.
2. World Health Organization. International Classification of Impairment, Disabilities, and Handicaps. Geneva: WHO, 1980.
3. Hulst R. Vox Nostra. Magazine of Disabled People International 4. December, 1992.
4. Finklestein V. Planning services together with disabled people. World Health Statistics Quarterly 1989;42:177–179.
5. Reed KL. History of federal legislation for persons with disabilities. Am J Occup Ther 1992;6(5):397–408.
6. Nagi S. An epidemiology of disability among adults in the USA. MMFQ/Health and Society 1976;54:439–467.
7. National Advisory Board on Medical Rehabilitation Research. National Center Medical Rehabilitation Research. Bethesda, MD: National Institutes of Health, 1992.
8. Pope AM, Tarlov AR, eds. Disability in America: Toward a National Agenda for Prevention. Washington, DC: National Academy Press, 1991.
9. Jette AM. Disablement outcomes in geriatric rehabilitation. Med Care 1997;35(6 Suppl.):JS28–JS37.
10. Koshel JJ, Granger CB. Rehabilitation terminology: who is severely disabled? Rehabil Lit 1978;39(4):103.
11. Verbrungge LM, Jette AM. The disablement process. Soc Sci Med 1994;38(1):1–14.
12. Gucionne AA. Physical therapy diagnosis and the relationship between impairments and function. Phys Ther 1991;71(7):499–504.
13. Jette AM. Physical disablement concepts for physical therapy research and practice. Phys Ther 1994;74(5):380–386.
14. Dekker J. Application of the ICIDH in survey research on rehabilitation; the emergence of the functional diagnosis. Disabil Rehabil 1995;17(3/4):195–201.
15. Driessen MJ, Dekker J, Lankhorst GJ, van der Zee J. Inter-rater and Intra-rater reliability of the occupational therapy diagnosis. Occup Ther J Research 1995;5(4):259–274.
16. Reed KL, Sanderson SR. Concepts of Occupational Therapy. Baltimore: Williams & Wilkins, 1980.
17. Department of National Health and Welfare and the Canadian Association of Occupational Therapy. Guidelines for the Client-Centered Practice of Occupational Therapy. (H39–33/1983E). Ottawa, Ontario: The Department, 1983.
18. Cunningham C, Horgan F, Keane N, et al. Detection of disability by different members of an interdisciplinary team. Clin Rehabil 1996;10:247–254.
19. Myers AM. The clinical Swiss army knife: empirical evidence on the validity of IADL functional status measures. Med Care 1992;30(5 Suppl):MS100.
20. Suzrez de Balcazar Y, Bradford B, Fawcett SB. Common concerns of disabled Americans: issues and options. In: Nagler M. Perspectives on Disability. 2nd ed. Palo Alto,CA: Health Markets Research, 1990.

The Models Base

CHAPTER 12

Why Study Models

Atkinson has suggested there are eight reasons to study models (1). First, models provide a link or bridge between theory and practice. Models suggest the order to decision making by providing an outline or sequence of steps to follow in translating the theoretical into the practical. Models suggest what is most important and what need not be addressed immediately. For example, a model using development as an organizing idea usually suggests which stage comes first or provides a list of tasks by age. Find the age group that most closely matches the developmental age of the client and start at that point. Thus, the model guides the practitioner from a maze of information to a specific reference point.

Second, models define and focus the area of interest to occupational therapy practitioners. Theories can be complex, but conceptual models can translate the abstract into understandable terms. Models can be used to present the complexities of the profession into a logical and explainable order that can guide everyday practice. Of course, the simplicity of the model depends on its purpose. Translating a practice model developed for a specific area of practice into terms for clinical practice is easier that translating a generic theoretical model for occupational therapy.

Third, models provide a framework for assessment, intervention, and evaluation. Models describe the concepts important to phenomena being explained. Concepts themselves and their interrelationships form the basis of the assessment process. An assessment instrument should be developed based on the concepts and their relationships as outlined in the model. The client should be assessed by measuring how well his or her performance does or does not agree with the concepts presented in the model. Based on the results of the assessment and the model's directions for preparing an intervention plan, the intervention can commence. Evaluation is completed based on the objectives of the model and expected outcomes.

Fourth, models contribute to a sound philosophical base for the profession. The philosophy of occupational therapy is based on organismic philosophy. Humanism and pragmatism are two schools of philosophy that figure prominently in the early models of occupational therapy. Systems and dynamic systems are currently being used. As a result, a common set of concepts frequently appear. Among these are occupation, environment, competence, adaptation, intrinsic motivation, purposefulness, and meaningfulness.

Fifth, through models a common vocabulary evolves to communicate ideas. Ideas or concepts are the framework for constructing a model and communicating the essence of model. As models are developed certain concepts and interrelationship between those concepts appear again and again. The concept of environment and the relationship of human interaction with the environment are examples. Various models discuss the environment using slightly different subdivision of the environment such as physical, social, economic, supraorganic environments but the central idea of humans interacting in an environment remains fairly constant. Another example is the subdivisions of occupational performance that an individual does. Subdivisions include self-care, self-maintenance, homemaking, child care, work productivity, leisure, play, recreation, rest, and others. Taken separately, the subdivision can be confusing; understood as variations of occupational performance areas reduces the confusion. Even the concept of occupational performance can be restated in similar ways such as occupational competence, occupational adaptation, or occupational mastery. All relate to the ideas of personal skill acquisition and achievement.

Sixth, models provide us with professional unity. In a profession such as occupational therapy, which can be applied to human problems in many diverse situations dealing with newborn infants to centenarians, the need for a common understanding and unity of thought may be particularly important. Many generic models of occupational therapy suggest the uniting ideas such as occupation as the major modality, occupation-ology as the knowledge base, rationale through individual meaning (meaningful) and social or shared purpose (purposeful), and individual action (motivation) through doing to achieve, master, or gain competence.

Seventh, common themes exist throughout all the models of occupational therapy practice. These themes include the concern for the individual person, the value of human occupation, the recognition of each human as a total entity, and the willingness to share professional knowledge to improve the lives of others. Values, attitudes, and ethics are not always spelled out in models. Such attributes are often assumed to be in place. Understanding the common themes reinforces that the shared philosophy of occupational therapists is much greater than that which separates us in the daily practice of the profession.

There should be consideration for the limits of models. For all the positive aspects of models, drawbacks do exist. Models can be used as if they were the ultimate gurus that answer all questions as to how occupational therapy should be viewed and practiced. Models are not, as Barnett alleges, "bibles" or "cookbooks" that include a proverb or recipe for all occasions to be followed as written without variation (2). Models are "guidebooks" to be used as helpers in organizing the practice of occupational therapy but not in dictating practice. Models can guide clinical reasoning, but the belief in the uniqueness of individuals precludes any model from having the solution to every problem. Learning from experience, the willingness to question the ordinary, and the desire to improve the profession's knowledge base are also important tools in the clinician's toolbox. Models should facilitate but not limit professional growth.

Second, models are sometimes used to form the boundaries of occupational therapy practice (3). If something does not fit neatly into an existing model currently being practiced, that something may be regarded as foreign and beyond the boundary or domain of practice in occupational therapy. Models should be viewed as inclusive, not exclusive. Occupational therapy practice should be responsive to the needs of persons in their environments, not the constraints of a model. Existing models may not fit the need for future situations. When a model does not address an identified problem, the practitioner must decide whether to revise the model, dispense with the model, or develop a new model. Limiting practice because of existing models does not serve either our clients or the profession of occupational therapy in the future.

Third, a single best model does not exist in occupational therapy theory or practice. Although the idea of "one size fits all" is appealing, the notion that one model fits all is inconsistent with the historical development of the profession. Occupational therapy has always addressed a variety of occupational problems in human life. Occupational problems have many possible solutions within the arena of human potential. Occupational therapy has been developed from many sources and resources to increase its potential for finding solutions to different humans' unique occupational problems. Models should suggest workable solutions for a variety of occupational problems, but any given model is not likely to have the answer to every occupational problem.

Finally, models—just as tools—should not be used indefinitely without a checkup and review. Tools need to be periodically assessed to determine if they are in good condition, and they should be repaired as needed to work properly for their intended purpose. A dull knife does not cut as well as a sharp one. Models also need to be checked and reviewed periodically to determine how they are performing. In any occupational therapy service program, the models used by that program need a schedule of review. Do the models being used still provide the best guidance or are there other models that might provide better guidance? If a model is worn out or has served its purpose, it should be retired. Out-of-date models can results in out-of-date practice.

SUMMARY

In summary, models provide many benefits to the profession of occupational therapy and to its practitioners. Models link theory and practice, and they define and focus the areas of concern for practice. Models guide the process of assessment, planning, implementation, evaluation, and revision. They provide a common language for discussion and communication and serve as a unifying framework within the profession. Simultaneously, models can be used to limit the profession and its practitioners by overzealous application and the failure to understand that models cannot address every problem. Models also should not be used as fences or boundaries to restrict practice nor as old familiar props that have outlived their usefulness. Models must be reviewed periodically to determine if they still provide the best advice or if other models might better guide current occupational therapy practice.

References

1. Atkinson K. Do we need to use models in occupational therapy practice? Br J Ther Rehabil 1995;2(7):370–374.
2. Barnett R. Knowledge, skills and attitudes; what happened to thinking? Br J Occup Ther 1990;53(11):450–456.
3. Feaver S, Creek J. Models for practice in occupational therapy: part 2. What use are they? Br J Occup Ther 1993;56(2):59–62.

CHAPTER 13

Models and Philosophy

There are two types of models used in occupational therapy: conceptual and practice. Conceptual models attempt to explain why whereas practice models explain how. It is important to know and be able to discuss both.

Models are devices for explaining phenomena. They may be complex or simple. Conceptual models in a profession are usually developed to explain ideas about why the profession works as it does. Practice models are used to explain how the ideas of the theoretical model can be implemented into a plan of action to provide services to clients. Implementation may occur in a variety of ways. Therefore, one theoretical model may be the basis for several practice models. Both conceptual and practice models, however, should be examined through research to determine how well they explain or implement the ideas proposed. Figure 13.1 shows the relations of the two types of models to each other.

The most important aspect of a conceptual model is the frame of reference. The frame of reference is based in philosophy. Philosophy attempts to describe or explain what we believe or value. Thus, philosophy is expressed in viewpoints, beliefs, values, and attitudes. There are two major philosophic views the have most influenced the development of occupational therapy. The two philosophic views are called organismic and mechanistic. Although organismic and mechanistic views tend to be opposites, the opposing views should not be interpreted as inherently good or bad but rather as different. Both viewpoints have contributed to the understanding of the humans and their environment. Table 13.1 is a list of concepts for both the organismic or mechanistic philosophies. No model incorporates all of the concepts. Instead, the model builder usually selected three or four of the concepts as a frame of reference for the proposed model. Nine of the concepts that appear frequently in occupational therapy models are described along with their counterparts.

LOCUS OF CONTROL

Most important is the concept of locus of control (1, 2). In the organismic school of thought, the individual is viewed as capable of initiating change from within. Change may be a result of growth, maturation, or learning. These processes provide the stimulation for action and behavior. This change process occurring within the person is called the internal locus of control. In contrast, the mechanistic school views the in-

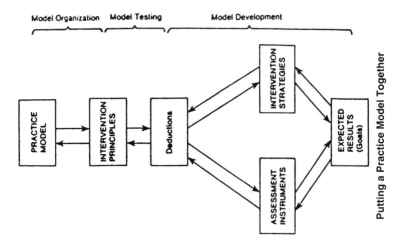

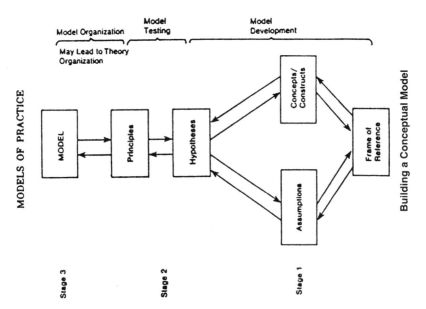

Figure 13.1. Building a model and putting it together. (From: Reed KL. Models of Practice in Occupational Therapy. Baltimore: Williams & Wilkins, 1984:18,20.)

Table 13.1. Metamodels: Contrasting Views Between Major Philosophies

Organismic	Mechanistic
1. *Internal locus of control* Activity generated from within; individual is active and dynamic	*External locus of control* Activity result of outside forces; individual is reactive, passive, and robotic
2. *Qualitative* Stages, levels, milestones, phases, ages, periods	*Quantitative* Cumulative effect
3. *End point* Fixed process	*No end point* Additive line or product
4. *Discontinuous change* Patterns of behavior irreversible	*Continuous change* Patterns of behavior are reversible
5. *Emergence of constructivism* Behavioral or functional change is a transformation and is irreducible	*Reductionistic* Any change in the organism can be reduced to more elementary form
6. *Holistic* Whole is different or greater than sum of parts	*Elementaristic* Whole is equal to the sum of parts
7. *Structure-function* Function determines structure	*Antecedent-consequent* All behavior caused by environmental forces
8. *Structural change* Change is determined by the form of the organization	*Behavioral change* Change is determined by efficient cause
9. *Open system* Interacts with the environment	*Closed system* Does not interact with the environment
10. *Age restriction* Chronological age is used as boundaries for stages or levels	*No age restriction* Chronological age is an increasing continuum of time
11. *Free will* Man is able to choose and exercise volitional control	*Determinism* All events follow natural laws which man does not control
12. *Universality* Behavior characteristics of all organisms	*Relativity* Behavior characteristics of individual only
13. *Heredity* Inherent, genetic, nature are primarily responsible for man's behavior	*Environment* Nurture is primarily responsible for man's behavior
14. *Rationalism* Reason is source of knowledge	*Expiricism* Experience is source if knowledge
15. *Man is responsible* Responsible for individual action	*Man is irresponsible* Is not responsible for self

continued

Table 13.1.   Metamodels: Contrasting Views Between Major Philosophies

16. *Steady state*
    Achieves balance in spite of input and output, a dynamic process
17. *Equifinality*
    Alternate route may have the same outcome
18. *Negentropy*
    Individual can increase amount of free energy
19. *Autonomous activity*
    Individual can initiate action

20. *Moral values*
    Have knowledge of right and wrong
21. *Symbolic activity*
    Individual seeks symbolic activity

22. *Critical periods*
    Certain times in development most favorable for learning
23. *Emotionalism*
    Feelings, affect, and mood are part of organism
24. *Monism*
    Mind and body are one
25. *Subjectivism*
    Concerned with inner processes of thought and feeling
26. *Tension seeking*
    Man seeks situations which increase tension in the body-need induction
27. *Fluid dimensions*
    of time and space
28. *Pull motivation*
    Emphasis on purpose, value, and needs, "carrot" theories
29. *Undirectional*
    Development of progression of complexity and expansion
30. *Present, future-oriented*
    Time perspective is looking ahead

Equilibrium
    Achieves balance through a static process
Finality
    The outcome is determined by initial conditions
Entropy
    Amount of free energy is limited

Dependent activity
    Individual is conditioned to do certain actions.
Amoral
    No need to know right and wrong

Nonsymbolic activities
    The environment controls the type of activity
Noncritical periods
    Learning is possible at any age

Unemotional
    Feelings, affect, and mood are not necessary
Dualism
    Mind and body are separate
Objectivism
    Concerned with external actions and responses
Tension reducing
    Man tries to reduce the tension which arises in the body-need reduction
Fixed dimensions
    of time and space
Push motivation
    Emphasis on drive, motive, and stimulus, "pitchfork" theories
Alternating directional
    Developmental progression and regression are equal possibilities
Past-oriented
    Time perspective is looking backward

From: Reed KL. Models of Practice in Occupational Therapy. Baltimore: Williams & Wilkins, 1984.

dividual as a passive entity that must be directed from an external source. Individual change is shaped and controlled by stimulation and influences that occur external to the individual. The individual changes as a result of action by persons and situations that did not occur from within the individual but rather from outside the individual. Thus, mechanistic philosophy is based on an external locus of control.

Examples of models based on internal locus of control are Piaget's stages of learning, Maslow's hierarchy of needs, and Gessell's stages of development. Notice that learning, needs, and developmental stages occur within the individual. Examples of models based on external locus of control are Skinner's operant conditioning (behavior modification) and Freud's psychoanalysis. Notice that the source of stimulation and influence is considered to be external to the individual. Most, but not all, occupational therapy models are based on the belief that humans are capable of internal locus of control.

RESPONSIBILITY VERSUS IRRESPONSIBILITY

Locus of control is related to another concept, responsibility (6). Organismic philosophy is based on the belief that a person is rational and thus capable of taking responsibility; that is, a person can think for him or herself, determine the results of actions, choose a course of action, and accept the consequences for that choice. This belief is illustrated in the social practice of encouraging the person to be responsible for individual actions. The objective of most laws in democratic societies is to correct or punish citizens for failure to control their own behavior. Mechanistic philosophy, on the other hand, is based on the belief that people are basically irresponsible and unable to direct individual behavior without an external source of assistance and control. In other words, a person must be told what to do and controlled to make sure the correct action occurs. Thus, laws in socialistic governments correct or punish citizens for failure to follow the party line. Thinking for oneself is considered impossible and/or highly undesirable because a person does not or should not initiate action but only should react to situations that already exist. Citizens who dare to "think for themselves" are likely to be punished severely.

Maslow's hierarchy of needs is an example of taking responsibility. The assumption is that a person can think or figure out how to satisfy the hierarchy of needs. In contrast, operant conditioning is based on external commands (stimuli) that require the individual to perform (response). No thinking or processing "in the little black box (brain)" is expected of the individual. The individual is to do as he or she is told—no more, no less.

FREE WILL VERSUS DETERMINISM

Taking responsibility is related to free will (5, 6). Free will is based on the assumptions that an individual is capable of choosing those activities and behavior that are needed or desired. In other words, each person is capable of guiding or directing the self through the use of volitional control. This capacity for self-direction is in contrast with the assumption of determinism. Determinism is based on the assumption that all facts and events are controlled by natural laws. By deduction, it follows that human behavior follows the same natural laws. Therefore, an individual's behavior and activity are directed by situations over which a person has little control. Thus, the individual is much like a pawn in a chess game who react to the actions of the king, queen, or bishop.

Volition is a key concept in Kielhofner's model of human occupation. Volition is concerned with internal dispositions and self-knowledge built on the individual's experience. In contrast, behavioral control models are based on determining in advance which behaviors are socially acceptable and developing a plan to attain the desired results.

HOLISM VERSUS ELEMENTARISM

Holism is the assumption that the organism as a whole is different from the sum of its parts (1, 3). In other words, an individual has characteristics as a total human that are not present *per se* in any of the specific parts of the body. Mind and spirit are two examples. On the other hand, elementarism is the assumption that the organism is the exact sum of its parts. Thus, when all the elements of a person are put together, the total person can be observed; conversely, any part of a person can be observed by examining the elements in that part. Any part of a person's behavior can be studied by examining the elements or units that comprise the behavior. If elementarism is not possible, the element does not exist. Models based on the concept of elementarism have difficulty explaining mind, spirit, or spirituality.

EMERGENCE VERSUS REDUCTIONISM

Holism is often related to emergence. Emergence, or constructivism, is the process of changing the structure and function of the organism into something that did not exist before. The organismic model is based on the concept that as stages or levels of development occur, the resulting changes reorganize the total individual into a different system (1, 2).

In contrast, reductionism is the process of reducing any higher level or more complex action into a lower level or simpler action. The action may be a behavior or function. The reductionistic approach is basic to the mechanistic assumption that all matter can be changed from one form to another and back again. In physics and chemistry, the basic level is the atom and molecule; in physiology, the cell is a basic unit; and in behavior, a stimulus-response sequence is the basic unit. Again, stage theories such as those by Piaget and Erickson are examples of emergence whereas Freudian and Skinnerian theories are examples of reductionism. The biomedical model of disease and pathology is also based on reductionism (1, 2).

DISCONTINUOUS VERSUS CONTINUOUS CHANGE

Models based on discontinuity organize the changes observed in the individual into stages, levels, periods, milestone, phases, or ages (1–3). Each stage represents a distinct organization of the total individual into something that was not present before (see Emergence in the previous section). Thus, models based on the concept of development, growth, and maturation are mostly likely to be examples of the organismic model. Erickson's eight stages of life and Piaget's levels of cognitive adaptation are examples of discontinuity. Once a stage has been obtained, it cannot be lost or stolen.

In contrast, models based on the continuous approach promise that change is a steady, cumulative process that can move forward or backward in time. "Development" is simply the process of acquiring units of behavior that can also be lost. Continuous change is evident in the model of behaviorism. Change occurs whenever the environmental conditions are such that events prior to, or given after, a response alter the nature of that response. As a result, change can be increased or decreased, brought about or extinguished.

HEREDITY (NATURE) VERSUS ENVIRONMENT (NURTURE)

The organismic model is usually built on the assumption that heredity is a critical component in determining behavior (7). That is because heredity is controlled by genes and expressed through maturation, an internal process. Environment is considered to facilitate the maturation of behavior by some theorists such as Piaget. However, the structural organization of behavior is present at birth. Environment provides the activity to interact with the existing (internal) organization. Followers of the mechanistic model, in contrast, believe that environment or nurture is the key to building the behavioral repertoire. Behavior is acquired through socialization and training.

MONISM VERSUS DUALISM

A basic assumption of the organismic model is that the mind and body operate together and that there is no real distinction between the mind, body, and spirit (8). Thought and reason are not considered as separate functions but as expression of the whole of which thought and actions are aspects for discussion but within the individual person they operate as a whole.

In comparison, the mechanistic model is based on the assumption that the mind and body are separate. Body became the more important of the two because it could be studied objectively. Soma could be studied as a machine, but psyche could not and thus was often ignored. Furthermore, machines—and individuals—could be understood entirely with reference to internal energy sources.

OPEN SYSTEM VERSUS CLOSED SYSTEM

The problem of an energy source can be further discussed by examining the concepts of an open system versus a closed system (4). An open system maintains itself by exchanging matter with the environment and by continuously building up and breaking down components. Humans are considered to be open systems in the organismic model because each individual is capable of taking in nutrients and information, converting this into useful products, and putting out energy, responses, or waste. A constant interchange exists between the individual and the environment.

On the other hand, a closed system does not draw energy from the environment. Technically, no materials enter or leave. A human functions as if there was no need to interact with the environment for energy. Although no theory proposes that humans are totally closed systems, one view within the mechanistic model supports interaction only for the purpose of tension reduction. In other words, a person only interacts with the environment when tissue needs or bodily drives arise.

THE INFLUENCE OF THE META MODELS ON OCCUPATIONAL THERAPY

Occupational therapists began working within the organismic philosophy from the beginning on occupational therapy practice within the moral treatment approach and the theory of psychobiology developed by Adolph Meyer. Practice was concerned with organizing the individual's daily activities, treating the individual with respect, and promoting socially acceptable behavior. As the influences of Gazelle began to affect practice in the 1930s and 1940s, the organismic model remained although the focus of intervention changed to following stages of development.

In the late 1940s and 1950s, the pressure of medical specialization in rehabilitation and psychoanalytic theory began to push the organismic orientation into a second-rate position. Behavior was assessed in discrete units, such as range of motion in degrees, muscle strength in pounds, and analysis of specific past events. The concentration was on observable details and regressive behavior. As a result the whole person was sometimes ignored, and cognitive thought was considered unimportant. Practice was oriented to research methods designed to find the statistical laws of human behavior. Health was viewed as the absence of disease, injury, or trauma. The shift from organismic to mechanistic models became evident. During the 1960s and 1970s, occupational therapy in psychiatry began to resist the move to the mechanistic model. Developmental ideas began to reappear. At the same time, occupational therapy in physical dysfunction tried to embrace the mechanistic model. Thus, the neurobehavioral approaches, such as the biomechanical model, became popular. Some neurobehavioral and sensorimotor concepts also followed the reductionistic concept.

Beginning in the 1960s, however, there were a few examples of a resurgence of the organismic model. The occupational behavior model developed by Reilly is most notable. In the 1970s, there were more models based on development such as the recapitulation of ontogenesis and the individual adaptation model by King. The concepts of humanism, holism, competence, and occupation became, once again, more visible as concepts with influence in occupational therapy. Occupational therapists began to reassert their rightful heritage.

DISCUSSION

It should be apparent that conceptual and practice models must be consistent with either the organismic or the mechanistic frame of reference. In other words, philosophic views based on the organismic frame of reference do not mix well with those based on the mechanistic frame of reference. An example of the problem of mixing can be seen in Freud's work. Psychoanalysis is based on the mechanistic frame of reference. Of importance is Freud's concept of regression. In regression, a person reverts or returns to an earlier time frame in life and functions like he or she did during the original time frame. Thus, regression is an example of continuous change. At the same time, Freud discusses stages of psychosexual development. If the psychosexual stages of development are true developmental stages, then complete regression is not possible because stages imply discontinuous change, which is a concept based on the organismic model. In discontinuous change, the person cannot revert or regress to an earlier stage of development. Trying to reconcile the discrepancies in Freud's model of psychoanalysis has continued to its decline as a major model of human behavior.

A similar problem arises in practice with certain neuromotor models. For example, a person has a brain injury and is unable to perform many basic movements such as coordination for walking. Several popular models suggest starting the person at the beginning of movement patterns such as creeping to prepare for more complex patterns requiring higher levels of brain function. Thus, an adult is placed on the floor on hands and knees and encouraged to practice creeping in preparation for dynamic balance, posture, and walking.

If the practice model is based on a conceptual model that views change as continuity, then creeping is appropriate. However, if the practice model is based on the conceptual model of development, then creeping is inappropriate because developmental models are based on the assumption of discontinuity. A better approach might be to work directly with the problems that appear to impede progress toward improving balance and posture.

Also important to note is that interest in conceptual models changes over time. As shown in Figure 13.2, during the early part of 20th century, organismic models dominated. Then mechanistic models became dominant. Beginning in the 1960s a shift back to organismic models occurred. Shifting ideas about the philosophy of models should be expected in the future.

Finally, several other concepts distinguish organismic models from mechanistic models. Occasionally, such additional concepts may be useful in analyzing a particular conceptual model. These additional concepts are discussed in Appendix A.

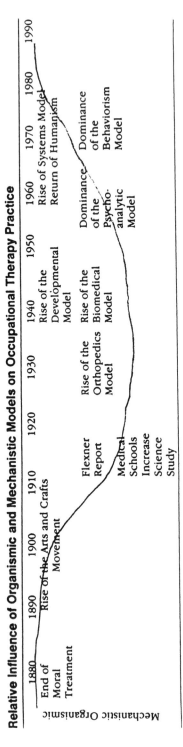

Figure 13.2. Relative influence of organismic and mechanistic models on occupational therapy practice. (Adapted from: Reed KL. Tools of practice: heritage or baggage? Am J Occup Ther 1986;40(9):601.)

References

1. Looft WR. Socialization and personality throughout the life span: an examination of contemporary psychological approaches. In: Baltes PB, Schaie KW. Life Span Developmental Psychology. New York: Academic Press, 1973:25–82.
2. Friedrich D. A Primer for Developmental Methodology. Minneapolis: Burgess Publishing, 1972:3–8.
3. Reese HW, Overton WF. Models of development and theories of development. In: Goulet LR, Battes PB. Life Span Developmental Psychology. New York: Academic Press, 1970:115–145.
4. Bertalanffy LV. General Systems Theory. New York: Braziller, 1968.
5. Solomon RC. Introducing Philosophy: Problems and Perspectives. 2nd ed. New York: Harcourt, Brace, Jovanovich, 1981.
6. Blackham HJ. Humanism. 2nd ed. New York: International Publications Service, 1976.
7. Thomas RM. Comparing Theories of Child Development. Belmont, CA: Wadsworth Publishing, 1979:29.
8. Lamont C. The Philosophy of Humanism. 6th ed. New York: Frederick Ungar Publishing 1982:12–14.

CHAPTER 14

Models of Health That Influence Occupational Therapy Practice

PHILOSOPHICAL BASE

As stated in the previous chapter, philosophy involves the critique and analysis of fundamental beliefs or values (1). Beliefs and values provide the foundation for all health care services, including occupational therapy. There are beliefs and values about how a person achieves and maintains health, how health is lost, and how professionals can help restore health. Most of the beliefs and values have existed for many hundreds of years and are not much affected by changing technology. The most comprehensive beliefs and values are called paradigms or world views. As discussed in the previous chapter, the two major world views are called organismic and mechanistic (2). The differences in beliefs and values will be illustrated further as the health modes are discussed and are summarized in Tables 14.1A through 14.1E.

MEDICAL OR PATHOLOGY MODEL

The medical or pathology model is the foundation of clinical medicine (3, 4). It focuses attention on assessing the symptoms of a disease or injury to determine what is not functioning. After the pathology has been pinpointed, treatment is begun to eliminate, neutralize, repair, or correct the existing pathology through the use of drugs (chemicals) and surgery.

The medical model is based on mechanistic philosophy. The human body is viewed as a machine that can be examined for problems, such as microorganisms or trauma, which cause fever, swelling, cuts, fractures, or other disturbances that the physician can treat. Thus, the role of the physician is to determine the problem and actively administer the solution or treatment. The role of the person seeking health service (patient) is to submit to the physician's authority and to follow the advice given.

Occupational therapists who work in hospitals and facilities that follow the medical or pathology model have three major problems in terms of philosophy. First, oc-

Table 14.1A.

	Biomedical Model	Biopsychosocial
Philosophical base	Mechanistic	Organismic
View of health	Absence of disease as measured by biological (somatic) variables	Involves an interaction of biological, psychological, and social factors
Strengths	Established cause of illness as pathogenic not political, economical, or spiritual	Includes psychological and social factors in health status assessment
Weaknesses	Disease-oriented, not person-oriented, based on reductionism	Difficult to measure psychological and social data

Table 14.1B.

	Chronicity	Holistic Health
Philosophical base	Mechanistic	Organismic
View of health	There is permanent disability and lack of health	A person functions as an integrated independent whole
Strengths	Recognizes long-term health problems	Recognizes interactive nature of person and environment as dynamic
Weaknesses	Depends on social attitudes and values that are not consistent with current knowledge; inconsistent in type of protection offered	Difficult to predict stressors and responses to stress

cupational therapists do not use their tools and skills to treat disease or injury. Rather, occupational therapists apply their tools and skills to the sequelae or residual effects of disease and injury. As a result, occupational therapists have only begun to help a client when the physician has nearly finished the use of medicinal tools and skills. Second, under the medical model, the person relinquishes self-control to the physician. Decision making and responsibility for actions are controlled by the physician. In contrast, occupational therapy was developed on the philosophy that a person can and should control the decision making and take responsibility for individual actions to the maximum degree possible. The client is caught in the middle. The physician

Table 14.1C.

	Milieu	Health Education and Prevention
Philosophical base	Organismic but is easily changed to mechanistic	Organismic
View of health	The total environment, human and nonhuman, promotes or diminishes health	Health is affected by heredity, physical environment, social conditions, health services, and personal actions
Strengths	Recognizes the role of the environment in producing behavioral change	Involves all factors that contribute to health and stresses prevention as well as intervention
Weaknesses	May lead to behavior control by others; behavioral change may be dependent on the particular environment	Creates logistic problems of coordinating variety of factors with varying attitudes, values, and willingness to act

Table 14.1D.

	Health Development	Wellness
Philosophical base	Organismic	Organismic
View of health	Involves a progression of stages from simple to complex in a particular sequence	All persons have a potential for wellness
Strengths	Focuses on capacities, function, and abilities	Attempts to describe health as more than lack of illness or absence of pathology
Weaknesses	Little consideration as to whether all steps in sequence are needed; not much information on development of adults of aged	Definitions of levels or degrees of health are difficult to develop and agree upon which in turn makes it difficult to accurately assess the level or degree

Table 14.1E.		
	Normality	Rehabilitation
Philosophical base	Mechanistic	Mechanistic, although may be presented as organismic
View of health	Is a statistical average	Involves reducing physical limitations and encouraging social conformity
Strengths	Easy to determine; has social and cultural recognition and support	Has government support for financial assistance
Weaknesses	No help in deciding what to do with those who cannot be average; what is average may change with age, custom, or social situation	Criteria for success are primarily work-oriented and controlled by professions

says "do this," but the occupational therapist says "the choice is yours." The occupational therapist can help by clarifying which activities the physician is directing and which activities the client still has to decide. The third problem relates to assessment. Physicians are concerned primarily with dysfunction and liabilities. Little attention is paid to the functional skills and behavior an individual may have. Abilities such as adaptation to or compensation for dysfunction can be overlooked, discounted, or ignored because the usual rule is to discharge a client if no cure can be achieved.

Occupational therapists, on the other hand, must be careful not to limit assessment to the dysfunctional aspects of occupations. The skills and behaviors that are functional can be used to assist in learning or relearning other occupational skills. For example, a young person whose neck is broken in a diving accident loses the use of both legs, part of the trunk, and part of the arms and hands. The person certainly has lost many functions, but can such an individual contribute anything to society as an independent person? To explore these possibilities, the occupational therapist must assess the potential functional abilities. Arms and hands can perform some functions and assistive devices with help. The neck and head are functional. With practice, the person can learn self-maintenance skills. Many desk or office jobs can be learned, as can writing, painting pictures, and doing sales jobs. Leisure skills can be achieved with some modifications. Ability can overcome or compensate for disability.

OCCUPATIONAL THERAPY AND THE BIOPSYCHOSOCIAL MODEL

The biopsychosocial model is an attempt to correct some of the limitations of the medical model. Specifically, the biopsychosocial model is designed to weigh the relative contributions of social and psychological as well as biological factors in determining the degree of health or illness and dysfunction (5). Health, disease, illness, and disability are defined in terms of the ability to function on a continuum, which ranges from total dysfunction and death to full functionality and health.

In contrast to the medical model, the biopsychosocial model is based on the organismic paradigm. The individual is viewed as a total organism with interacting systems, not as a collection of diseased or injured parts. Social and psychological factors are seen as important sources of information in addition to the biological. Furthermore, the person is considered to have an active role rather than a passive one in determining whether to seek medical assistance and how much.

Initially, the biopsychosocial model seems to be a substantial improvement over the medical model. However, occupational therapists must be aware that the model provides little if any support for the role of occupations (self-maintenance, productivity, and leisure) in promoting or maintaining health and function. The primary contribution of the biopsychosocial model is the acknowledgment that health is more than the mere absence of disease.

Another problem that has hampered acceptance of the biopsychosocial model is the difficulty in quantifying intrapersonal and interpersonal data. Biological or physiological data can be measured by scientific instruments with finely calibrated scales. Emotions, values, interests, interaction skills, and roles are more difficult to measure because they rely on human decision rather than on mechanical devices. Furthermore, little consideration is given to the role of environment in health development and maintenance. In summary, although the concept of the biopsychosocial model is encouraging, it is not broad enough to encompass all aspects of human function.

OCCUPATIONAL THERAPY AND CHRONICITY

The chronic or impaired model of health is based on the concept of permanent handicap. Usually, the handicap is the result of a disorder acquired at birth or the residual effect of an illness or injury (6). The model is based primarily on the mechanistic view, and the locus of control tends to be external.

Perhaps, at first glance, the chronic or impaired model does not appear to be a health model at all because some aspect of health is missing. Otherwise, the person would not be disabled. Such is the position that many disabled people face. Society views them as lacking some degree of health and, therefore, not able to participate in socially expected behavior, such as employment and self-care activities.

Chronicity, therefore, is a socially defined indicator of health status rather than a biological one. The locus of the control is external to the individual; thus, the model is based on the mechanistic view. The social definition of health includes being able to perform those occupations and tasks that society expects or encourages. If a person with a disability can demonstrate the ability to perform self-maintenance, productive tasks, and leisure occupations, then society tends to accept the person as healthy and a member of normal society. If such performance is not demonstrated, the person's health is questioned and his or her social status is marginal. For many of the people seen by occupational therapists, the major problem is to achieve an acceptable level of health by demonstrating the ability to perform in spite of limitations. Such limitations include problems in cognitive and psychosocial functioning, as well as sensory or motor functioning. Many persons labeled as retarded or chronically mentally ill face the same problems of demonstrating ability to perform as a person who is blind or confined to a wheelchair. The major problem with the chronic or impaired model is that society tends to be narrow-minded and prejudiced in its beliefs and values concerning chronic limitation. Furthermore, judgments are based often on intuition rather than fact. One result is that some disabled people such as those who are blind or wheelchair users, are never given the chance to show the skills they have. Others whose disability, such as deafness, cannot be seen may be expected to perform normally.

Another result is the tendency of society to vacillate from overprotection to underprotection. A disabled person may be denied a job because the employer fears the person may be injured further. At the same time, society reduces the amount of the person's disability payments because the social viewpoint is that everyone should "pay his or her own way" if possible. Vacillation may occur in leisure activity as well. A disabled person may be encouraged to attend a social event only to find that the building is inaccessible. A third result of social definition and opinion is the slowness of change. Scientists and professionals may have found and dispelled many myths, but the facts are slow to change social attitudes. For example, people with Down syndrome, a genetic disorder, are considered still to be severely retarded and die at an early age. The truth is that the intelligence is not as limited as thought 20 years ago, and modern medicine can cure many of the respiratory diseases that once took the lives of many people with Down syndrome early in life.

OCCUPATIONAL THERAPY AND HOLISTIC HEALTH

Holistic health is based on the assumption that a person functions as an integrated whole in relation to the environment (7). The whole includes physical, emotional, intellectual, social, spiritual, and lifestyle dimensions. The environment includes internal (body) and external (human and nonhuman) aspects. Holism is based on a philosophical assumption that the whole is more than just the sum of its parts and thus cannot be divided into pieces for separate analysis, but must be analyzed in total because all dimensions or systems interact and are interdependent on each other. The concept of holism is consistent with the organismic view because, ultimately, the person determines the state of health and not the physician or other professional. Thus, health becomes a dynamic process that is not limited by the presence or absence of disease but involves the interacting systems of the body and a relationship to the external world as well.

Holistic practitioners look for signs of stress as the symptom of ill health. Stress is anything that upsets the balance of the systems, creates conflict within the self, and leads to disintegration of the whole. The role of the practitioner is to help the person identify the existence of stress and to assist in planning a program to reduce or eliminate the stress. Thus, the practice of holistic health depends on the person to be motivated and actively involved in the process of therapy. Ultimately, the person must use the resources available to obtain and maintain health.

Holistic health has several attractive features for occupational therapists. The belief that a person should be treated as a whole is very consistent with the philosophy of an occupational therapist, which states that therapists work with the whole person. The concept of balance is also familiar. Occupational therapists have been concerned with balancing occupational tasks. Integration has been a central theme in occupational therapy to explain how a person functions.

The attractive features, however, must be weighed against the problems. Holism in practice is a difficult concept to actualize. Assessment becomes complex when information from such diverse systems as motor and spiritual are analyzed together. Problem solving becomes more difficult and time-consuming also. An intervention program must be developed with the person's full understanding because the person, not the therapist, will be the primary implementor. Such planning requires attention to details that a therapist might take for granted. Learning about stress and stressors is another potential problem. Potential stressors include almost everything and everybody a person encounters directly or indirectly. What distresses one person might never distress another person. What distresses a given person at a particular time or event might not cause distress in another situation. In other words, all health professionals, including occupational therapists, must learn more about the nature of stress, types of stressors, responses to stress, and techniques or methods for reducing or eliminating stress before the holistic health model can become useful for a large segment of the population.

OCCUPATIONAL THERAPY AND MILIEU

The milieu model is based on the concept of using the environment to promote health and effect change in health status. Milieu therapy is an attempt to organize the physical and social environment into a therapeutic situation that will increase health status and health behavior (8). The primary goal is to change socially unacceptable behavior into socially acceptable behavior.

Conceptually, the milieu model is based on organismic philosophy. There is a recognition that the person can become responsible for changing or controlling self-behavior. At the same time, however, the professionals tend to control the environment in such a manner that the person must act in accordance with the professional's plan. Thus, the philosophy of the milieu model is organismic, but the implementation becomes mechanistic. As a result, the locus of control shifts from self to other.

The milieu model has been identified and recognized in the area of mental health. However, the model may be operating in many physical rehabilitation programs without being identified. Anywhere in which the architectural design, equipment used, and staff organization are planned to facilitate certain behavior and discourage other behavior, the milieu model probably is being used. Formal recognition may be less important than awareness. The key question is how much control the person has over the changes in behavior and function. If the person can leave or refuse to participate without jeopardy of position or status, the locus of control remains with the self. When others control the leaving or participating, the program probably is operating from a mechanistic view. The result may be behavior control but not behavior change. Another possibility is behavior change within the environmental setting that does not carry over to another environment. In other words, the person performs as expected by the professionals in their environment, but in the community or at home, the person performs in terms of self or family expectation.

The latter example is common in rehabilitation programs. A client learns to become independent in self-care activities using more adapted equipment and is discharged. In a follow-up visit, the client or family indicates that none of the adapted equipment is being used and most self-care is being performed by the family. The client has not forgotten how to be independent, but the environmental expectation has changed. In the rehabilitation center, independence was expected; at home, dependence is expected. Either the client must change the home environment or the therapist must help change the family's expectations if the independent performance of self-care is to continue beyond the rehabilitation facility.

OCCUPATIONAL THERAPY AND HEALTH EDUCATION AND PREVENTION

The health education and prevention model involves the recognition of the effects of heredity, physical environment, social conditions, available health services, and personal actions on health (9, 10). Education and prevention are accomplished by increasing the amount or improving the quality of action and resources. Actions include personal practices that prevent unnecessary disability and death, prompt use of health services when needed, carrying out diagnostic treatment and procedures, and participation in health program development. Resources include health education, finances, preparation and distribution of health personnel, facilities, equipment, and legislation (9).

Health education and prevention as a health model is based on the organismic model of self-responsibility. However, more than one's self must be involved to implement many of the actions. Unity of action is difficult because values, goals, interests, habits, and other influences on health vary widely.

Therapists can help educate for health and prevent disability because they have useful information on developmental assessment, work simplification, work efficiency, architectural barriers, adapted equipment and aids, work habits that protect joints and muscles, avocational interests for retirement planning, and many other tools and techniques. The message can be spread through inservice and continuing education, consultation, speeches to clubs and community organizations, booths at fairs or in public buildings, pamphlets, folders, booklets, audiovisual aids, articles in popular magazines, and presentations on radio and television. These ideas are all in addition to service programs.

The problem with the health education and prevention model is largely concerned with logistics. There is a tendency to plan larger projects that can be accomplished. A small education and prevention program that meets the needs for a few people may be better than a large program that rarely meets anyone's needs.

OCCUPATIONAL THERAPY AND HEALTH DEVELOPMENT

Development is a biological concept that pertains to the progression from earlier to later stages in an individual's life (11, 12). The process usually involves the joining of complete skills and behavior. For example, first, the child has limited organized movement pattern, then movement is organized through the arms but the legs are disorganized. Next, movement is organized using the hands and knees. Finally, motor organization permits the child to walk on two feet, leaving the arms free to engage in other pursuits. Other aspects of development can be assessed and measured by determining the progression of skill development and approximate age of normal occurrence. Intervention begins at the point at which an individual does not perform the next step in the sequence. Theoretically, each step, in turn, is practiced until mastery is obtained.

Development is consistent with the organismic view because maturation and growth are innate properties of the individual. Occupational therapists have found developmental progression a useful concept in analyzing performance and planning intervention programs because of the sequential steps that suggest what to do and when to do it (13). The assumption is that normal progression denotes and promotes health.

The problem with the developmental approach to intervention is the reliance on progressing from step to step without considering other factors. One of these factors includes deciding if all steps are essential to achieving mastery. Is it essential to creep or crawl for a certain length of time in order to walk? Some studies have suggested that certain children do not creep or crawl before walking, but they do learn to walk.

Another factor to consider is whether practice in one sequential step may interfere with performance in a later step. In this case, consider the child with cerebral palsy who has been practicing movement on hands and knees. The knees and hips are flexed or bent in this movement, but while walking, the knees and hips are usually extended or straight. If contracture (tightness) occurs in the flexed knees and hips, walking will be difficult. The occupational therapist would consider eliminating movement on hands and knees because this movement pattern is rarely used as an adult. Time could be spent in promoting balance and coordination in the upright position for sitting, standing, and walking.

Finally, development progression may be useful in planning programs for children and adolescents, but most development stages end at the adult level or provide few subdivisions between the age range of 21 to 101 years. As a result, the therapist must either use another health model for planning intervention or add to knowledge about adult and aging development.

OCCUPATIONAL THERAPY AND WELLNESS

Wellness frequently is associated with health. Defining wellness, however, is complex. There appear to be three uses of terms, which include 1) wellness as the polar opposite of illness; 2) wellness as a graduated scale with illness; and 3) wellness as a partially or nearly separate dimension from illness, as illustrated in Figure 14.1 (14).

Wellness as the opposite of illness probably is the most commonly accepted definition by the public. Basically, a person is either sick or well. When a person

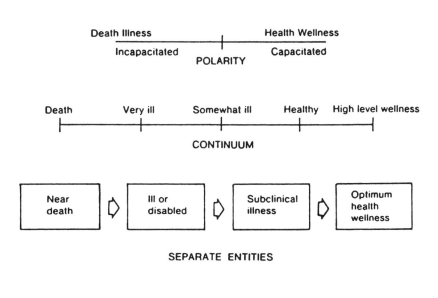

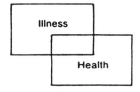

INCOMPLETE SEPARATE ENTITIES

Figure 14.1. Models of wellness.

is sick, the social custom is to send a "get well" card. Parsons uses the either-or concept in his definition of health as the "state of optimum capacity" and illness as an "impairment to capacity" (15). A person is either able to perform required roles and tasks effectively and is healthy and well, or he or she is unable to perform effectively and is impaired or ill.

The polar view of wellness and illness typically is a static view of health. There are no points in-between and thus no range of health; that is, there is no more well than ill nor more ill than well. Capacity to perform roles and tasks becomes a total criterion also. There is no degree of capacity or incapacity.

The second definition of wellness uses a graduated scale, as suggested by Dunn in his work on high-level wellness (16). The scale is a continuum from death to peak wellness with such subdivisions as serious illness, minor illness, and good health in-between. Wellness as a continuum still uses polar points but adds graduations in-between.

One problem with scaling is defining what each point on the scale represents. For example, what is the actual difference between good and peak wellness?

Separate dimensions was the third definition of wellness. Jahoda has suggested that wellness and illness are separate dimensions of health and that a person may experience varying conditions of wellness or health as well as varying conditions of illness or disability (17). A person's total health status or level of wellness is determined by the actions of the person who may be able to perform some behaviors but not others that are a part of the normal routine. The advantage of the separate view is that it permits assessment of wellness aspects apart from illness aspects. For example, a person who is paralyzed from the waist down may continue to have medical problems with urinary infections. However, the person may be quite capable of maintaining home, job, and community activities. Illness is present but so are several aspects of health and wellness.

All three aspects of wellness have two factors in common. All are based on the organismic view, and all propose an optimum or utopian view of health in which all aspects of the person function to the maximum potential. This potential may be called high level wellness, self-actualization, optimal functioning, or optimum health. All refer to the attempt to define a utopian or ultimate level of health as a goal or outcome to be achieved or toward which to strive. The problem is the difficulty in arriving at a definition that is acceptable and observable to more than one person. Health has many facets, with illness and wellness being only two such facets. A few others are capacity–incapacity, ability–disability, function–dysfunction, and assets–limitations. Wellness may have a high social value, but its application is difficult to actualize.

OCCUPATIONAL THERAPY AND NORMALITY

Many factors that are related to health, such as caloric intake, drugs prescribed, and types of diseases, can be measured in terms of norms or averages (3). These norms are based on a statistical measurement technique called central tendency, which groups an item such as weight so that approximately 68% of the people will find their weight to be in the middle range. The other 32% will be above or below that middle range. The concept of normality is reinforced strongly in North American society. Being normal or average is considered a desirable goal in society because the individual then "fits in" with others.

The normality model of health is based on the mechanistic view. Society, not the individual, determines what is normal. One of the problems with this health model is that what exists becomes the criterion for normality, even though the norm may be objectionable. For example, statistics show that most women who work receive lower wages than men. Therefore, according to the averaging mode, it is normal for women to receive less pay for their work than men, even though the women may be doing exactly the same work as the men. Anyone who objects to this arrangement would be upsetting the status quo and thus would not be considered normal.

Another problem is that what is normal and average in one segment of society may be considered not normal by another segment. The most common example is the teenage behaviors that occur in each generation that drive their parents to distraction. The occupational therapist must be alert so that the individual is not assessed as abnormal because the behavior is not common according to the therapist's standard. The same precaution applies to selecting an outcome or goal of intervention. Not every client has to become one of the 68% or average. Some clients may be unable to reach the norm, others do not want to reach the norm, and still others may select to reach beyond the norm.

OCCUPATIONAL THERAPY AND REHABILITATION

The rehabilitation model of health is not really a separate health model. It is presented because occupational therapists will incur the rehabilitation model many times in practice and thus should be familiar with the basic rationale. Also, the federal government has strongly supported the model.

Rehabilitation has been defined since 1942 as the "restoration of the handicapped to the fullest physical, mental, social, vocation and educational usefulness of which they are capable" (18). The rehabilitation model has two types. One type is an extension of the biomedical model. The physician looks for problems that can be corrected or improved through the use of drugs or surgery. The goal is to decrease limitations of structure and function in the body. This type may be called biorehabilitation.

The second type is an extension of several socially oriented models that stress capacity to perform roles and exhibit behavior consistent with social demands. Rehabilitation counselors, social workers, and psychologists frequently use the second type of rehabilitation, called social rehabilitation.

Both types of rehabilitation are based on the mechanistic model and focus on the productive or work-oriented goal. The person is expected to conform to the rehabilitation specialist's criteria as to what constitutes a successful rehabilitation. Conformity, not individual style, is the key to receiving rehabilitation services.

The problem with the rehabilitation model is the concern with achieving results that allow the professional to close the file and discharge the client either as fully rehabilitated or as unable to benefit from service. The latter category is for people who cannot or do not conform and perform to expectations set by rehabilitation personnel. In other words, the person must fit the program; the program does not adjust beyond present limits to accommodate the client. Occupational therapy should be concerned with meeting the client's needs, not having the client meet the therapist's needs.

In summary, no perfect or ideal model of health exists for occupational therapists to follow. Rather, occupational therapists must select the best aspects from the health models that most closely fit the beliefs and values of occupational therapy. Ultimately, occupational therapy may need to develop its own definition of health in which the performance of occupations is viewed as the central measure of health status.

References

1. American Heritage Dictionary. Boston: Houghton Mifflin, 1975:985.
2. Pepper SC. World Hypotheses. Berkeley: University of California Press, 1942.
3. Offer D, Sabshin M. Normality. New York: Basic Books, 1974.
4. Leifer R. In the Name of Mental Health: Social Functions of Psychiatry. New York: Science House, 1969.
5. Engel SL. The need for a new medical model: a challenge for biomedicine. Science 1977;196:129–136.
6. Commission on Chronic Illness. Prevention of Chronic Illness. Cambridge: Harvard University Press, 1957:4.
7. Tubesing NL. Whole Person Health Care: Philosophical Assumptions. Hinsdale, IN: Society for Holistic Medicine, 1977.
8. Cumming J, Cumming E. Ego and Milieu. New York: Atherton Press, 1967.
9. Sullivan D. Model for comprehensive systematic program development in health education. Health Educ Rep 1973;1:4–5.
10. Commission on Chronic Illness. Prevention of Chronic Illness. Cambridge: Harvard University Press, 1957:3–15.
11. Flapan D, Neubauer PB. Issues in assessing developing. Child Psychiatr 1970;9: 669–687.
12. Friedrick D. A Primer for Developmental Methodology. Minneapolis: Burgess, 1972.
13. Llorens L. Application of a Developmental Theory for Health and Rehabilitation. Rockville, MD: American Occupational Therapy Association, 1967.
14. Wu R. Behavior and Illness. Englewood Cliffs, NJ: Prentice Hall, 1973.
15. Parson T. Definitions of health and illness in the light of American values and social structure. In: Jaco EG. Patients, Physicians and Illness. New York: Free Press, 1958:165–187.
16. Dunn HL. High Level Wellness. Arlington, VA: RW Beatly, 1961.
17. Jahoda M. Current Concepts of Positive Mental Health. New York: Basic Books, 1958.
18. Symposium on the Process of Rehabilitation. National Council on Rehabilitation, Washington, DC, 1944.

CHAPTER 15

Understanding Conceptual and Practice Models

Because concepts form the framework of theoretical models, looking for concepts is a logical starting point. Concepts are usually noun or adjective-noun phrases. Occasionally, a preposition also appears as in activities of daily living, the verb form appears such as adapts, or an adverb form appears such as holistically. Some common concepts in models of occupational therapy are occupation, occupational performance, occupational competence, person or individual, role, skills, tasks, environment, context, adaptation, adaptive behavior, adaptive response, learning, developmental sequence, sensorimotor, cognition, psychosocial, self-care, activities of daily living, work, productivity, leisure, and play. Sometimes, a concept is presented with a definition such as: Occupations are the ordinary and familiar things that people do everyday (1). Most often, concepts are presented with a description such as: Occupation occurs routinely in a person's everyday life. Sometimes, several concepts appear in a short sentence such as: A person adapts to the environment through occupation. This short sentence includes four concepts: person, adapts (adaptation), environment, and occupation. The sentence is also an assumption because it is a broad general statement. Concepts often appear in statements of assumption. Assumption statements are easiest to find when they begin with key words such as assume, assumption, axiom, axiomatic, belief, believe, idea, maxim, postulate, predicate, premise, principle, propose, proposition, theory, theorize, theoretical, and viewpoint. An example might be as follows: This model is based on the belief that each person should be treated holistically. Holism is thus a concept in the model.

Concepts can also be divided into major and minor. Major concepts form the central focus of the theoretical model. Most often, there are three major concepts. In complex models, there may be three concepts, each of which can be further divided into three, making a total of twelve concepts. Occasionally, there are two, four, or five major concepts, but the most common number is three. Major concepts are often presented first in a description of the model and appear frequently in the discussion of the model.

Minor concepts are used to support, illustrate, and explain the major concepts. The number of minor concepts depends on the complexity of the model. There may be only five or six minor concepts or there may be as many as thirty. At some point, the number of minor concepts becomes difficult to understand and relate to the major concepts. When too many concepts exist, the model becomes too complex for practical use. Almost always, a suggestion is made to the author of the model that simplification is needed.

To learn about a new model, the best approach is to identify as quickly as possible the major focus or assumption and the three major concepts. Usually, an understanding of the three major concepts and their interrelationship will provide a good basic understanding of the model. For example, a simple explanation of Ayres' model of sensory integration is the understanding that she assumed the "near" senses were more important in organizing and integrating in the nervous system than the "far" senses. "Near" senses usually require direct contact by the person's body with the source of information or stimulus. "Far" senses, such as vision and hearing, provide information without direct contact. Ayres proposed there are three key "near" senses: proprioception, tactile, and vestibular. These three senses are the major focus of discussion about the model of sensory integration and form the basis for practice using the sensory integration model. Practice is thus based on how to help the person achieve sensory organization and integration of the proprioceptive, tactile, and vestibular senses into the nervous system to facilitate learning and performance of daily tasks. With this quick overview, a student or therapist should understand that learning about the model of sensory integration will require considerable attention focused on the function of the proprioceptive, tactile, and vestibular senses and how they are integrated into the nervous system. To practice occupational therapy using the model of sensory integration will require learning to use the assessment instruments that identify deficits in sensory integration and to use the equipment and teaching techniques which best facilitate sensory integration.

Thus, in practice models, assessment instruments measure the concepts to confirm their existence or lack of same. Equipment and teaching techniques are designed to facilitate the attainment of the concept to some level of performance. In research models, concepts often become the variables that are manipulated by the research design.

Visual illustrations of the concepts can also help keep the important ones in mind. Figure 15.1 illustrates the three major sensory concepts and their interaction to obtain sensory integration. The three overlapping circles are called a Venn diagram, name for the person who first described the use of the diagram. Venn diagrams can be used to advantage in visualizing a model and for comparing one model to the next using the same visual illustration. Therefore, a Venn diagram will appear with each discussion of a model in the section.

Models can also be categorized by their major domain of concern—in other words, their most important organizing idea. Table 15.1 outlines the major domain of concern, and Table 15.2 chronologically lists the models by year of the original publication. In Chapter 17, eight models currently being used are briefly discussed, and in Chapter 18, eight recently developed conceptual models are

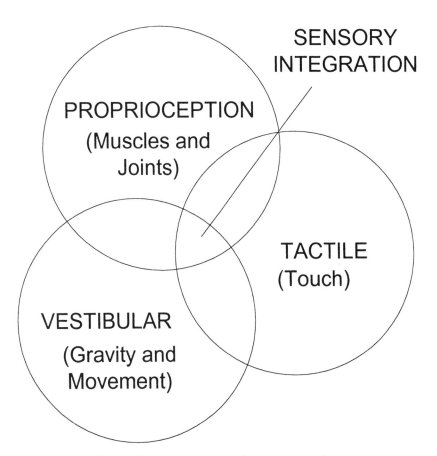

Figure 15.1. Major concepts of sensory integration.

Table 15.1. Models of Occupational Therapy by Domain of Concern

Adaptation Frame of Reference

Individual adaptation—Lorna Jean King
Temporal adaptation—Gary Kielhofner
Individual adaptation through occupation—Kathlyn Reed
Spatial–temporal adaptation—Eleanor Gilfoyle and Ann Grady
Occupational adaptation—Jeanette Schkade and Sally Schultz

Context/Ecology Frame of Reference

Ecological systems model—Margot Howe and Anne Briggs
Multicontext treatment approach—Joan Toglia
Ecology of human performance—Winnie Dunn, Catana Brown, Ann McGuigan
Person–environment–occupation model—Mary Law et al.

Occupation/Activity

Philosophy of occupational therapy/habit training—Adolf Meyer and Eleanor
    Clarke Slagle
Invalid occupation—Susan Tracy
Therapeutic occupation—William R. Dunton, MD (OT founder)
Occupational behavior—Mary Reilly
Model of human occupation—Gary Kielhofner
Activities model—Simme Cynkin
Model of occupational functioning—Catherine Tombly

Occupational Performance and Competence

AOTA educator model/Uniform Terminology
Client-centered practice—Task force of the Canadian Association of
    Occupational Therapy
Person–environment–occupational performance model—Charles Christiansen
    and Carolyn Baum
Occupational performance process model—Virginia Fearing, Mary Law, and
    Jo Clark
Occupational competence model—Helene Polatajko
Enablement model—Rose Martini, Helene Polatajko, and Ann Wilcox

Developmental Frame of Reference

Neurobehavioral model—Barbara Banus
Spatiotemporal adaptation—Eleanor Gilfoyle and Ann Grady
Facilitating growth and development—Lela Llorens
Recapitulation of ontogenesis—Anne Mosey
Group development—Anne Mosey
Human development through occupation—Patricia Clark (Allen)

Prevention

Prevention—Ruth Brunyate Weimer

Productivity

Graded occupation—Herbert Hall, MD (OT leader)
Preindustrial training—Thomas Kidner, AIA (OT founder)

continued

Table 15.1. Models of Occupational Therapy by Domain of Concern

Play/Leisure

Play as exploratory learning—Mary Reilly
Playfulness—Anita Bundy

Sensorimotor

Sensory skills
 Perceptual motor—A. Jean Ayres
 Sensory integration—A. Jean Ayres
Motor learning and motor control
 Contemporary task-oriented approach—Virgil Matheowetz and Julie Bass
  Haugen
Neurodevelopmental
 Reflex therapy—Mary Fiorentino
 Sensorimotor therapy—Margaret Rood
Biomechanical approach
 Biomechanical or restoration—Bird T. Baldwin, Psychologist (OT leader)
 Reconstruction—William R. Dunton (OT founder)
 Orthopedic model—Marjorie Taylor (OT Reg.)
 Kinetic occupational therapy—Sidney Licht, MD (OT leader)

Cognitive

Reeducation—George Barton
Cognitive disorders—Claudia Allen
Perceptual cognitive rehabilitation—Beatriz Abreu

Psychosocial

Object relations—H. Azima (psychiatrist)
Communication process—Gail and Jay Fidler
Doing and becoming—Gail Fidler
Activity therapy—Anne Mosey
Biopsychosocial model—Anne Mosey
Group work—Sharon Schwartzberg and Margot Howe

Professional Development

Clinical reasoning—Joan Rogers
Occupational science—Elizabeth Yerxa and Florence Clark

Table 15.2.   Models by Year of Major Publication

Year	Model
1910	Invalid occupation—Susan E. Tracy, Nurse Graded occupation—Herbert J Hall, MD
1911	Therapeutic occupation—William Rush Dunton Jr, MD
1918	Biomechanical or restoration model—Bird T. Baldwin (psychologist who started OT Dept at Walter Reed General Hospital)
1919	Reconstruction therapy—William Rush Dunton Jr, MD Reeducation—George E. Barton, architect
1922	Philosophy of occupation therapy—Adolph Meyer, MD Habit training—Eleanor Clarke Slagle, OT Reg
1925	Preindustrial training—Thomas B. Kidner (manual education teacher and architect)
1934	Orthopedic model—Marjorie Taylor, OT Reg
1947	Kinetic model—Sidney Licht, MD
1954	Sensorimotor therapy—Margaret Rood, OTR, RPT
1958	Perceptual motor development—A. Jean Ayres, OTR
1959	Object relations—H. Azima, MD
1961	Reflex development—Mary Fiorentino, OTR
1963	Communication process—Gail Fidler, OTR and Jay Fidler, MD
1966	Recapitualization of ontogenesis—Anne Mosey, OTR Occupational behavior—Mary Reilly, OTR
1968	Sensory integration—A. Jean Ayres, OTR
1970	Group development—Anne Mosey, OTR
1972	Prevention—Ruth Brunyate Weimer, OTR
1973	Activity therapy—Anne Mosey, OTR
1974	Play model—Mary Reilly, OTR Biopsychosoical model—Anne Mosey, OTR Program educator model—AOTA
1976	Human development through occupation—Patricia Nuse Clark (Allen), OTR Facilitating growth and development—Lela Llorens, OTR
1977	Temporal adaptation—Gary Kielhofner, OTR
1978	Activities model—Simme Cynkin, OTR Doing and becoming—Gail Fidler, OTR Individual adaptation—Lorna Jean King, OTR
1979	Neurobehavioral model—Barbara Banus, OTR Uniform terminology model—AOTA
1980	Model of human occupation—Gary Kielhofner, OTR Personal adaptation through occupation—Kathlyn Reed, OTR
1981	Spatiotemporal adaptation—Eleanor Gilfoyle, OTR and Ann Grady, OTR
1982	Clinical reasoning—Joan Rogers, OTR Ecological systems model—Margot Howe, OTR and Ann Briggs, OTR
1983	Client-centred practice—Task Force of the Canadian Association of Occupational Therapy
1985	Perceptual cognitive rehabilitation—Beatriz Abreu, OTR Cognitive disability—Claudia Allen, OTR Group work—Sharon Schwartzberg, OTR and Margot Howe, OTR

continued

Table 15.2.   Models by Year of Major Publication

1988	Occupational form and occupational performance—David Nelson, OTR
1989	Occupational science—Elizabeth J. Yerxa, OTR and Florence Clark, OTR
1991	Person–environment–occupational performance model—Charles Christiansen, OTR and Carolyn Baum, OTR
1992	Occupational adaptation—Jeanette Schkade, OTR and Sally Schulz, OTR
	Multicontext treatment approach—Janet Toglia, OTR
	Occupational competence model—Helene J. Polatajko, OT(C)
1994	Ecology of human performance—Winnie Dunn, OTR Catana Brown, OTR, Linda H. McClain, OTR, and Kay Westman, OTR
	Contemporary task-oriented approach—Virgil Mathiowetz, OTR and Julie Bass Haugen, OTR
1995	The enablement model—Rose Martini, OT(C), Helene J Polatajko, OT(C), and Ann Wilcox
	Model of occupational functioning (ends-means)—Catherine A Trombly, OTR
1996	Person-environment-occupation model—Mary Law, OT(C), Barbara Cooper, OT(C), Susan Strong, OT(C), Debra Stewart, OT(C), Patricia Ribgy, OT(C), and Lori Letts, OT(C)
1997	Occupational performance process model—Virginia Fearing, Mary Law, OT(C), and Jo Clark
	Playfulness—Anita Bundy, OTR

Table 15.3. Summary of Basic Concepts in Occupational Therapy Models

DEFICIT STATE		DIRECTION		MEDIUM		PROCESS	
dysfunction	which	improved	through	occupation	which	selected	based
disorder	can	increased	the use	environment	is . . .	purposeful	on. . . .
disability	be . . .	developed	of . . .	activity		picked	
handicap		prevented				goal	
illness		cured				-directed	
impairment		overcome					
limitation		ameliorated					
sickness		reduced					
unhealthy		maintained					
developmental delay		remediated					
loss of roles		rehabilitated					
condition		habilitated					

PERSONAL EXPERIENCE		COGNITIVE STATE		INTERNAL STATE		EXTERNAL STATE	
skills	which. . . .	engage	a person's	learning		social norms	or which is
abilities		employ		attention		environment	consistent
interests		direct		curiosity		demands &	with . . . .
knowledge		occupy		doing		limitations	
attitudes		take up		sense of			
aptitudes				exploration			
values				participation			

OUTCOME/GOAL/CRITERIA							
adaptation or adjustment		independence		reeducation		self-actualization	leading
function		performance		rehabilitation		well-being	to. . . .
habilitation		quality of life		restoration		wellness	
health		recovery					

presented along with a brief description, major concepts, significant interactions, assessment, intervention, and at least one Venn diagram.

Yet another way to view models is by a diagram of the common thought processes used to construct such models. Table 15.3 provides an outline of the thought process. The thought process is that a *deficit state* can be *changed* (direction) through the use of a *medium* which is *processed* based on specified *personal experience* in a *cognitive state, an internal state and/or an external state* which leads to an *outcome, goal, or criterion.*

The next chapter discusses some models that are not part of occupational therapy practice but are commonly confused with occupational therapy practice. These models are discussed to assist in discriminating what is and is not occupational therapy knowledge and practice.

CHAPTER 16

Models Discarded by Occupational Therapy

As a profession evolves, many models may surface to be explored and analyzed. Some will be discarded because they do not fulfill the promise of the original concepts forming the core of professional practice. Others must be discarded because current realities make implementing the concept impractical. This chapter reviews some of the models that do not fulfill the promise of occupational therapy in today's world. The models are shown in Figure 16.1.

OCCUPATIONAL THERAPY VERSUS IDLENESS AND BUSY WORK

In the papers read at the first annual conference for occupational therapy in 1917, there are several references to the word "idleness." Herbert J. Hall, for example, says, "It seems clearer now than ever before that idleness, long continued, is a menace, not only to the proper functioning of the body, but also the morale and the spirit of the individual" (1). The remedy was work in occupations that ranged from service to the institution to arts and crafts. The initial benefit was supposed to be that occupations killed time and were diversionary. In other words, occupational therapy could be used to provide busywork, keeping patients busy doing something rather than nothing.

Elizabeth Upham admits that "in certain advanced and chronic cases, this is all that can be claimed" (2). Of course, certain disorders, such as tuberculosis, were treated in the early 1900s by sending the person to the hospital or sanitarium to rest. Today, however, few people can afford a long rest, and few disorders need to be treated by prolonged bed rest as a result of new drugs and surgical techniques.

The problem is that providing busy work and diversion continues to be identified with occupational therapy. Such identification is no longer of value to the profession. A busy occupational therapist and modern health care center cannot afford the luxury of providing, or paying someone to provide, patients with busy work and diversion from idleness. If a hospital has patients who need diversional activities, technical personnel with the assistance of volunteers can provide prepackaged or simple craft projects. Outpatients or other persons living in the community can be directed to hobby shops, community projects, and

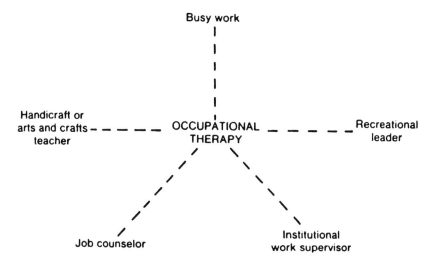

Figure 16.1. Discarded models of occupational therapy.

adult education for instruction in diversional arts and crafts. Occupational therapy does not have a role in providing busy work or diversional activity to simply kill time.

OCCUPATIONAL THERAPY VERSUS VOCATIONAL TRAINING

A common error made by people unfamiliar with occupational therapy is to assume that the word "occupation" is synonymous with the word "vocation." Thus, these people reason that occupational therapy must be concerned with helping people find jobs. Of course, the interpretation is not accurate. Occupational therapists are not employment counselors, job placement specialists, or vocational counselors.

Occupational therapists are interested in the person's ability to engage in productive work and may assist the individual to gain basic productive skills. However, the role of occupational therapy is much broader than the attention to productive skills alone. Attention also is paid to self-maintenance and leisure needs and skills. Nevertheless, it is true that occupational therapists may work in settings that stress productive work, such as sheltered workshops. Their function may include teaching and assessing a certain number of work skills. The primary difference between employment counselors and occupational therapists is the ability of therapists to teach and assess self-maintenance and leisure skills as well as to help the individual learn to balance the three occupational areas for better life adjustment and satisfaction.

OCCUPATIONAL THERAPY VERSUS HANDICRAFT TEACHING

One of the media that occupational therapy has used for many years is arts and crafts. Many specific arts and crafts, such as weaving, ceramics, and woodworking, have properties and processes that can be used to help clients to follow directions, use judgment, channel aggression, or cooperate with others.

The problem is that some institutions have hired occupational therapists solely to teach handicrafts. Patients or residents indicate which art or craft they wish to learn, and the occupational therapist teaches this handicraft. No individual treatment plan with specific goals or objectives is developed.

The use of occupational therapists to teach handicrafts is expensive and does not use the occupational therapist's knowledge and skills to full advantage. Many persons without a degree in occupational therapy are excellent craftsmen and artists with good teaching skills. Such persons can be assigned to occupational therapy if professional supervision is needed. However, the occupational therapist should not be employed primarily to teach handicrafts. The only exception might be teaching a particular craft to a person who needed to learn a leisure time skill to maintain a level of independent functioning. Otherwise, occupational therapists use arts and crafts only when such handicrafts provide a task that will facilitate a person to learn or gain a certain occupational goal.

In summary, occupational therapists are not handicraft teachers for disabled, ill, or injured persons. All use of handicrafts in occupational therapy is goal-directed according to a treatment plan. Teaching the handicraft is a means to an end, not the end in itself.

OCCUPATIONAL THERAPY VERSUS RECREATIONAL PROGRAMS

Occupational therapy has included some use of sports and table games as part of the media employed for numerous purposes. For example, a baseball game provides a group activity where cooperation is needed to have an effective team. Games, such as checkers or tic-tac-toe, require attention and visual perceptual skills. All games require that a person learn the rules and abide by them. Thus, games can be analyzed for the useful properties and selected when these properties assist a person to learn or relearn a specific performance skill. However, recreational games are not taught for the sake of teaching the game. An occupational therapist, therefore, should not be employed as a recreational leader whose primary purpose is to develop a schedule of recreational activities for a group of people who might otherwise have nothing interesting to do. The services of an occupational therapist should be used to develop and implement programs based on assessed needs of an individual person or group of persons with similar needs for occupational skill development.

A recreational activity program could be implemented by persons with knowledge of a variety of sports and table games but with limited professional training.

The occupational therapist may provide supervisory skills, or a qualified therapeutic recreation specialist may be hired.

In summary, the occupational therapist should not be employed as a recreational leader who plans a schedule of "fun and games" activities. The occupational therapist uses recreational games only when such games are part of the activities that may assist a person or persons to gain specific goals as outlined in a plan for that person or persons.

OCCUPATIONAL THERAPIST VERSUS CONSTITUTIONAL WORK SUPERVISOR

When occupational therapy was developing in the early 1900s, institutions, especially psychiatric hospitals, assigned patients to perform work needed to maintain the hospital functions. Some of the work included activities that could be done in an occupational therapy clinic, such as weaving material, making brooms, sewing, mending and washing clothes, and making pottery. The institution could save money by having the work done within the institution, patients had something to keep them occupied, and patients did not have to be paid.

Although the work was ostensibly for good of the patients, the needs of the institution often came before the needs of the patients. Occupational therapists could find themselves being directed by the institution to assign patients to work activity for the purpose of getting the work done, not on the basis of meeting a planned goal in the patient's treatment program.

In the early 1970s, a human rights movement was begun to make illegal the practice of using patients as cheap, captive labor to accomplish the institution's work. This legal opinion has forced institutions and some occupational therapists to rethink the role of occupational therapy in such institutions. In essence, occupational therapy should not be used as a means of accomplishing service or work for the institution. Occupational therapy must provide a service to a patient based on the assessment of that patient's needs. The patient's needs, not the institution's needs, should be the focus of any activity that person does. The institution should not expect to get its work done by the patients, nor should the institution have the occupational therapist demand that a patient perform services primarily to benefit the institution.

References

1. Hall HJ. Renumerative occupations for the handicapped. Mod Hosp 1917;8:383–386.
2. Upham EG. Some principles of occupational therapy. Mod Hosp 1917;8:409–413.

CHAPTER 17

Models Currently
in Practice

HABIT TRAINING—ADOLF MEYER AND ELEANOR CLARKE SLAGLE

Frame of Reference

Habit training is the oldest model of occupational therapy practice. It was developed by Slagle and Meyer in 1913–14 while both were at the Henry Phipps Clinic at Johns Hopkins in Baltimore (1, 2). Today, much of the idealogy of habit training has been integrated into every mental health setting to the extent that identification with occupational therapy may be difficult to pinpoint. Nevertheless, occupational therapy—in cooperation with the nursing profession—organized habit training, and it remains today but the label has been lost.

Assumptions

Habit training is a practice model based in part on the idea developed during the arts and crafts movement that life should be simplified and become as routine as possible. A second major organizing idea is based on Adolf Meyer's concept of disorganized habits as a major cause of the behavior seen in schizophrenia. Meyer saw the behavior of persons with schizophrenia as indicative that occupational cycles had become unbalanced or out of balance. This unbalance resulted in loss of the organizing and stabilizing (and therefore healthful) effects of work, play, rest, and sleep. The lack or loss of balance of occupation was evidence by the disorganized or disordered habits displayed by the person with schizophrenia.

Concepts

Habit training is based on the concepts of balance, order, and sequence of occupational cycles and habit forming as a learning process (Figure 17.1). A balance of occupational cycles includes alternating cycles or rhythms of work, play, rest, and sleep over time such as a 24-hour day. The belief is that each person should have occupations that are orderly, sequenced, scheduled, patterned, or routine. This belief was developed into a practice model by scheduling cycles of occupations into a 24-hour day, which becomes the treatment plan. For each patient, a schedule is developed

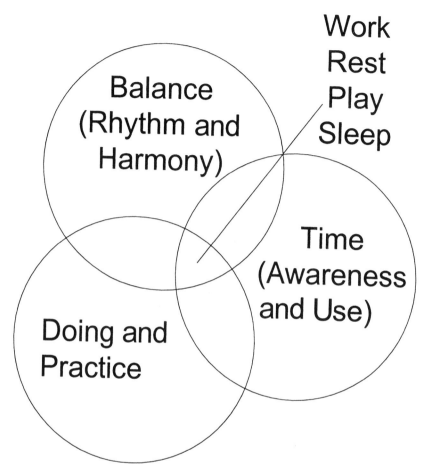

Figure 17.1. Habit organization by Adolph Meyer.

that is organized, orderly, sequenced, and patterned. The schedule may be individualized or part of a group plan. When a person follows the 24-hour schedule of occupational cycles over time (days, weeks, and months), the schedule becomes habitual.

Expected Results

Clients were expected to organize or reorganize their lives according to a schedule and to do what was expected of them according to the scheduled event or task. Normal or acceptable social behavior was expected. At the same time, clients were expected to control abnormal or unacceptable behavior.

Assessment

The behavior (occupational habits) could be assessed and documented by having a person record (or someone else) record what he or she was doing (occupying the time) at regular time intervals, such as 15 minutes or hourly, for one or more days. Examples include a person who spends most of the day in bed sleeping but wanders around much of the night, another person who sits for hours "looking out the window" or perhaps hallucinating, and a third person who aimlessly moves about or talks frequently most of the time. All the examples lack the regular cycles of work, play, rest, and sleep, which are assumed to provide the order and sequence of occupational cycles.

Intervention Strategies

As a practice model, habit training involves establishing a schedule of occupational cycles into an orderly pattern and teaching patients/clients to follow the schedule until it becomes a habit and thus habit formation has occurred (Figure 17.2). Intervention is aimed at assisting the individual to establish and maintain (habit formation) an occupational cycle that is orderly and scheduled throughout the day and from one day to the next. Initially, the person may be placed with a group of patients/clients who all have the same schedule, but as the person improves, the schedule is changed from group to individual activity.

Analysis

Although the term habit training may not be used today, the concept is very much in evidence. Almost all treatment centers provide a basic schedule of activities or "things to do." Patients/clients are expected to follow this basic schedule. As they improve, the schedule is modified to provide more individualized activities. If a treatment center did not have a basic schedule, the facility would be considered to be "warehousing" the patients/clients.

OCCUPATIONAL BEHAVIOR MODEL—MARY REILLY

Frame of Reference

Mary Reilly began publishing her study of occupations in 1966 (3). She suggested that occupation should be studied primarily in the behavioral sciences such as psychology, sociology, and anthropology. Specific areas of study include developmental, achievement, and role theory (Figure 17.3) She also suggested that the term occupation encompasses a broader definition than "work for pay." One's occupations include anything that engages one's time, energy, and resources.

Occupational behavior is based on Meyer's and Slagle's work but expands the emphasis on developing a conceptual model that can be studied and researched

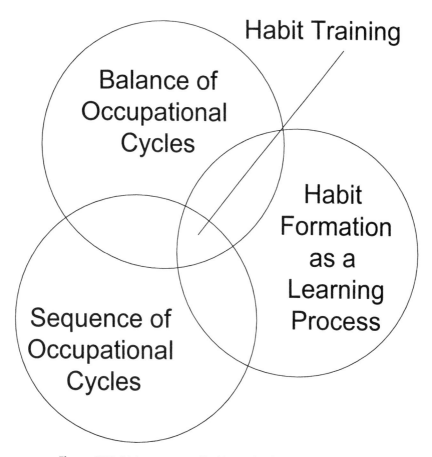

Figure 17.2. Major concept of habit training by Eleanor Clarke Slagle.

as well as applied in practice. Reilly is primarily responsible for increasing the profession's interest in model building.

Assumptions

Inherent in occupation is: 1) some motive, purpose, or reason for engaging or doing something; 2) some level of interest in or awareness of what one is doing; and 3) some level of ability, aptitude, or skill in actually doing the occupation. Thus, models concerned with the concept of occupation address the issues of why people engage in occupation, when individuals develop the ability or learn to perform certain occupations, and what happens to occupational performance if the abilities or skills are not developed or learned.

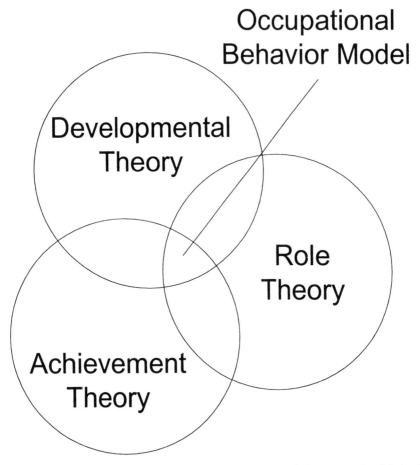

Figure 17.3. Theoretical influences on the development of the occupational behavior model.

Reilly believed that humans have a vital or inherent need for occupation because, through the use of occupations, human beings could master, alter, and improve the environment. Furthermore, she thought that society and culture determined the specific occupations that an individual would learn. Therefore, her
model of occupational behavior is based on the assumption that occupations are
developmentally acquired (4). As Figure 17.4 shows, occupational behavior is
concerned with the developmental continuum of play and work that contributes
to the level of competence, achievement, and occupational role that a person will
attain.

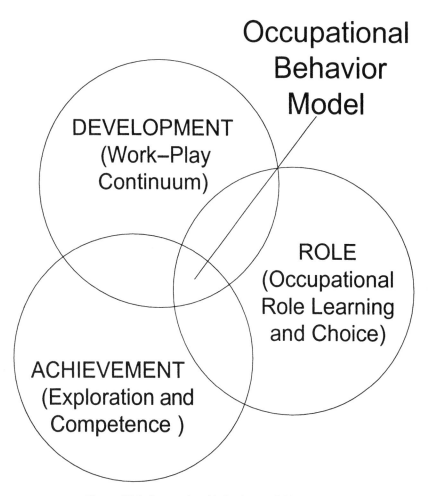

Figure 17.4. Occupational behavior model by Mary Reilly.

Concepts

Competence is described as having sufficient or adequate behavior to meet the demands of the situation. Achievement is a specified level of success, attainment, or proficiency. There are three occupational role systems: gender identification, group membership, and occupational behavior. Specific occupational roles are not limited to paid employment and, therefore, can include housewife, student, preschooler, volunteer, or retiree.

Expected Results

Reilly proposed that the role of occupational therapy is to prevent and reduce the incapacities in occupational behavior that result from illness. In other words, the job of occupational therapy is to activate the residual forces within the individual so that the person can carry on the daily activities required by his or her role in society. The person could contribute to the process of therapy and should not be a passive recipient of service. Therapy should be directed toward individual achievement. Reilly is well-known for her statement that "Man, through the use of his hands as they are energized by mind and will, can influence the state of his own health" (5). She means that the individual possesses the inner resources to regain health. The job of the therapist is to tap the resources and facilitate the individual's participation in self-controlled recovery.

Assessment

Reilly did not develop any specific assessments herself, but several of her students did. Probably the best known is the Interest Check List by Matsasuya (6).

Intervention Strategies

Although the emphasis in the occupational behavior model is on building occupational behavior and performance, Reilly recognized that occupational behavior does not exist in a vacuum and that health involves a dynamic balance between work, play, rest, and sleep. Therefore, a complete therapy program would provide opportunities for practicing life skills in a balanced pattern of daily living, which takes into account individual interests and abilities and tailors events to age, sex, and occupational roles.

Analysis

Reilly began the modern emphasis on organizing the ideas about occupation and occupational therapy into recognizable conceptual and practice models. She updated much of the thinking expressed by Meyer and Slagle. She also encouraged students to explore the meaning and purpose of occupation in daily life.

MODEL OF HUMAN OCCUPATION—KIELHOFNER, BURKE, IGI, AND OTHERS

Frame of Reference

One of Reilly's student's, Gary Kielhofner, expanded the concept of occupation further by suggesting that occupation be studied as an open system that interacts with the environment by the process of input, throughput, output, and feedback (7). In other words, a person is changed by the environment and, in turn, can cause change in the environment. The process is interactive, not unidirectional.

Assumptions

The human system is assumed to be a dynamic, changing, open system that interacts with the environment based on analysis of the volitional, habituation, and mind–body subsystems (see Concepts). Human occupation can be analyzed into three occupational forms: work, play, and daily living tasks. Human occupation is performed in three contexts or environments: temporal, physical, and sociocultural. In other words, human occupational performance is the result of the dynamic and meaningful interaction between occupational form, context, and human system.

Concepts

Kielhofner's model of human occupation proposes three subsystems that form a hierarchy loosely correlated with age (Figure 17.5). First is the volition subsystem, which guides the choices of action through personal causation, valued goals, and interest. Second is the habituation subsystem, which is comprised of habits and internalized roles. Habits and roles function to maintain action. Third is the performance subsystem, which produces action through skills, including physical, cognitive, and social skills. Change in the system (individual) is the result of the interaction of the three subsystems to produce the motives of exploration, competency, and achievement that lead to occupational functioning (Figure 17.6).

Expected Results

According to Kielhofner, occupational therapy is useful in assisting an individual to make the transition from one stage or subsystem to the next. Also, occupational therapy may be helpful in reorganizing the system (individual) to facilitate adjustment to the environment and restore a normal course of occupational development (8).

Assessments

Kielhofner and his students have developed several assessments. Among them are the Occupational Performance History Interview (9).

Planning and Intervention

The practice model is based on the concept of occupational dysfunction, which may occur when a person does not use his or her capacities to respond according to society's expectations or when personal behavior results in loss of meaning, hope, habits, and/or roles. Assessment involves examining the strengths and limitations of the person's system organization, environmental influences on occupational behavior, and the person's system dynamics when engaged in occupation within the individual's environment.

Intervention includes increasing the strengths of the person's system organization, using occupational form to promote change and using context and environment to organize occupations.

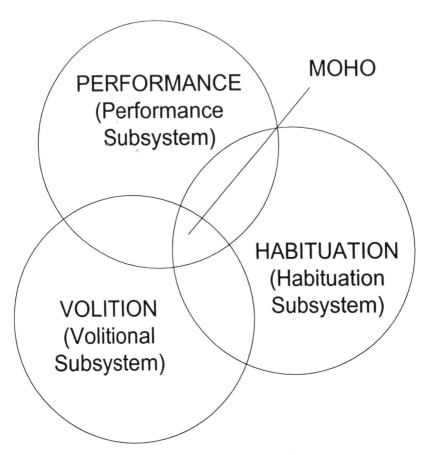

Figure 17.5. Model of human occupation (MOHO) by Gary Kielhofner.

Summary

The model of human occupation is a complex model with many minor concepts. Over the years since the model was originally published in 1980, concepts have been added, such as occupational form and the importance of concepts changed.

BIOMECHANICAL MODEL

Frame of Reference

The biomechanical approach, also called the kinesiological model, is based on the application of kinetics and kinematics to movement of the human body by the muscles and skeleton. As such, the biomechanical approach is organized in the

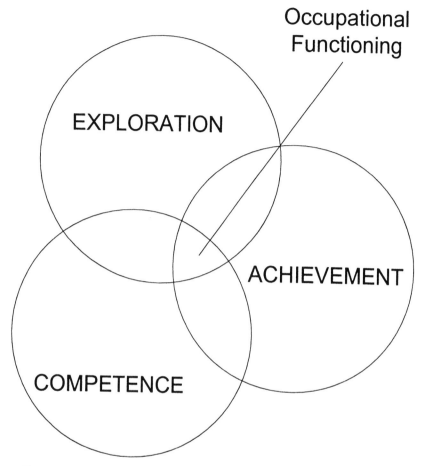

Figure 17.6. Levels of occupational functioning by Gary Kielhofner and colleagues.

logic of the mechanistic philosophy. Human movement and equilibrium are reduced to the mechanical principles involved in the action of physical forces, levers,
and torques on the body and how these physical forces (weights of objects), levers
(bones and joints), and torques (muscles) affect the extent and quality of the movement and equilibrium. The study of mechanical physics is useful to understanding and applying the biomechanical approach.

Typical disorders to which the biomechanical approach has been applied include
fractures, amputation, traumatic injuries, burns, and motor unit and nerve disorders
(10). Specific diagnoses include rheumatoid arthritis, Guillain-Barré syndrome, mus-
cular dystrophy, stroke, Parkinson's disease, and other orthopedic conditions.

Assumptions

The primary assumptions incorporated in the biomechanical approach are based on physics. The body functions like a machine and thus can be studied as a machine.

Concepts

The important concepts are range of motion, muscle strength, and physical endurance (Figure 17.7). *Range of motion* is the arc of movement through which a joint can move. Passive range of motion means the arc of movement through which an external power source, such as a therapist, can move the joint. Active range of motion is the arc of movement the individual can move the joint by voluntary effort. *Muscle strength* is the degree of muscle power when movement is re-

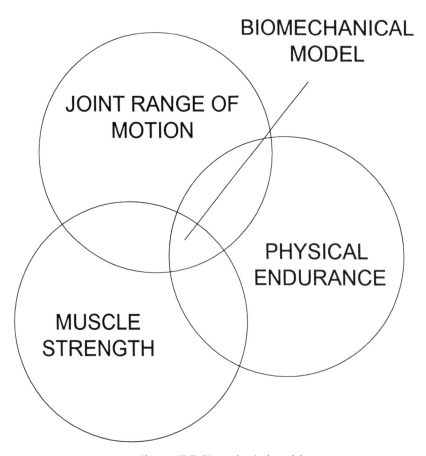

Figure 17.7. Biomechanical model.

sisted with weight or gravity. *Physical endurance* involves the sustained cardiac, pulmonary, and musculoskeletal exertion over time.

Important secondary concepts are balance and equilibrium and joint stability and mobility. Balance and equilibrium involve the position and maintenance of head, neck, trunk, and limb alignment when body weight is shifted using protective or equilibrium reactions. Joint stability involves the integrity of the joint structures to maintain position under load. Joint mobility involves the ease with which the joint moves from one position to another.

Expected Results

Expected results are an increase in the range or arc of motion of individual joints, an increase the strength of individual and groups of muscles, an increase physical endurance and prevention of deformity, or a decrease in the effects of deformity, when and where possible. In instances in which the individual cannot perform part or all of a movement or task, assistive technology may be provided to reduce the effects of disability

Assessment

Joint range of motion is measured using a goniometer (protractor with extended arms). Several normative value charts are available.

Muscle strength testing is measured either manually or with a dynamometer. Measurement may be for a single maximum effort or an average of several efforts.

Physical endurance is measured in the amount of time a person can sustain activity and/or performance of selected tasks. Activity level may be minimal, moderate, or maximum.

Posture and equilibrium are measured using the following methods. Standing posture is measured using a plum line or by taking a photograph against a background grid. Symmetry of posture can be observed or examined against a background grid. Equilibrium can be measured using a tilt board or by walking on a straighten line or within a certain set of lines.

Joint stability is measured usually by manually moving the joint in a pattern of motions while pulling and pushing (stretching and compressing) the joint and joint structures. It is also measured by observing the joint under load (weight).

Joint mobility is measured by manually moving the joint in a pattern of motions while observing whether the movement is smooth and easy to move or whether there is resistance to movement possibly caused by adhesions or contractures.

Planning and Intervention

Techniques frequently considered in planning intervention are isolated or coordinated movements, rhythmical or arrhythmical movements, linear or diagonal movements, reciprocal (symmetrical) or asymmetrical movements, movements to

SECTION IV / THE MODELS BASE

increase or maintain range of motion, and movements against maximum resistance or maximal repetitions (10). Dutton also suggests that isolate, rhythmical, linear, and reciprocal movements increased range of motion and maximal resistance are most easily accomplished through therapeutic exercise (enabling activities), whereas coordinated, arrhythmical, diagonal, and asymmetrical movements; maintenance of range of motion; and maximal repetitions for endurance are more easily achieved through purposeful activity. In other words, there is a progress from easier to more difficult movements, range of motion, and endurance. When the client is only capable of isolate, rhythmical, linear, and reciprocal movements, exercise and other enabling activities should be used. As the client progresses, coordinated, arrhythmical, diagonal, and asymmetrical movements can be attained, purposeful activities should be incorporated. The same logic is applied to increasing versus maintaining range of motion and increasing strength versus improving endurance.

Analysis

Analysis of the biomechanical approach suggests three ideas should be kept in mind if the approach is applied in an occupational therapy service program. First, the biomechanical approach does not automatically provide the client with much opportunity to plan and participate in the process of therapy. The role of the client in the biomechanical approach can be totally passive. Occupational therapy personnel must be creative in finding ways to increase the client's active participation.

Second, the client is likely to display noncompliant behavior because his or her role is largely passive.

Third, the biomechanical approach does not incorporate the strengths of occupational therapy service delivery. It is, however, attractive to occupational therapy personnel because it is does provide many of the adjunctive methods and enabling activities that are useful during the acute phase of treatment. In addition, other health care personnel, especially physical therapists and physiatrists, understand the biomechanical approach and its language because they use the approach extensively. Communication between health care team members is often facilitated by use of the biomechanical approach or by adapting the language of another approach to the biomechanical frame of reference.

NEURODEVELOPMENTAL THERAPY

Frame of Reference

Neurodevelopmental therapy, called also neurodevelopmental treatment, NDT, or Bobath approach, was developed originally by Karl Bobath, a neurophysiologist, and Bertha Bobath, a physical therapist, to treat children with cerebral palsy (11). Later, they applied the principles to persons with hemiplegia poststroke (12). The model is based on neurophysiology. Development applies only to the assumption of how the nervous system matures. There are no true stages of development in the model, and no attempt is made in therapy to facilitate development of any specific motor milestone. Primary work on the model was done from the 1940s through the 1960s.

The originating ideas are from the English neurologist, J. Hughlings Jackson. Jackson proposed that the nervous system is organized hierarchically beginning with the spinal cord as the lowest level; moving next through the brainstem, cerebrum, and midbrain; then to the subcortical or basal ganglia area; and finally to the cerebral cortex or highest level. Therefore, motor control follows the same sequence. Motor control is concerned with reflexes, reactions to movement, synergies, and mass movement patterns.

Assumptions

The nervous system is assumed to be organized into a series of levels of control with each succeeding or higher level having control over all preceding or lower levels. In other words, a hierarchy is assumed starting with the spinal cord and ending with the cortex.

The brain, especially the cortex, contains centralized programs that control muscle activation patterns, muscle tone, and posture. Thus, control is organized from the top down.

The central programs are based on reflexes and reactions. Primitive reflexes occur first and influence muscle tone and postural control. They are inhibited by the righting and equilibrium (automatic) reactions. The result is an organized nervous system capable of increasing complex movement patterns.

A separation of reflex and voluntary movement exists. Voluntary movement occurs after the primitive reflexes are inhibited and the righting and equilibrium reactions are facilitated.

In either congenital or acquired injury, there is a release of abnormal reflex patterns of posture and movement from inhibit or control. Higher centers of control either have not taken over control (congenital) or have been damaged resulting in loss of inhibition over the lower centers (acquired).

Treatment on the injured brain is based on the five assumptions (8). The first is that foundation skills should be remediated first. Foundation skills include midline symmetry, righting reactions, trunk rotation, and others related to facilitating normal posture and movement. Second, normal movement is learned through experiencing what normal movement feels like (feedback). Third, postural control or stability is essential for movement (mobility). Fourth, normal movement requires normal muscle tone. Normal movement cannot be imposed on abnormal tone. Fifth, the central programs in the brain can be modified through experience with normal movement patterns.

Concepts

The primary concepts are motor patterns or synergies, postural reflexes and reactions, and muscle tone (Figure 17.8). Normal and abnormal motor patterns and muscle synergies are groups of muscle that work or respond together to create total flexion or extension of an arm or leg more readily than would otherwise be possible. In abnormal conditions, motor patterns and synergies are present in greater or lesser amounts than would be expected. Postural or attitudinal reflexes are involuntary, stereotyped responses to a stimulus related to the position of the head and/or body to gravity and horizontal or vertical planes. These reflexes are assumed to contribute to the developmental of postural control. Postural control is the use of automatic re-

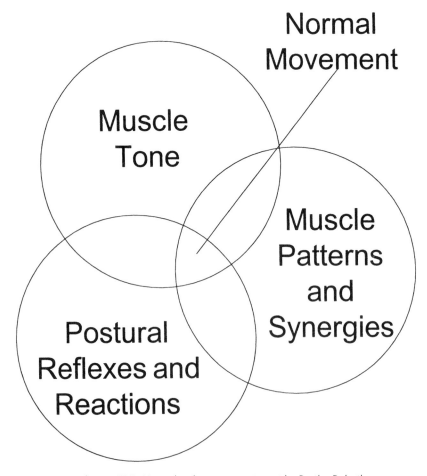

Figure 17.8. Neurodevelopment treatment by Bertha Bobath.

action patterns, including righting and equilibrium reactions as well as postural sets, to maintain posture, balance and equilibrium, and positioning. Muscle tone is defined as the slight degree of contraction that muscles maintain when inactive. Normal muscle tone keeps muscles in good condition and makes it possible for them to respond. In abnormal movement conditions, muscle tone also affects the quality of the movement by decreasing to create floppy tone or increasing to create spasticity.

Expected Results

Expected results are to modify the response of the central nervous system by breaking up abnormal motor patterns synergies and inhibiting abnormal tone and primitive reflexes, thereby achieving a balance between muscle groups and a decrease in the effects of abnormal tonal influences on automatic responses and movement patterns.

Areas of Assessment

Movement patterns and synergies are usually observed as the person stands or moves. For example, the flexion synergy of the arm in a person with hemiplegia shows the characteristic flexed elbow less than 90° with the wrist flexed and the fingers curled into the hand. An extension pattern exists as well. Reflexes and reactions are measured by the presences or absence of primitive, righting, and equilibrium reflexes and reactions. Muscle tone is measured in subjective values of normal, low or flopping, and high or spastic. Postural control is measured by observation and the results of reflexes, reactions, muscle tone, and synergies.

Planning and Intervention

Therapy is planned and implemented on the basis of facilitation and inhibition. Facilitation, to make easier, is designed to increase the likelihood of a normal muscle contraction or a "mature" righting or equilibrium reflex response. Inhibition, to make harder, decreases the likelihood of an abnormal muscle contraction or primitive reflex response by encouraging the higher centers of the brain to dampen or override the effects of the lower centers. Facilitation and inhibition are accomplished through the use of handling techniques that are the manner in which the therapist uses the hands to stop abnormal tone and movement and to encourage active normal tone and movement. Key points of control are the specific hand placements on the client's trunk and limbs used to change muscle tone and quality of movement.

Analysis

In recent years, the idea of a strict hierarchy identical for everyone has been replaced with the notion of distributed control within the nervous system, degrees of freedom of movement determined by joint positions and environment demand

(Figure 17.9). Therefore, some of the assumptions on which neurodevelopmental therapy is based have been challenged. Another problem is the lack of application from therapy into functional activities of daily life. Motor patterns or synergies are rarely used in performing activities of daily living. Almost always the patterns are varied to perform a specific skill. Inhibiting primitive reflexes does not automatically generate normal movement. A third problem for occupational therapists is to remember that neurodevelopmental therapy was developed within a mechanistic view. Clients can easily become, to the therapist, so many primitive reflexes with abnormal tone and motor patterns. The individual client as a person can be lost. In fact, intervention can be done to the client in such a manner as to avoid speaking to the client beyond saying hello and good-bye. Occupational therapy practition-

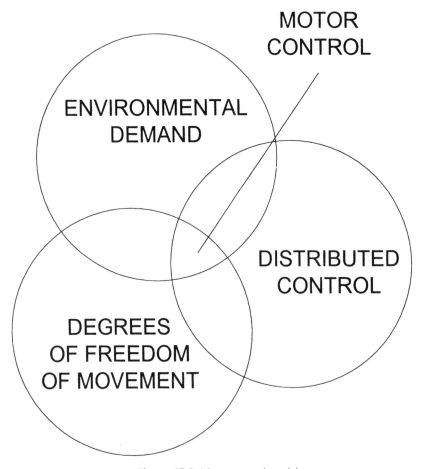

Figure 17.9. Motor control model.

ers must try to humanize the intervention as much as possible. Nevertheless, the Neurodevelopmental therapy model remains extremely popular with practitioners in occupational and physical therapy as well as in speech pathology. Continuing education courses on neurodevelopmental therapy are usually well attended.

COGNITIVE DISABILITY—CLAUDIA ALLEN
Frame of Reference

The cognitive disability model is based on the work of Piaget, a developmental psychologist, who described the sensorimotor period of the development in a hierarchical sequence. Allen stated that the model is designed to deal with the problems often ignored by other models such as changes in ability to function that would happen regardless of disability, difficulties in the capacity to learn, and the existence of chronic mental disorders (13). Examples of diseases and disorders causing chronic mental disorders are Alzheimer's disease and other dementias, traumatic brain injury, delirium multiple sclerosis, Parkinson's disease, schizophrenia, affective disorders, mental retardation, and cerebral palsy (10).

Assumptions

Allen listed six assumptions about cognitive disability that can be used to guide the evaluation and treatment (13).

1. A mental disorder's severity can be judged by the consequences it has on a person's capacity to think, do, and learn.
2. Mild mental disorders can be compensated for by learning psychological substitutes for normal mental processes.
3. Severe mental disorders can be associated with limited mental abilities that can not be corrected by what the person says or does.
4. Severe mental disorders can be compensated for by providing environmental substitutes for normal mental processes and identifying normal processes that can still be used.
5. The remaining mental abilities can be engaged to do realistic activities that are meaningful to the client, practical for caregivers, and sustainable over time.
6. When people are unable to learn to use psychological compensations effectively, environmental compensations can improve the quality of life of persons with cognitive disabilities and their long-term caregivers.

Concepts

The major concepts are related to the cognitive levels, performance modes, and activity analysis (Figure 17.10). Six major categories are used to describe the levels of function and performance. *Automatic actions* are those that a person does while conscious

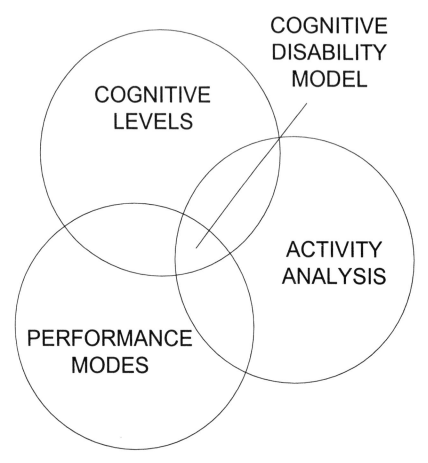

Figure 17.10. Cognitive disability model by Claudia Allen.

and responding to internal stimuli. *Postural actions* are those that a person initiates as gross body movement and which may be unusual postures. *Manual actions* are those a person does with the hands to manipulate objects, but the manipulations may be repetitive or pointless actions. *Goal-directed actions* are those a person does to engage in purposeful activity to achieve a short-term goal. *Exploratory actions* are those a person does to solve problems by trial and error. *Planned actions* are those a person does when he or she can anticipate the effects of future actions and can think abstractly.

Expected Results

The cognitive disability model is designed to provide environmental compensation for people with severe cognitive or mental disorders. By interpreting changes in performance to the cognitive disability of such people, the practitioner is able to help them find alternative strategies for managing disability.

Assessment

Assessment involves the use of the Allen Cognitive Level Screen (ACLS), which uses leather lacing to obtain an initial estimate of the client's ability to function. The Larger Allen Cognitive Level Screen may be used for those with visual impairments. For assessment of activities of daily living, the Routine Task Inventory is available (14).

Planning and Intervention

Although called the Allen Diagnostic Module, the Module actually provides interventions based on the level of function. For clients functioning at a low level, there are sensory motor stimulation activities. For clients functioning at the moderate to high level, the Module contains craft projects that can be used to continuously evaluate learning skills and adaptive potential to changes in the environment (15).

Analysis

Allen comments that environmental compensations, techniques used to compensate for decreased cognitive functioning, cannot be generalized to a wide range of situations or activities. Usually, environmental compensations are specific to the environment in which the client most frequently functions. One of the problems with teaching compensation in a hospital is that generalization to the home environment is low at best. Compensation skills need to be learned where they are needed. If they are needed in the home environment, they need to be learned in the home.

SENSORY INTEGRATION MODEL—A. JEAN AYRES

Frame of Reference

Sensory integration was introduced by Ayres in 1968 (16). Many of the ideas had developed from her earlier work on perceptual motor problems associated with visual and motor disorders (17). The theory is based on the contributions to the developmental approach made by Gesell and Piaget, sensory stimulation and deprivation made by Harlow, Held, and others, and neurophysiologic concepts organization by Rood. The focus of this model is on how the brain processes sensation and organizes a response.

Sensory integrative (or integration) dysfunction is Ayres' concept, which identifies children who have difficulty integrating sensory information. She assumed that the lack of sensory integration is associated with learning problems identified in education as learning disabilities in which students are behind two grades or more in academic performance of one or more subjects. Ayres paid particular attention to sensory development and organization and the impact possible disorganization of sensory information has on the developing nervous system.

Assumptions

Like neurodevelopmental treatment, the model of sensory integration is based on the assumption that the nervous system is organized in an orderly, predictable sequence in which higher levels control lower levels. A comparison of these orderly sequences is provided in Figure 17.11. One major difference is that sensory integration is a true developmental approach in which each developmental stage assimilates and builds on the previous one. Furthermore, Ayres assumed that early development was preprogrammed into the human brain at conception but ontogenetic or individual experience is necessary for the full expression of the inherent developmental tendencies. Finally, when the development of the brain deviates from normal development, the resultant behavior is often reminiscent of lower level functioning (18).

Sensory integration was assumed to result in perception and other synthesis of sensory data that enable a person to interact effectively with the environment, especially the academic environment. Through sensory integration, the person is able to make adaptive responses. Without sensory integration, the person is unable to make adaptive responses. The most important sensory data come from vestibular, proprioceptive, and tactile information (Figure 17.12). The vestibular data provide information about space, gravity, and motion that enable postural responses. Vestibular, proprioceptive, and tactile data provide information for mo-

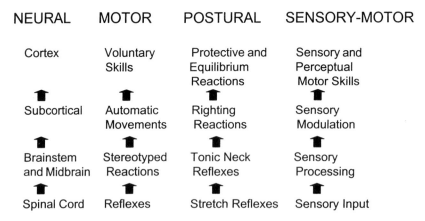

Figure 17.11. Hierarchical models of stepwise progression of anatomical, postural, and sensory motor models. (Adapted from: Horak FB. Motor control models. In: Forsberg H, Hirschfeld H. Movement Disorders in Children. Basel: Karger, 1992:23.)

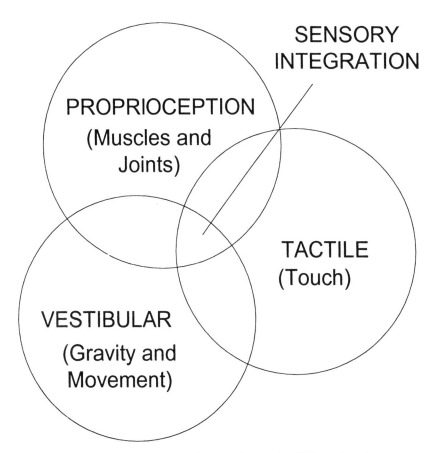

Figure 17.12. Major concepts of sensory integration (SI) by A. Jean Ayres.

tor planning and the development of a body scheme. Vision evolved through association with the vestibular, locomotor, and oculomotor processes. Thus, the development of the visual system depends on the development and function of the vestibular system (19).

Ayres defined occupational therapy as a profession that employs a purposeful activity to help the client form adaptive responses that enable the nervous system to work more efficiently (20, p. 183).

Concepts

Sensory integration is the ability to organize sensory information for use (18). Sensory integrative dysfunction is an irregularity or disorder in brain function that makes integrating sensory input difficult (20, p. 184). Sensory integrative therapy is treatment involving sensory stimulation and adaptive responses to it according to the child's neurologic needs (20, p. 184). An adaptive response is an appropriate action in which the individual responds successfully to some environmental demand (20, p. 181).

The primary problems defined in sensory integrative dysfunction include eight types. *Vestibular-bilateral disorder* is caused by underreactive responses and is characterized by shortened duration postrotary nystagmus, poor integration of the two sides of the body (body scheme) and brain, and difficulty learning to read or compute. *Overactive or hyperactive vestibular disorder* is exemplified by a child who has a vestibular system that is overresponsive to vestibular input and thus responds by being insecure or intolerant to movement. *Developmental dyspraxia or apraxia* is a brain dysfunction that hinders the organization of tactile, and sometimes vestibular and proprioceptive, sensations and thus interferes with the ability to motor plan. *Gravitational or postural insecurity* is abnormal anxiety and distress caused by inadequate modulation or inhibition of sensations that arise when the gravity receptors of the vestibular system are stimulated by head position or movement. *Tactile defensiveness* is the tendency to react negatively and emotionally to touch sensations. *Visual perception problem in space and form* is difficulty comprehending the dimensions of space and the relationship of the body to space (20). *Unilateral disregard and dysfunctions of the right hemisphere* is described as a tendency of the child to avoid moving into the left side of space (in relation to the body) or incorporating the left side of the body space into the environmental scheme. *Auditory language disorder* is described as involving problems in postural and bilateral integration, praxis, and visual perception (18).

Expected Results

Sensory integrative therapy is designed to provide sensory stimulation and promote adaptive responses according to the child's neurologic needs to organize the central nervous system. Specific outcomes depending on the sensory integrative problem might be a more accurate body percept (less clumsy), reduced hyperactivity and more purposeful activity in a child with vestibular-bilateral disorder, better ability to move in vertical and horizontal space in a child with overactive vestibular disorder, improved motor planning in a child with developmental dyspraxia, improved postural and equilibrium reactions in a child with gravitational or postural insecurity, normalized touch system in a tactilely defensive child, improved visual perception in a child with visual perception problems in space and form, better ability to localize and identify sound in a child with auditory language disorder, and improved cerebral processes for speaking, reading, writing, and using tools.

Evaluation

The primary assessment instrument is the *Sensory Integration and Praxis Test* (SIPT) published in 1991 (21). This assessment instrument replaces the *Southern California*

Sensory Integration Test (SCSIT) published in 1980 and the *Southern California Postrotary Nystagmus Test* (SCPNT) published in 1975. The SCSIT contains several assessment units that were previously published separately. These older assessment instruments are likely to still be found in occupational therapy service programs but should not be used in client assessment because their normative values have been re-standardized. The SIPT is primarily designed for children with learning disabilities.

Planning and Intervention

Planning is based on the results of the SIPT and other data available from assessments administered by other sources. The primary intervention strategies involve providing a play area with equipment designed to facilitate or inhibit vestibular, proprioceptive, and tactile stimulation. In addition, strategies are used to encourage the integration of primitive reflexes and activation of righting and equilibrium reactions by positioning and vibration to encourage contraction of extensor muscles. Examples of equipment are scooter board, swing bolster, platform swing, ramp, net suspended from a hook, inflatable plastic shapes and balls, buoy, jungle gym, and vestibular boards. Activities might include swinging, spinning, sliding down a ramp, holding onto a bolster upside down, balancing on a ball while sitting, balancing on a rocking vestibular board while standing, "driving" through an obstacle course on a scooter board, or climbing a jungle gym.

Usually, the child is allowed to choose the activity on the assumption that the child's nervous system will seek the stimulation needed to organize it. The practitioner may guide the selection of activity and control the time period. For new activities, the practitioner may provide assistance to get started and suggest play themes such as "flying an airplane" while holding onto a bolster, to maintain interest.

Analysis

Sensory integration is based on development as a hierarchical process in which successive stages of sensation integrate lower levels of the central nervous system to promote adaptation to the environment. As stated in the discussion of neurodevelopmental treatment, newer models of motor control suggest that a fixed hierarchical progression of the nervous system control does not occur. Ayres, however, in recommending intervention suggested that the individual child pick the activity to integrate that child's nervous system. Therefore, the assumption of fixed hierarchy is actually being applied to the individual. From the practitioner's standpoint, the same fixed hierarchy for everyone simplifies intervention because the same plan can be used for everyone with adjustment made only for where the individual level of current function occurs. In the individualized hierarchy, each person must be examined individually to determine how that person's nervous system is functioning and adjusting intervention accordingly. The challenge to the practitioner is to find the right sensory mix of stimulation and inhibition for each person.

SUMMARY

The current models of practice have a history of practical application and have withstood the test of time. Each is rooted in models and theories that preceded. The question is whether they meet the demands of practice today or whether newer models will do a better job of providing practitioners with the best options for meeting the needs of clients and the expectations of the health care industry. Several newer models are presented in the next chapter.

References

1. Slagle EC. The occupational therapy program in the state of New York. J Men Sci 1934;80:639–649.
2. Meyer A. Philosophy of occupation therapy. Arch Occup Ther 1922;1(1):1–10.
3. Reilly M. A psychiatric occupational therapy program as a teaching model. Am J Occup Ther 1966;20:61–67.
4. Reilly M. The education process. Am J Occup Ther 1969;23:299–307.
5. Reilly M. Occupational therapy can be one of the great ideas of 20th century medicine. Am J Occup Ther 1962;16:1–9.
6. Matsasuya J. The Interest Checklist. Am J Occup Ther 1967;21(6):323–328.
7. Kielhofner G, Burke JP. A model of human occupation. Part 1. Conceptual framework and content. Am J Occup Ther 1980;34:572–581.
8. Kielhofner G, Burke JP, lgi CH. A model of human occupation. Part IV. Assessment and intervention. Am J Occup Ther 1980;34:777–88.
9. Kielhofner G, Henry A. A User's Guide to the Occupational Performance History Interview. Bethesda, MD: American Occupational Therapy Association, 1995.
10. Dutton R. Clinical Reasoning in Physical Disabilities. Baltimore: Williams & Wilkins, 1995.
11. Bobath B. Abnormal Postural Reflex Activity Caused by Brain Lesions. London: William Heinemann Medical Books, 1965.
12. Bobath B. Adult Hemiplegia: Evaluation and Treatment. London: William Heinemann Medical Books, 1970.
13. Allen CK. Cognitive disability frame of reference. In Neistadt M, Crepeau EB. Willard and Spackman's Occupational Therapy. 9th ed. Philadelphia: Lippincott, 1998: 555–557.
14. Allen CK, Earhart CA, Blue T. Occupational Therapy Treatment Goals for the Physically and Cognitively Disabled. Rockville, MD: American Occupational Therapy Association, 1992.
15. Allen CK, Earhart CA, Blue T. Allen Diagnostic Manual. Colchester, CN: S & S/ Worldwide, 1993.
16. Ayres AJ. Sensory integrative processes and neurophysiological learning disabilities. In: Hellmuth J. Learning Disabilities. Vol. 3. Seattle: Special Child Publications, 1968: 41–68.
17. Ayres AJ. Methods of evaluating perceptual motor dysfunction. In: Proceedings: World Federation of Occupational Therapists, 3rd International Congress, New York, American Occupational Therapy Association, 1962:113–117.

18. Ayres AJ. Sensory Integration and Learning Disorders. Los Angles:Western Psychological Services, 1972:4–7.
19. Ayres AJ. Sensorimotor foundations of academic ability. In: Cruickshank WM, Hallahan DP. Perception and Learning Disabilities in Children. Vol 2. Syracuse, NY: Syracuse University Press, 1975:301–358.
20. Ayres AJ. Sensory Integration and the Child. Los Angeles: Western Psychological Services, 1972, revised 1980.
21. Ayres AJ. Sensory Integration and Praxis Tests. Los Angles: Western Psychological Services, 1991.

CHAPTER 18

Models Being Explored and Developed

The models discussed in this chapter are in various stages of development, but each shows promise of becoming important to the practice of occupational therapy.

THE CONTEXTUAL FRAME OF REFERENCE

Ecology of Human Performance—Dunn, Brown, and McGuigan, 1994

The major assumption of the ecology of human performance model, which was first published in 1994, is that human behavior or performance can be best understood by examining the relationship of the context, the person, and the task (2). The major concepts, therefore, are the context, person, and task and their relationship to human performance (Figure 18.1). The context has two parts: the physical, temporal, social, and cultural elements of the environment and the phenomenological experience of the person. The person is an individual with unique skills and abilities. The task is whatever the person is expected to perform or wants to perform. By integrating the nature of the context, the person's skills and abilities, and the specific task, a performance can be evaluated and recommendations for change be suggested.

No specific assessments have been developed to directly measure the concepts within the model. Five types of interventions have been outlined according to concepts to create a practice model. The interventions are as follows:

1. Establish or restore the persons's skills and abilities.
2. Change or alter the context to a different situation so that the person is able to perform.
3. Change or adapt the existing context or change the task demands to better fit the context.
4. Prevent maladaptive performance from occurring.
5. Create contexts that promote more adaptive or complex performance.

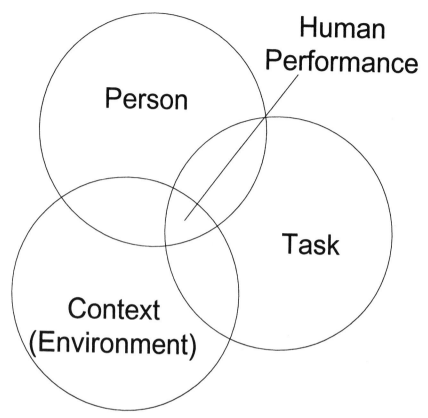

Figure 18.1. Ecology of human performance based on Dunn, Brown, and McGuigan.

OCCUPATION/ACTIVITY FRAME OF REFERENCE

Model of Occupational Functioning

The model of occupational functioning was proposed in 1995 as Trombly's Eleanor Clarke Slagle lectureship (3). The focus of the model is on practice in physical disability because that is the author's area of practice, but the concepts are not limited to physically disabled persons. This model could be discussed in the occupational performance section, but because the discussion in centered on occupation, it is discussed in the occupation and activity frame of reference section. Three concepts are discussed in detail: a proposed hierarchy of occupational functioning (sometimes called occupational performance), occupation-as-ends, and occupation-as-means (Figure 18.2).

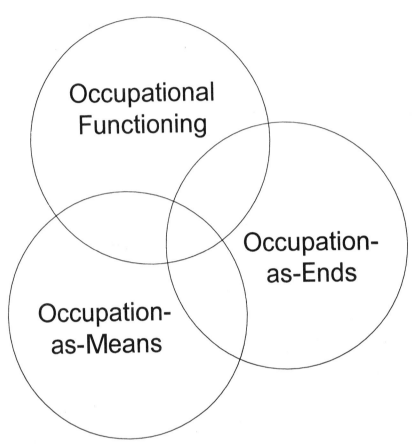

Figure 18.2. Model of occupational functioning based on Trombly.

The idea that a hierarchy of stages exists that leads to occupation has been proposed before by Levine and Brayley (4) and Christiansen and Baum (5, 6). Trombly's hierarchy is more extensive because eight levels are proposed: a sense of competence and self-esteem, life roles, tasks, activities, abilities and habits, developed capacities, first-level capacities, and cognitive–neuromuscular substrate (genetic endowment). Trombly prefers to explain occupation from the top-down approach as opposed to a bottom-up approach. Thus, definitions begin with the goal or outcome. "A competent person has sufficient resources to interact effectively with the physical or social environment and to meet the demands of a situation. A *sense of competency* is highly associated with feelings of *self-efficacy*" (3, p. 961).Trombly does not define life roles, but states that she prefers to categorize roles from the point of view of the person, such as roles relating to self-achievement or productivity, roles that are self-enhancing or add pleasure to a person's life, and roles that maintain the self–including family preservation and home maintenance. *Life roles* encompass *tasks* and *activities*. *Tasks* are defined as being comprised of activities, but she points out that some *tasks* are essential to a *life role* and must be mastered whereas other tasks are variable depending on how the person chooses to interpret the life role. For example, the life role of a mother has many variations depending on the expectations of the socioculture and the individual. *Activities* are smaller units of behavior than tasks. For example, peeling potatoes is considered an activity within the task of preparing dinner. *Abilities* are described as the skills one has developed through practice. *Abilities* underlie many different activities and include such items as hand-eye coordination. *Abilities* are derived from *developed capacities* a person gains through learning or maturation. *Developed capacities* are gained from learning and maturation and thus are refinements of biological capacities called *first-level capacities*. *First-level capacities* are reflex-based responses or subroutines underlying voluntary movement, which in turn is derived from a person's *genetic endowment*. Reflexive grasp and release are given as examples of first-level capacities.

The hierarchy of stages leading to competency and occupational performance are seen as operating in a nesting of levels of occupation. For example, the life role of a homemaker involves doing laundry (task), which in turn may require hanging up clothes (activity), which depends on dexterity for handling the clothes pins (ability), which in turn is based on grasping to hold (developed capacity), which is determined by reflexive grasp (first-level capacity), which is part of neuromuscular substrate.

Trombly equates occupation-as-end to the levels of roles, tasks, and activities in the model. The three levels have a goal or purpose that is accomplished through the use of abilities and capacities. According to Trombly, occupation-as-end is purposeful—that is, organizing—by nature. Many writers in the occupational therapy literature have suggested that purposeful occupation-as-end enabled a person to organize behavior, to schedule a day or to bring order to one's life. Occupation-as-end is also meaningful because it is perform within activities or tasks the person sees or determines are important. "Only meaningful occupation remains in a person's life repertoire" (3, p. 963). Meaningfulness is based on the person's beliefs and values, which are based on those of the family and culture. Meaningfulness is also based on the person's sense of what is important. Thus, the individual determines the meaningfulness of any occupation-as-end. Meaningfulness is strongly associated with motivation.

The therapeutic principles for the occupation-as-end are derived from cognitive information processing and learning theories. Occupations are analyzed to ensure they are within the capabilities of the client who is aware of the purpose for doing any activity or task within a given occupation. The therapist organizes the activities or tasks to be learned so that the person will succeed, provides the feed-

back to ensure successful outcome, and structures the practice to promote improved performance and learning (3, p. 964).

Occupation-as-means is considered to be the therapy used to bring about
changes in impaired occupational functioning. Often, occupation at this level is
limited to very simple behaviors. Trombly suggests occupation-as-means is equivalent to purposeful activity as defined in the position paper adopted by the American Occupational Therapy Association (7). The practitioner analyzes the occupation to determine what responses are needed to challenge the person to perform
at the next level and then offers the client the opportunity to engage in potentially
therapeutic occupation. In other words, occupation-as-means is based on the assumption that a given activity within a task or occupation has purposefulness such
as a healing property that will change organic or behavioral impairments and that
practitioners can identify through activity analysis.

Meaningfulness in occupation-as-means seems to relate to basic values held by
the person in a manner similar to meaningfulness in occupation-as-end but is
probably less profound. The meaningfulness is more likely to be an emotional
value that provides an interesting or creative experience. Nevertheless, the meaningfulness is still dependent on the individual. In therapy sessions, the therapist
and the client must have an exchange of information sufficient to construct the
meaning of an activity to determine the meaningfulness within the context of culture, life experiences, and current life situation.

OCCUPATIONAL PERFORMANCE AND/OR COMPETENCE MODEL

The Person–Environment–Occupation Model of Occupational Performance—Law and Colleagues

The person–environment–occupation (PEO) model, published in 1996, proposes to describe the interactions between person, occupation, and environment
as they contribute to occupational performance throughout the life span and to
determine the amount of overlap or congruence called person–environment–occupation fit (8). Five concepts are necessary to understand this model: person,
environment, occupation, occupational performance, and person–environment–occupation fit (Figures 18.3 and 18.4). Person is defined as "a unique being who assumes a variety of roles simultaneously" (4, p. 15). Environment includes cultural, socioeconomic, institutional, physical, and social considerations.
Occupation is "groups of self-directed, functional tasks and activities a person engages in over the lifespan" (8, p. 16). Within the concept of occupation is an assumption that activity, task, and occupation are a sequence in which activity is
considered to be the basic unit of a task and a task is a set of purposeful activities. Occupational performance is the "dynamic experience of a person engaged
in purposeful activities and tasks within an environment" (8, p. 16). Occupational performance in this model becomes a complex concept affected and

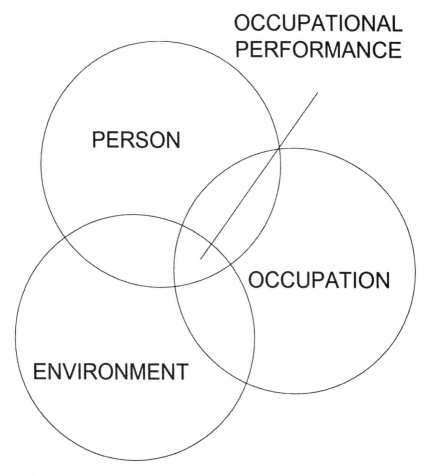

Figure 18.3. Person–environment–occupation model based on Law and colleagues.

changed by individual skills, occupation demands, and environmental supports and barriers.

The unique feature of this model is the concept of person–environment–occupation fit and assumptions about how the concept works. The concept is illustrated by using Venn diagrams. The more the circles of person, environment and occupation overlap, called congruence, the more harmoniously they are assumed to be interacting. "The outcome of greater compatibility is therefore represented as more optimal occupational performance" (8, p. 17). Congruence is also assumed to vary over the life span as ongoing development occurs.

For some clients, the goal may not be total congruence but rather a shift from

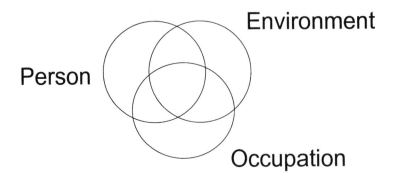

Good Congruence or Fit

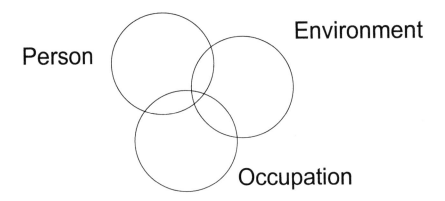

Poor Congruence or Fit

Figure 18.4. Examples of person–environment–occupation fit.

more congruence of, for example, occupational and environment to more congruence of person and environment. The Venn diagram can also illustrate this goal by increasing the overlapping circles of person and environment and decreasing the overlapping circles of occupation and environment.

Because this model is new, specific assessments have not been developed. The authors suggest using several assessments developed outside the field of occupational therapy. Only two assessments developed by occupational therapists are mentioned: the Canadian Occupational Performance Measure (COPM) and the Safety Assessment of Function and Environment for Rehabilitation (SAFER) (9, 10). Intervention can target the person, occupation, and environment as a three-part focus or on any two, depending on the needs of and demands on the client for better occupational performance.

ADAPTATION AS A FRAME OF REFERENCE

Occupational Adaptation—Schkade and Schultz

The model of occupational adaptation, published in 1992, is based on the idea that occupation is a primary means of achieving individual adaptation (11). Individual adaptation is viewed as both a state of being and a process. Thus, the occupational adaptation of the individual can be examined at a given point in time, over a specified period of time, or over a lifetime.

There are five general definitions: occupation, adaptation, the state of occupational adaptation, the process of occupational adaptation, and mastery. "*Occupations* are activities characterized by three properties: active participation, meaning to the person and a product that is the output of a process" (11, p. 831). "*Adaptation* is a change in [the] functional state of the person," which occurs as the person learns to master an occupation (11, p. 831). *Occupational adaptation* (*the state*) is a state of competency in the performance of occupation toward which a person aspires.

The process of occupational adaptation is more complex. "*Occupational adaptation* (*the process*) is the process through which the person and the occupational environment interact when the person is faced with an occupational challenge that calls for an occupational response reflecting an experience of relative mastery" (11, p. 831). Notice there are three more concepts, occupational challenge, occupational response, and relative mastery, embedded within the definition of occupational adaptation that must be defined to properly understand the definition. The problem of understanding the process of occupational adaptation is similar to looking up a word in the dictionary only to discover that several words in the definition must also be looked up in order to understand the original word. When faced with such a problem, one should continue reading and then come back to see if explanations or definitions are forthcoming later in the article or chapter.

The concept of mastery is not defined as a general concept by Schkade and Schultz although several concepts associated with mastery are used in the model such as relative mastery, desire for mastery, press for mastery, and demand for mastery. Mastery is a motive usually related to achieving a level, typically high, of functioning or performance in a skill or task recognized by the person and the environment as meeting certain preset criteria (12). In the model of occupational adaptation, the most important concept related to mastery is relative mastery, defined as occurring when the response of the person to the challenge to perform some task or role meets a criterion judged efficient, effective, and satisfying to the self and society.

Efficient relates to use of time and energy, effective relates to the production of the desired results, and satisfying relates to pleasing the self and society (11, p. 835).

The model focuses on three elements: person, occupational environment, and interaction (Figure 18.5). Each of the three elements in turn has additional concepts. There are eleven concepts related to person, two related to occupational environment and four related to interaction. However, the concepts related to person are all concerned with mastery, adaptive mechanisms, and functioning or performing.

The person is composed of three systems, sensorimotor, cognitive, and psychosocial, which are uniquely configured for each person as a result of genetic, environmental, and experiential and phenomenological subsystems. The occupa-

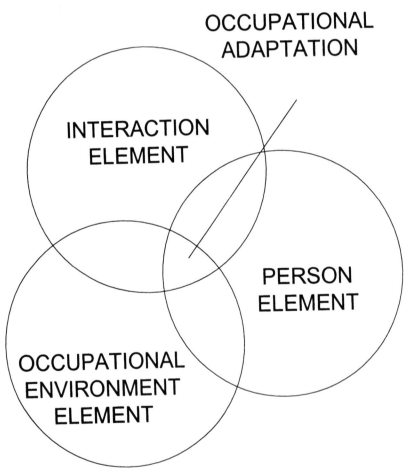

Figure 18.5. Occupation adaptation based on Schkade and Schultz.

tional environment is the context in which occupations occur such as work, play, leisure, and self-maintenance. The occupational environment is also comporised of three systems: physical, social, and cultural. The influences exerted by the occupational environment create the external role expectations.

The interaction element encompasses the occupational challenge, the occupational role expectations, and the occupational response. An occupational challenge is a process or series of steps a person chooses to go through to meet a particular purpose or goal, or the environment expects the person go through these steps to master some objective. The occupational challenge often requires learning new skills or using those skills to solve a new (to the person) problem. The occupational role expectations are the result of the combination of internal expectations (personal) and external expectations (occupational environment) for occupational performance. The occupational response is the action (occupational activity) of the person as he or she attempts to achieve relative mastery of the occupational challenge presented by the occupational environment.

The practice model "emphasizes the creation of a therapeutic climate, the use of occupational activity, and the importance of relative mastery" (13, p. 917). The focus of treatment is "affecting the patient's internal ability to generate, evaluate, and integrate adaptive responses in which relative mastery is experienced" (13, p. 917). These concepts are seen in Figure 18.6.

Assessment is based on the Guide to Practice (13, p. 925), which includes three areas: occupational adaptation data gathering, occupational adaptation programming, and evaluation of the occupational adaptation process. Each has a series of questions that the occupational therapist must answer in preparation for developing an intervention program.

Intervention involves improving occupational adaptation through occupational activities, occupational readiness, occupations of daily living, and a therapeutic climate. *Occupational activities* are "discrete activities that are occupational" (i.e., active, meaningful, and process-oriented with a tangible or intangible product) and are incorporated into treatment because they can promote the occupational adaptation process. *Occupational readiness* includes skill-based activities and other such interventions that focus on change in the person systems in preparation for occupational activities (e.g., the use of preparatory techniques, instruction, or assistive devices necessary for the patient to engage in occupational activity). *Occupations of daily living* are the unique patterns of occupations in which the person regularly engages as a result of the interaction between his or her occupational environments and related occupational roles. *Therapeutic climate* is the product of an interdependent exchange wherein the therapist, as the primary facilitator, functions as the agent of the patient's occupational environment and the patient functions as the agent of his or her unique person system. The climate defines the role of each party, the goal of therapy, and expected outcome so that both parties are empowered to make their optimal contribution.

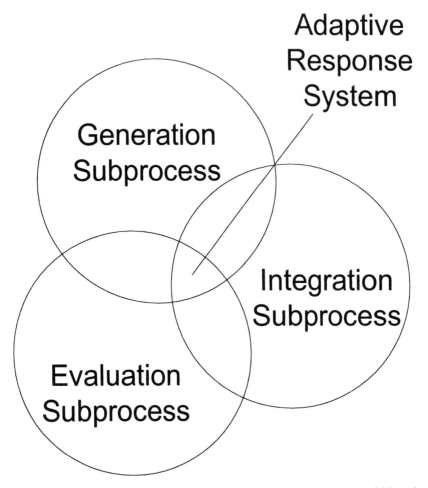

Figure 18.6. Adaptive response system in the occupational adaptation model based on Schkade and Schultz.

COGNITIVE FRAME OF REFERENCE

Multicontext Treatment Approach—Toglia

The previous models are broad and general in their assumptions, concepts, and application. In contrast, the multicontext treatment approach is primarily directed toward cognitive functions. No specific attempt is made to address motor or psychosocial skills although these areas of function may indirectly benefit from cognitive retraining.

The multicontext treatment approach, first published in 1991, is based on the dynamic interactional model of cognition (14). Thus, a model of treatment used in occupational therapy is based on a model developed by persons who are not occupational therapists. The three major concepts of the dynamic interactional model are the person, environment, and task (Figure 18.7).

Person factors that interact during information processing and learning include the following: structural capacity, strategies, metacognitive processes, and specific learning characteristics such as past knowledge, motivation, and emotions. Structural capacity is the physical limitation in the amount of information that a person can process at any given time. Processing strategies and behaviors are the "organized approaches, routines, or tactics which operate to select and guide the pro-

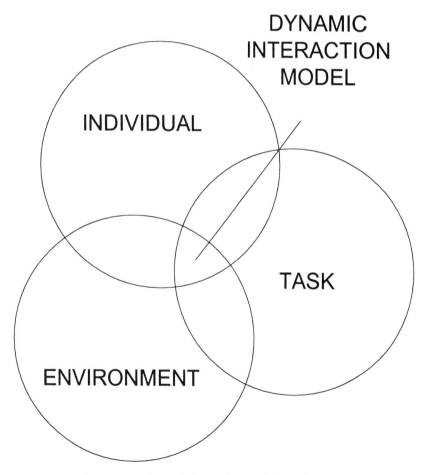

Figure 18.7. Dynamic interaction model based on Toglia.

cessing of information" (14, p. 108). Metacognition is the "knowledge and regulation of one's own cognitive processes and capacities" (14, p. 109).

Knowledge can be divided into two types, procedural and declarative. Procedural knowledge is knowing how to perform or what to do in a particular situation, which is acquired through practice and feedback. Declarative knowledge is knowing facts, which is acquired when new information stimulates connections to prior knowledge. The person's motivation and emotional states influence the extent to which information is processed and monitored.

Environmental factors include social, physical, and cultural. The type of environment the person is in may influence the individual's ability to process information and adapt to demands. The social environment, which includes the people with whom the individual interacts, is considered especially important because of the belief that "much of learning and higher cognitive skills are mediated through social interaction" (14, p. 111). The physical environment includes the objects and materials surrounding the person. The cultural environment includes the expectations and values accepted by the cultural group. More familiar environments facilitate better cognitive functioning (14).

The task factors are divided into two aspects: surface characteristics and conceptual characteristics. Surface characteristics include such observable data as the number of items, their spatial arrangement, presentation mode, directions, type of stimuli, variable attributes such as color or shape, and active movement and postural requirements. Conceptual characteristics cannot be directly observed because they are the underlying skills and strategies the person used to perform the task as well as the meaning of the task.

The practice model is based on the dynamic interaction model, which views learning as an interaction between internal (person) and external (task and environment) variables (15). Problems in processing information and learning are assessed by analyzing the dynamic interaction between person, task, and environmental variables and factors. Three assessment instruments are available: the Contextual Memory Test (16), the Toglia Category Assessment (17), and the Dynamic Visual Processing Assessment (18). In addition, the Guidelines for the Analysis of Surface Task Parameters appears in Neistadt and Crepeau (15, p. 559).

Treatment is aimed at systematically changing the variables of the environment and task to increase the person's ability to process, monitor, and use information. In Toglia's article, she states there are five components that are important to the process of generalization which is defined as the "ability to apply what has been learned . . . to a variety of new situations and environments" (19, p. 505). The five components are as follows: use of multiple environments, identification of criteria for transfer, metacognitive training, emphasis on processing strategies, and use of meaningful activities. In Neistadt and Crepeau, the five treatment components are listed as 1) specifying a processing strategy for transfer, 2) task analysis and establishment of criteria for transfer, 3) practice application of the strategy in multiple environments, 4) metacognitive training, and 5) individual characteristics related to motivation and active participation (15).

Toglia comments that the multicontext treatment approach is time-consuming to plan and provide treatment because the treatment must be tailored to the clients previous interests and experience (15). Thus, the same deficit may be treated differently because of the individual differences. Some preliminary research studies are listed, but detailed studies need to be done.

MOTOR CONTROL AND MOTOR LEARNING

Contemporary Task-oriented Approach— Mathiowetz and Bass Haugen

Over the years, there have been three models of motor control (reflex, hierarchical, and systems) and two models of motor learning (developmental and learning). These models have lead to three categories of practice models (muscle reeducation, neurodevelopmental, and motor relearning). The neurodevelopmental model was further divided into several approaches known by a technique name and the person who created the technique (Sensorimotor by Margaret Rood, Proprioceptive Neuromuscular Facilitation [PNF] by Margaret Knott and Dorothy Voss, Movement Therapy by Signe Brunnstrom, and Neurodevelopmental Treatment by Karl and Bertha Bobath).

The contemporary task-oriented approach (20), presented in 1994, is based on a dynamical systems model of motor control and ecological approach to perception and action (21). A key assumption is that the central nervous system is organized in a heterarchial arrangement as opposed to a hierarchical. Hierarchial organization is created by designating several levels that must be followed in sequence without variation because each is subordinate to the one above it. Heterarchial organization emerges from the interaction of various elements or subsystems; thus, there is no absolute order of command that allows the subsystems to vary the order of control with the task requirement. The assumption of heterarchy leads to the second assumption, which is that the person interacts with the environment and thus responds to changes in the environment as opposed to the idea that the central system development will "unfold" as maturation progresses without regard to the external environment. A third major assumption is that learning seems to occur best when the whole task is practiced in a variety of contexts or environments with less verbal feedback as opposed to practicing one activity of a task over and over in the same environment while receiving detailed feedback from a coach or therapist.

Important concepts include *heterarchy,* which has already been defined; *attractor,* which is a "preferred, but not obligatory, pattern of behavior that emerges from the interaction of a unique person with a particular task and environment" (21, p. 158); *control parameter,* which is a variable that acts as an agent to cause transition (phase shift) behavior from one preferred form to another and therefore facilitate the reordering of behavior; *phase shift,* which is the transition from one preferred coordinated pattern to another; and *degrees of freedom,* which are elements or variables that are free to vary in response to the task being performed. Other concepts are *knowledge of results* (KR), which is the awareness, by the person, of the outcome of movement in relation to the goal; *self-organization,* which is the ability of the person system and its subsystems to organize spontaneously from the dynamic interaction of the subsystems without any representation, prescription, or motor program; *collective variable,* which is the fewest number of variables or dimensions that can be used to describe a unit of behavior in quantitative terms, effector with the element in an open-loop control system that carries out instructions from the executive center; and *high-dimensional system,* which is complex-system composed of many elements such as subsystems, variables, dimensions, and degrees of freedom.

A practice model based on the contemporary task-oriented approach should be using the top-down approach; that is, it should start with occupational and role performance and then look at the subsystems as indicated. The person should assist in the identification of problems and tasks used in planning intervention. There are many assessments that can be used. Some of those recommended for assessment of dexterity are the Minnesota Rate of Manipulation Text, The Purdue Pegboard Test, the Box and Block Test, Nine-Hole Peg Test, and Jebsen Test of Hand Function. Analyze the results in terms of what personal characteristics and environment factors are hindering performance.

The client should be an active participant in the intervention phase as well as in the planning phase by identifying tasks of interest and importance. Intervention should be based on an active learning approach that encourages the client to experiment with movement and that provides various opportunities to practice because different environments provide different challenges even if the same task is being performed. The practitioner should help the person find the optimal strategy for achieving functional goals based on that person's unique system and subsystem. To increase the degree of difficulty and enhance performance, alter or change the task requirements and/or the environment. Help the client alter personal characteristics and environmental factors that are hindering performance. Assist the client to develop more efficient movement strategies.

This conceptual model and suggestions for practice are important. The model strongly suggests that previous practice models have been based on incorrect ideas of how the nervous system works. If practitioners actually have been fully implementing the older practice models, they have been doing their clients a disservice. If they continue to practice out-of-date approaches when newer information is available, their practice is unethical. The real question though can only be answered by observing and videotaping actual intervention sessions. Some practitioners say they are practicing one way, but actually they are practicing another.

PLAY/LEISURE MODELS

Playfulness—Bundy

The playfulness model, published in 1997, is based on three concepts: intrinsic motivation, internal control, and freedom to suspend reality (Figure 18.8). Intrinsic motivation "refers to some (unnamed) aspect of the activity itself, rather than to an external reward, that provides the impetus for the individual involvement in the activity" (22, p. 53). Internal control "suggests that the individual is largely 'in charge' of his or her actions and at least some aspects of the activity's outcome" (22, p. 53). Freedom to suspend reality "means that the individual chooses how close to objective reality the transaction will be" (22, p. 53). A fourth

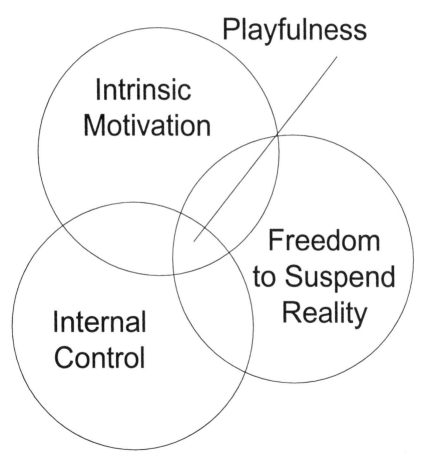

Figure 18.8. Model of playfulness based on Bundy.

concept is called the play frame, derived from the larger concept of frame. Frame as described by Bateson is used to describe

> any social situation [which] can be "defined" in accordance with basic principles that will affect and control the ways in which people involve themselves with and experience that situation. These "definitions" are frames. Note that the term is used here specifically to refer to the perceived and experienced organization, the agreed-upon "frame" within which people function. (23, p. 298)

In a play frame, the player gives cues to others about how they should act toward the player. A good player must be able to both give and read the cues.

As Bundy points out, one difference between play and other occupational areas such as self-care and work is that the latter are often obligatory and extrinsically motivated whereas play is self-chosen and intrinsically motivated. In play the process of doing is often more important than the product or outcome. This emphasis on process separates play from some of the constraints of self-care and work. There are fewer right and wrong ways to play and the person is able to try different approaches to the play situation that might quickly be stopped if tried with self-care or work occupations.

Play is not often assessed—even in children. Bundy suggests the lack of assessment may be owing to lack of assessment instruments. To partially remedy that lack of play assessments she developed a test of playfulness (ToP) with input from other occupational therapists. The scale is described in Parham and Fazio (22, p. 58–60). Three scales, extent, intensity, and skillfulness, are used to measure the 24 items. When each item is scored and categorized into perception of control, source of motivation, and suspension of reality, a fourth scale of playful versus nonplayful is determined.

As this review of the playfulness model is being written, no practice model of intervention based on the playfulness model has yet been published. The case studies suggests that intervention should be directed at play activity, which would lead to scoring toward more internal perception of control, more intrinsically based source of motivation, and more freedom to suspend reality, which would increasingly tilt the total score toward playful on the playful/nonplayful scale (22, pp. 60–65). The exact nature of such play and examples of play activities are not described.

The theoretical model of playfulness seems to provide the information necessary to create a practice model. Assessment is available and the criteria for increasing playfulness have been identified. What remains is to provide examples of play activities that might be structured by making them available in the environment or by using therapist direction to facilitate the three potential goals of increasing internal perception of control, increasing intrinsic modification, and increasing a sense of freedom to suspend reality. There may also be specific approaches to encouraging the play frame.

PROFESSIONAL DEVELOPMENT

Occupational Science—Yerxa and Clark

The occupational science model, first published in 1989, has a different purpose than the others. The model is not designed to guide practice but rather to guide the development of occupational therapy as an academic discipline. To many occupational therapy practitioners, the idea of an academic model for occupational therapy seems ridiculous. Occupational therapy is a practice-oriented discipline designed to help people cope with the problems of performing the occupations of daily living. The statement is correct and necessary but not sufficient. Occupational therapy must also survive and fit into the academic community because the profession selected colleges and universities as the location for educational programs for occupational therapists. Thus, the education program must be accepted in the higher education environment or the profession must develop another means of educating practitioners. Over the years, the occupational therapy education program has been located in the Agriculture and Mechanical College; College of Physicians and Surgeons; College of Medicine; College of Liberal Arts; College of Education; College of Letters, Arts, and Science; and the School of Auxiliary Medical Services (24). In other words, the education program of occupational therapy was placed in whatever college or school would accept the program. Even 20 years later, the crazy quiltwork of occupational therapy education programs continued including School of Health Sciences, School of Allied Sciences and Arts, School of Allied Health Professions, Division of Health Related Professions, College of Home Economics, School of Health and Social Services, School of Associated Medical Sciences, College of Human Resources Development, and others (25). Some of these arrangements probably did little to help the development of occupational therapy as an academic discipline. Better knowledge about the academic underpinnings of occupational therapy might have helped the educational program find a better placement in the academic community such as in the College of Social Sciences or as a separate college or school of occupational therapy.

The other major purpose for the occupational science model is to provide a basic science for occupational therapy that studies humans as occupational beings (26, p. xiv). The concept of basic science is used in academia to distinguish between fields that study a field to gain knowledge about a phenomena such as occupation and an applied field, which is focused on the application of knowledge to particular problems such as adaptive strategies for coping with changes in occupational performance due to a disorder. Basic science adds to the body of knowledge in the discipline. That knowledge may have application in practice but also may add to the knowledge and skills necessary to better study the discipline.

In Clark, Wood and Larson discuss occupational science in relation to three major concepts: occupations, adaptation, and cultural themes such as cultural place (Figure 18.9) (27). Occupations are defined as "the daily activities that can

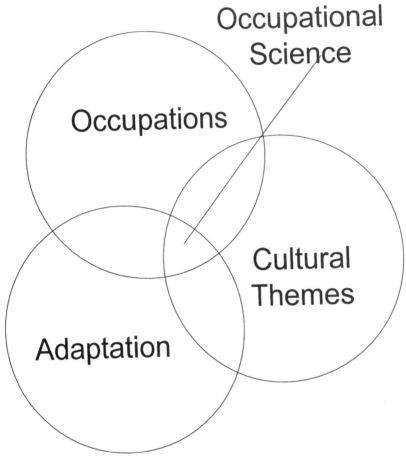

Occupational
Science

Occupations

Cultural
Themes

Adaptation

Figure 18.9. Major concepts in the occupational science model based on Yerxa and Clark.

be named in the lexicon of the culture and that fill the stream of time" (27, p. 13). Adaptation is defined as "a process of selecting and organizing activities (or occupations) to improve life opportunities and enhance quality of life according to the experience of individuals or groups in an ever-changing environment" (28, p. 44).

Culture is defined by Reber as "[t]he system of information that codes the manner in which the people in an organized group, society or nation interact with their social and physical environments . . . and thus is a . . . set of rules, regulations, mores and methods of interaction within the group" (29). There are many culture themes. One is cultural place, which is defined as "the place in which development occurs, the ecology and locally adapted environment which includes meanings, beliefs, values and conventional practices learned and shared by members of a community" (20, p. 390).

Key to the research efforts using the occupational science model is the tripart orientation to occupation (26). Namely, the occupation can be studied through form, function, and meaning. Form is studied by directly observing aspects of occupation such as the environmental context in which the occupation is performed and demands of the tasks within the occupation. Function involved the ways in which occupation serves adaptation by acting to promote the person's health. Of course the opposite is occupations that compromise health and thus are not adaptive or may be maladaptive. Meaning is the significance of occupation within the context of a person's life and in the culture in which the person lives. Meaning can be derived through the symbolism expressed by the culture such as a highly valued occupation like successful athlete, through a person's emotions such as writing as a means of expressing grief, and through the sense of one's self as an owner of occupation such as opera singer or ditch digger.

Johnson suggests occupational science can be of benefit to occupational therapy is four ways (31): 1) by adding to the development, creation, testing, and expansion of the body of knowledge, 2) by providing a sense of achievement and feeling of power that comes from participation in a common goal and vision, 3) by achieving a new sense of meaning and satisfaction derived from the challenges and the commitment of testing our commitment to enrich all people's lives through occupation, and 4) by promoting content and methodologies that address meaning and outcome using occupation.

References

1. Representative Assembly. Position Paper: Occupation. Am J Occup Ther 1995;49(10), 1015–1018.
2. Dunn W, Brown C, McGuigan A. The ecology of human performance: a framework for considering the effect of context. Am J Occup Ther 1994;48:595–607.
3. Trombly CA. Occupation: purposefulness and meaningfulness as therapeutic mechanisms. 1995 Eleanor Clarke Slagle Lecture. Am J Occup Ther 1995;49(10):960–972.
4. Levine RE, Brayley CR. Occupation as a therapeutic medium. In: Christiansen C, Baum C. Occupational Therapy: Overcoming Human Performance Deficits. Thorofare, NJ: Slack Inc., 1991:591–631.
5. Christiansen C. Occupational therapy: intervention for life performance. In: Christiansen C, Baum C. Occupational Therapy: Overcoming Human Performance Deficits. Thorofare, NJ: Slack Inc., 1991:4–43.
6. Christiansen C, Baum C. Person–Environment Occupational Performance: a conceptual model for practice. In: Christiansen C, Baum C. Occupational Therapy: Enabling Function and Well-Being, Thorofare, NJ: Slack Inc., 1997:47–70.
7. American Occupational Therapy Association. Position Paper—Purposeful Activity. Am J Occup Ther 1993;47:1081–1082.
8. Law M, Cooper B, Strong S, et al. The Person–Environment–Occupation Model: a transactive approach to occupational performance. Can J Occup Ther 1996;65(1):9–23.

9. Law M, Baptiste S, Carswell A, et al. Canadian Occupational Performance Measure. 2nd ed. Toronto: Canadian Association of Occupational Therapists Publications, 1994.

10. Oliver R, Blathwayt J, Brackley C, Tamaki T. Development of the Safety Assessment of Function and the Environment for Rehabilitation (SAFER) tool. Can J Occup Ther 1993;60(2):78–82.

11. Schkade JK, Schultz S. Occupational adaptation: toward a holistic approach for contemporary practice, part 1. Am J Occup Ther 1992;46(9):829–837.

12. Reber AS. Dictionary of Psychology. 2nd ed. London: Penguin, 1995:437.

13. Schultz S, Schkade JK. Occupational adaptation: toward a holistic approach to contemporary practice, part 2. Am J Occup Ther 1992;46(10):917–925.

14. Toglia JP. A dynamic interactional approach to cognitive rehabilitation. In: Katz N. Cognitive Rehabilitation: Models for Intervention in Occupational Therapy. Boston: Andover Medical Publishers, 1992:104–143.

15. Toglia JP. The multicontext treatment approach. In: Neistadt ME, Crepeau EB. Willard and Spackman's Occupational Therapy. 9th ed. Philadelphia: Lippincott, 1998:557–559.

16. Toglia JP. Contextual Memory Test. Tucson, Therapy Skills Builders, 1993 (Now part of the Psychological Corporation, San Antonio, TX.)

17. Toglia JP. Dynamic Assessment of Categorization Skills: Toglia Category Assessment. Pequanrock, NJ: Maddax Inc, 1994.

18. Toglia JP, Finkelstein N. Test Protocol: The Dynamic Visual Processing Assessment. New York: New York Hospital-Cornell Medical Center, 1991.

19. Toglia JP. Generalization of treatment: a multicontext approach to cognitive perceptual impairment in adults with brain injury. Am J Occup Ther 1991;45(6):505–516.

20. Mathiowetz V, Bass Haugen J. Motor behavior research: implications for therapeutic approaches to central nervous system dysfunction. Am J Occup Ther 1994;48(8): 733–745.

21. Bass Haugen J, Mathiowetz V. Contemporary task-oriented approach. In Trombly CA. Occupational therapy for Physical Dysfunction, 4th ed. Baltimore, Williams & Wilkins, 1995:157–185.

22. Bundy AC. Play and playfulness: what to look for. In: Parham LD, Fazio LS. Play in Occupational Therapy for Children. St. Louis: Mosby, 1997:52–66.

23. Reber AS. Dictionary of Psychology. 2nd ed. London: Penguin, 1995.

24. American Occupational Therapy Association: Schools offering courses in occupational therapy. Am J Occup Ther 1955; 4:182.

25. American Occupational Therapy Association. Occupational Therapy Education Programs. Rockville, MD: The Association, 1975.

26. Zemke R, Clark F. Preface. In Zemke R, Clark F. Occupational Science: The Evolving Discipline. Philadelphia: F.A. Davis, 1996:vii–xviii.

27. Clark F, Wood W, Larson EA. Occupational science: occupational therapy's legacy for the 21st century. In: Neistadt ME, Crepeau EB. Willard and Spackman's Occupational Therapy. 9th ed. Philadelphia: Lippincott, 1998:13–21.

28. Frank G. The concept of adaptation as a foundation for occupational science research. In: Zemke R, Clark F. Occupational Science: The Evolving Discipline. Philadelphia: F.A. Davis, 1996:47–55.

29. Reber AS. Dictionary of Psychology. 2nd ed. London: Penguin, 1995:177.

30. Clark F, Ennevor BL, Richardson PL. A grounded theory of techniques for occupational storytelling and occupational story making. In: Zemke R, Clark F. Occupational Science: The Evolving Discipline. Philadelphia: F.A. Davis, 1996:373–392.
31. Johnson JA. Occupational science and occupational therapy: an emphasis on meaning. In: Zemke R, Clark F. Occupational Science: The Evolving Discipline. Philadelphia: F.A. Davis, 1996:393–397.

The Knowledge Base

CHAPTER 19

Knowledge Sources in Occupational Therapy

The knowledge of occupational therapy covers a wide variety of diverse information. Figure 19.1 illustrates some of the major aspects of the diversity. The wide variety is in part to be expected of an applied discipline but more significant is the wide variety of occupations in which humans can participate. Although much intervention is focused on the occupations that are commonly or routinely done, occupational therapy technically could assist human beings in the performance of any occupation. Any occupation covers a wide field. Studying all that information requires more knowledge of where to locate information than is necessary for many fields. Practicing physicians, for example, have one major source of information, an electronic database named MEDLINE. For the technologically challenged, there is a paper version titled *Index Medicus.* Most of the questions a doctor wants answered can be located in MEDLINE or in a few comprehensive textbooks. For occupational therapy practitioners, there is no "one source fits all." Therefore, occupational therapists must be more aware of where various sources of information came from originally and how to locate information from those sources. This chapter is designed to help start the process of learning where to look and how to help the librarian offer better guidance.

BIOLOGICAL SCIENCES

Biological sciences are perhaps the most direct. Anatomy is the study of structures and interrelations of the structures in the body. For a review of the location of the pisiform bone and its relation to the hamate and triquetrum, a basic anatomy textbook or textbook on the hand rehabilitation should provide the information and illustrations. Physiology is the study of the function of the body. To review the functions of the liver and kidney, locate a basic physiology textbook. Questions regarding anatomy and physiology are fairly easy to answer.

Kinesiology is the study of human movement. Questions about specific muscle action, how a joint works, the role of tonic versus phasic muscles, and standing balance are most likely to be answered by books discussing kinesiology. Basic anatomy and physiology books will probably not provide the detailed information needed for subjects in kinesiology asked by occupational therapy students, prac-

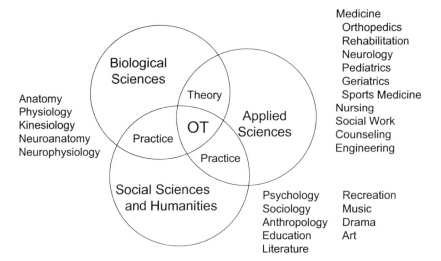

Figure 19.1. Body of knowledge in occupational therapy.

titioners, or researchers. On the other hand, measurement of joints, goniometry, and measurement of muscle strength, dynamometry, may be discussed in some kinesiology books but more likely in textbooks on physical therapy and rehabilitation or occupational therapy textbooks on physical disabilities. Other possibilities are orthopedic textbooks and disability evaluation textbooks in occupational medicine. Now, the complexity becomes more apparent. Ask a simple question, such as "What is the accepted range of motion of the elbow?", and four choices are provided in response. Welcome to the world of occupational therapy information.

Neurology, neuroanatomy, and neurophysiology textbooks will provide more detailed information on the structure and function of the nervous system. The location and role of the spinal tracts will be explained in more detail in neurology textbooks than anatomy or physiology texts. For even more detail, select a neuroanatomy or neurophysiology text.

SOCIAL SCIENCES, HUMANITIES, AND ARTS

Psychology, the study of human behavior, is a primary source of information for occupational therapists. Subjects such as personality, attitudes, emotions, feelings, perception, motivation, mind, individual differences, and group dynamics are good topics for psychology textbooks. Libraries that use the Library of Congress system for cataloging will have psychology texts and sometimes the psychology journals under the call letters BF. These letters are easy to remember because of B.F. Skinner, the psychologist who popularized behavioral psychology.

Measurement, assessment, and evaluation of human behavior are also subjects in psychology. Looking for information on reliability and validity? Any textbook on psychological testing will include a chapter or two on reliability and validity. Need the name of the test publisher for the Miller Assessment of Preschoolers? Try a book that lists published tests such as *Tests* (1) or *Tests in Print* (2). Of course, if the test is not published by a commercial publisher, these books will not help. They will not list a source for the Jebsen Hand Function Test (also known as the Jebsen-Taylor Hand Function Test, Jebson, Jepson, and other variations). However, a test kit is available from the catalog Sammons Preston (3). So, another good source of information on occupational therapy subjects is commercial catalogs. At conferences, it is a good idea to pick up any catalog that might be helpful. The price is right—free.

Psychology textbooks are also reliable sources of information on interviewing, observation, and test administration and scoring procedures. Much of the classic work on tests and measurements is in the psychology literature. For occupational therapists interested in developing, revising, or renorming existing assessment, the psychology literature provides many resources.

Also in the section with psychology are the philosophy textbooks. This is because psychology was part of philosophy at the beginning of the 1900s. The philosophy section is a good place to look for issues such as humanism, holism, free will, emergence, and monism, which form many of the basic philosophic assumptions in the field of occupational therapy. There are introductory textbooks for people who never took a basic course in philosophy; these books include information about many occupational therapists. Two of the major philosophers who influenced occupational therapy will also appear in other sources. William James was a philosopher and a psychologist, which was common in his day; therefore, information on James and on pragmatism often appears in history of psychology textbooks as well as in philosophy books. John Dewey, the other philosopher who influenced occupational therapy, is also known for his influence on American education. Information about John Dewey appears in many textbooks dealing with public education in America, especially at the beginning of the 1900s.

Sociology is the study of human society and social relations. Sources of information include topics of interest to occupational therapists such as role behavior and theory, the structure and function of institutions, human values, human ecology, social control, social conflict, socialization, family and family life, deviance, and social behavior, all of which are topics covered in sociology. Anthropology studies human origins and culture. Topics of interest to occupational therapists are acculturation, culture and personality, cultural patterns, cultural traits, cultural diversity, ethnography, ethnogeography, social anthropology, folklore, and rituals.

Architecture may seem an unusual subject to include in the information sources for occupational therapy, but actually there are many points of connection. Architects are concerned with the built environment, the use of physical space, and how these relate to human activity. The built environment involves design, composition, and construction. John Ruskin, William Morris, George Barton, and Thomas Kidner were all trained as architects. All had an understanding of manual education, which stressed drawing and construction. Ruskin liked gothic art and design in buildings whereas Morris was more interested in the interior design of wallpaper and furniture. The design of space can facilitate group interaction or encourage individual primacy. Lack of space restricts access by wheelchairs as do stairs. Rooms can be organized to facilitate group interaction by placing the chairs around small tables or to discourage group interaction by placing the chairs against the wall. Architects and occupational therapists are both interested in how humans use the space around them and how the environment shapes behavior.

Education provides several important areas of information to occupational therapists. Teaching, instruction, and learning methods are particularly important. The methods and techniques involved in demonstration, role-playing, simulation, exploration and discovery, problem solving, decision making, practice, and repetition are all examples. Educational methods and techniques are used every day by practitioners working with clients as well as by educators.

Many of the creative arts provide information for intervention: recreation, music, art, dance, drama, and psychodrama. The subject matter is usually easy to identify, but resources written for intervention are limited. There are not many books that discuss the application of the arts to intervention, but there are articles. Some older articles appear in both *Occupational Therapy and Rehabilitation* (*OT&R*) from 1922 to 1951 and the *American Journal of Occupational Therapy* (*AJOT*). The only source of indexing for all of *OT&R* and *AJOT* from 1947 to 1965 is in OT BibSys from the American Occupational Therapy Foundation. Access requires an institutional membership such as a hospital or university or an individual account. From 1966 to the present, AJOT has been indexed in the MEDLINE database.

APPLIED SCIENCES—MEDICINE

Medical libraries have sections for textbooks on orthopedics, rehabilitation, neurology, pediatrics, geriatrics, sports medicine, psychiatry, and cardiology. Other sections do exist as well, but the topics listed here are the most relative to occupational therapy.

Orthopedics includes disorders of the skeletal system, which includes subsections for hand, wrist, shoulder, head and neck, hip, knee, and foot. There are subsections for disorders such as arthritis, amputations, polio and post-polio, and osteoporosis. Rehabilitation appears in two sections of medicine. General social rehabilitation and assistive technology appear in one section and physical therapy and rehabilitation appear in another. In the National Library of Medicine (NLM) classification, check both WB 320 and WB 460.

Neurology includes all basic textbooks in neurology as well as books on specific structures such as the basal ganglia or cerebellum. Specific disorders include stroke, brain injuries, Parkinson's disease, multiple sclerosis, coma and stupor, epilepsy, and pain. In addition most textbooks on speech and language are cataloged under neurology. The NLM classification is WL. One peculiar cataloging problem exists. Textbooks considered to be concerned with brain injuries are cataloged in WL. However, some textbooks considered to be concerned with head injury are cataloged in WE (orthopedics) because head is a name for a skeletal part. Brain, however, is considered neurology. Mostly, brain injuries—whether resulting from closed or open causes—are now cataloged in neurology.

Pediatrics is a separate section. In the NLM classification, the call letters are WS. All aspects of pediatrics are included, such as developmental disabilities, cerebral palsy, learning disabilities, hyperactivity, attention deficit disorders, and sensory integrative dysfunction.

Geriatrics is organized with chronic diseases in the NLM classification with the call letters WT. All aspects of geriatrics are covered although subjects such as dementia and Alzheimer's disease are considered mental health subjects in the NLM classification system and thus are cataloged in psychiatry and mental health. Especially useful in the geriatric section are the books on assessment of the elderly.

Sports medicine often appears with the sports section, which is GT in Library of Congress section. Many medical libraries still use some Library of Congress sections because they provide better cataloging choices.

Mental health and psychiatry often comprise a large percentage of textbooks in a medical library. Also, remember that mental retardation is cataloged in mental health and psychiatry. Thus, books on schizophrenia, bipolar disorders, personality disorders, autism, and Aspergers will be cataloged within the call letters WM.

NURSING, PHYSICAL THERAPY, SOCIAL WORK, AND SPEECH PATHOLOGY

Nursing has the most professional literature of any health care field other the medicine. Much of the information from nursing is potentially useful. The philosophy of nursing comes from the same concerns that developed occupational therapy. Nursing is also concerned with humanitarianism, humanism, and holism. The primary difference is nurses' focus on caring whereas occupational therapy practitioners focus on occupation. Several of the nursing diagnoses are similar to those in occupational therapy such as coping skills, growth and development, home maintenance, impaired mobility, chronic pain, self-care deficit, low self-esteem, impaired swallowing, and others. A list is provided in Table 19.1. Subspecialties within nursing that are particularly useful to occupational therapists are rehabilitation nursing, occupational nursing, pediatric nursing, and community health nursing.

Physical therapy does not share a common heritage with occupational therapy. Physical therapy began in the United States as an assistant field to orthopedics and

Table 19.1. Nursing Diagnoses Which Overlap with Occupational Therapy

Activity intolerance	Mobility, impaired physical
Activity intolerance, potential	
Adjustment, impaired	Noncompliance (specify)
Anxiety	
	Pain
Body image disturbance	Pain, chronic
	Parental role conflict
Communication, impaired verbal	Parenting, altered
Coping, defensive	Parenting, altered, potential
Coping, family: potential for growth	Personal, identify disturbance
Coping, ineffective family: compromised	Post-trauma response
Coping, ineffective family: disabling	Powerlessness
Coping, ineffective individual	
	Role performance, altered
Decisional conflict (specify)	
Denial, ineffective	Self-care deficit, bathing/hygiene
Disuse syndrome, potential for	Self-care deficit, dressing/grooming
Diversion, activity deficit	Self-care deficit, feeding
Dysreflexia	Self-care deficit, toileting
	Self-esteem disturbance
Family processes, altered	Self-esteem, chronic low
Fatigue	Self-esteem, situational low
Fear	Sensory-perceptual alterations (specify)
	Sexuality patterns, altered
Grieving anticipatory	Skin integrity, impaired
Grieving, dysfunctional	Skin integrity, impaired, potential
Growth and development, altered	Social interaction impaired
	Social isolation
Health maintenance, altered	Swallowing, impaired
Health-seeking behaviors (specify)	
Home maintenance management, impaired	Thought processes, altered
	Trauma, potential for
Hopelessness	
	Unilateral neglect
Infection, potential for	
Injury, potential for	Violence, potential for
Knowledge deficit (specify)	

developed within the biomedical model. Physical therapists can share information on pathokinesiology. Their knowledge base is more extensive than that of occupational therapists in relation to motor control disorders, delayed motor development and learning, and techniques for remediation of the disorders and delays. Most neurodevelopment techniques were developed by physical therapists. Knott and Voss, Brunnstrom, and Bobath were physical therapists. Rood was both an occupational and a physical therapist. In addition, as mentioned in the section on activities of daily living as a concept, the original activity of daily living scales were created by physical therapists. Occupational therapy personnel can use the knowledge from physical therapy to assist clients to improve their performance of all occupations in daily life including but not limited to activities of daily living.

Social work shares with nursing and occupational therapy the common heritage of humanitarianism, humanism, and holism. Hull House was primarily a social service project. Social workers organize information about local and national resources, advocacy, and group behavior. Social workers can be allies with occupational therapists in helping clients return successfully to the community, ensuring knowledge and access to community resources.

Speech pathology provides information on cognitive perceptual tasks especially in regard to right hemisphere lesions. Other topics include dysphasia, apraxia of motor actions, and communication systems. Speech pathologists and occupational therapists can share knowledge of assistive devices and on helping clients learn to use assistive technology effectively.

ENGINEERING AND TECHNOLOGY

Engineering is a vast source of information on how to make and improve assistive technology. Information on mechanical and electrical technology is most often useful. Rehabilitation engineering combines both aspects and is particularly useful in relation to building and creating assistive technology from better wheelchairs to better motion analyzers. Increasing the use of computers and computer technology increases the opportunities for engineers and occupational therapy personnel to join talents to improve resources for persons with disabilities.

ORTHOTICS AND PROSTHETICS

The literature on orthotics is particularly useful to occupational therapists in relation to splints. The improvement in splinting materials has revolutionized the making of splints. Splints can be made quickly for temporary use and for tryout to determine the best permanent splint for a person. However, the changes in prosthetic limbs is also important to occupational therapy practice because amputees are able to use their prosthetic devices to perform many occupations that were difficult or impossible just a few years ago. There are many aspects of choosing and selecting the best prosthesis for a client where the occupational therapist and prosthetist can work together.

BUSINESS AND MANAGEMENT

The first information occupational therapists borrowed from business were work efficiency and task analysis to achieve work simplification, motion economy, and job analysis. Frank and Lillian Gilbreath were early specialists in work efficiency. Mr. Gilbreth was even given honorary membership in the National Society for the Promotion of Occupational Therapy (4). Although Mr. Gilbreth died in 1924, Mrs. Gilbreath maintained her interest in work efficiency for persons with disabilities.

Management literature obviously provides good sources for management issues including organization of services, supervision, employee performance evaluation, leadership, and organizational planning.

GOVERNMENT

The federal government is one of the largest publishers in the world. In each area of the country, government depository libraries receive publications according to a profile. Of most interest to occupational therapists are those related to health, delivery of health services, and occupational health and safety. Government publications can be bewildering. The classification system used to organize government publications is different from both the National Library of Medicine and the Library of Congress systems. A librarian knowledgeable about government documents is essential to help locate many of the sources. The Internet can also provide access to government publications.

VOCATIONAL REHABILITATION

Vocational rehabilitation literature is useful for subjects related to learning and returning to work. Information is available on testing for vocational readiness, physical capacities, and functional assessment. Job training is another area. Supported employment, job coaching, and sheltered workshops are some of the topics. Occupational therapists have been interested in prevocational assessment and training for many years. Legislation related to vocational rehabilitation has had an impact on occupational therapy as well. The history of the relationship between vocational education and occupational therapy provides the answers to the uneasy relationship in the United States between vocational rehabilitation and occupational therapy.

Additional information on locating sources is also discussed in Chapter 31 on sources of professional literature.

References

1. Sweetland RC, Keyser DJ. Tests: A Comprehensive Reference for Assessments in Psychology, Education, and Business. 3rd ed. Austin, TX: Pro-Ed, 1991.
2. Murphy LL, Conoley JC, Impara JC. Tests in Print IV: An Index to Tests, Test Reviews, and the Literature on Specific Tests. Lincoln, NB: Buros Institute of Mental Measurements, 1994.
3. Sammons Preston, P.O. Box 5071, Bolingbrook, IL 60440-5071.
4. NSPOT: List of members. Proceedings of the First Annual Meeting of the National Society for the Promotion of Occupational Therapy. Towson, MD: The Society, 1918:7.

The Skills Base

CHAPTER 20

Therapeutic Roles and Functions

Thomas has suggested there are five roles that a helping professional such as an occupational therapist can perform (1). These are clinician–behavior changer, consultant–educator, broker–advocate, research–evaluator, and caretaker–caregiver. The first four were originally described by Fischer for social caseworkers, but the concepts apply equally well to occupational therapists (2). A sixth role has also been added to complete the role complex. This role is counselor–mentor. These six roles are illustrated in Figure 20.1.

CLINICIAN–BEHAVIOR CHANGER

The clinician–behavior changer provides therapy, behavior change, crisis intervention, advice, and counseling. The goal is to attend directly to problems in the individual's functioning (or individual and family or support unit) by applying any number of individually oriented change strategies related to prevention, development, remediation, environment adjustment, or maintenance. As an occupational therapist, the clinician–behavior changer has addressed one of the three outcomes: diversion, expression, or skill building. This role is the most common role taught in occupational therapy education programs, sometimes almost to the exclusion of the other roles.

The occupational therapist often performs several roles within the clinician–behavior changer. These include interviewer, assessor, planner, negotiator, advisor, decision maker, role model, problem solver, and communicator (3). As an interviewer, the therapist established a working relationship with the client and a beginning knowledge of the individual and his or her perceived strengths and concerns. The initial interview often set the stage for the therapeutic change relationship. Thus, the interviewer should consider how to approach the client and what information to obtain first. As an assessor, the therapist identifies the client's skills, problems, and abilities to form a baseline for intervention. The assessor needs to know what information to obtain beyond the initial interview and what types of assessment strategies and instruments will best provide that information. As a planner, the therapist explores the options available in relation to client needs. The options must be considered on the basis of objectivity and realism. A planner must

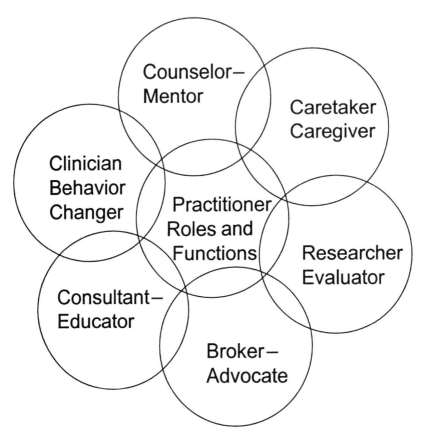

Figure 20.1. Therapist's roles and functions.

analyze the current data, look into the future, think about possible outcome scenarios, and consider which scenario is most like the client's perspective. As a negotiator, the therapist must be able to exchange ideas with the client, the client's support system such as family members, the physician, and other health care team members. Mutual decision making, agreement on a plan, resolving differences, and motivating the client and others are important aspects of the negotiation role.

The advisor role in client management entails imparting information that may be useful to the client. Advising is based on the therapist's knowledge and skills. Because occupational therapists are concerned with all aspects of daily living, the therapist needs to have knowledge about a wide range of topics and basic skills in most aspects of daily living tasks. As a decision maker, the therapist most often must assist the client and other caregivers to select or choose from a range of options that may be limited to two choices (such as blue or brown shoes) or involve choosing from several choices. Another aspect of the decision-making role is to choose when the client does not have the knowledge or skills to select—for example, selecting the best practice model on which to base the client's intervention program. Role model is another role that therapists may assume. Therapists can adopt roles to achieve empathy with their clients in order to better understand the situation and problems clients face. Therapists can also provide role models for clients and other caregivers by doing and talking about the tasks than are necessary to the caregiver role. Of course, therapists may also act as a role model to assist the client in learning to react and cope with a situation; for example, the therapist may act as a personnel manager in a job interviewing situation. Finally, the therapist is a problem solver. Problem solving is usually done with the client so the client can participate and learn from the process. Other problem-solving situations may involve the other team members to determine, for example, the best seating system for a person with a curved spine.

Communicator is one of the most important roles the therapist must assume. As a communicator the therapist must be able to speak and write effectively. Speaking is required in working with clients, their support system, and with other health care professionals. Speaking is often required to report what the therapist is doing with the client and how the client is responding. Writing is necessary to record and document the data from the assessment, intervention plan, intervention management, and discharge. Therapists must be able to write in the client's chart the information necessary to provide a legal record and to satisfy the reimbursement agency or service provider payer.

CONSULTANT–EDUCATOR

The role of consultant–educator involves teaching, consultation, goal setting, interpretation, and supervision. In this role, the occupational therapist may function to provide information, interpret rules or regulations, teach individuals, groups, or families, and transmit knowledge through audiovisual or written publications. The role may be provided to clients, consumers, community leaders, staff members, other professionals, or occupational therapy students and personnel. Thus, the occupational therapist could teach parents how to use toys to promote development, help colleagues with problems in their own practice, provide training to teacher or nursing aides, set the goals for professional education, interpret certain laws and policy regulations such as the Americans With Disabilities Act to local business, or provide consultation to a local industry on ways to prevent hand injuries. Fischer states that two general types of knowledge are required to function in this role: a substantive body of knowledge (e.g., knowledge of many toys that have been analyzed for their attributes in relation to developmental tasks and stages) and a way of communicating or teaching the knowledge. Certain steps can be identified in the process. One, become familiar with the target system (client, agency, business, educational institution), its structure, strengths, and problems.

Two, establish a working relationship by identifying functions and purposes and developing rapport and mutual trust. Three, attempt to alleviate anxieties and guilt over previous difficulties that may have occurred as the client, agency, business, etc., tried unsuccessfully to achieve a desired result. Four, describe and explain basic principles and procedures of the approach to be used. Five, present alternative methods for dealing with the problem; use a variety of means for teaching, including direct explaining, modeling, role-playing, and using audiovisual media. Six, help establish a specific program to meet the needs of the situation. Seven, conduct one or more follow-up sessions to provide supportive help, deal with further problems, and evaluate the success of the approach.

The major advantage Fischer reports for promoting the role of consultant–educator is to teach other professionals (nurses, teachers) and nonprofessionals (family members) who come into direct contact with consumers to identify and correct minor problems in occupational performance.

BROKER–ADVOCATE

The third role is broker/advocate, which is based on the idea of mediating between the individual and social institutions to secure assistance and access to resources from the social institutions. Although social workers do much of the broker–advocate functions such as obtaining proper medical care, housing, and financial aid, occupational therapists can also help. Consumers may need help in dealing with a local grocery store that is not as accessible to persons with limitations or changes in mobility as it might be. Motorized carts reduce the amount of walking required, which in large stores can be nearly a quarter of a mile. Wider aisles and less items placed in the aisles can facilitate movement. Making the most common sizes available within reach of a seated individual is another accessibility option. Many times, accommodating persons with disabilities requires more cognition than expensive remodeling of the physical environment. Many barriers to accessibility are more mental than physical.

There are two principles types of broker advocacy: individual and group. Individuals usually require broker advocacy owing to laxness or illegalities on the part of lower-level personnel in government or private agencies. The occupational therapist may be able to go directly to a supervisor or manager to address the problem of lack of service, denial of service, demeaning or harassing service, or illegal demands before service is rendered.

Group broker advocacy usually involves establishing or maintaining an action group to represent the interests of persons who are disadvantaged by age, social situation, and/or health status. The occupational therapist can act as a spokesperson to articulate an individual's needs, as a provider of factual knowledge, as an advice giver or consultant, as a specialist in "objectifying" or clarifying viewpoints and goals, as a public relations specialist to spread the word about the groups, or as an organizational specialist in setting up and maintaining the group as a cohesive and vibrant group.

Fischer outlines six aspects of the broker–advocate role. These are provision of material aid, mediation and liaison, referral, resource location, problem identification, and aggressive representation of the client's rights.

RESEARCH–EVALUATOR

Fischer suggests there are six ways in which research can be useful to a profession: One, select and use principles of behavior change that have been experimentally validated as underpinning for the development of intervention procedures. Two, use rigorous criteria to evaluate research from other areas that may not be primarily concerned with intervention (e.g., social psychological research, neurophysiological research, or cognitive thinking research). Three, use rigorous criteria to evaluate procedures from intervention systems from within and without social work as a basis for considering selection and use of those procedures for occupational therapy. Four, study comparisons between procedures derived from different orientations to determine which is most effective with a particular client or problem. Five, conduct ongoing objective evaluation of intervention with each and every client. Six, provide overall evaluation of effectiveness, using controlled group experimental studies.

CARETAKER–CAREGIVER

The fifth role suggested by Thomas is that of caretaker–caregiver (1). The function of the caretaker–caregiver is to care for the needs and/or safety of those who cannot care for themselves or who are a danger to themselves or others. Examples include persons with dementia or persons who cannot walk or use a wheelchair due to muscle weakness or atrophy. The role entails locating resources that can provide help and/or providing direct services such as educating the family in how to provide a safer environment to reduce the changes of unsafe conditions. The home can have many unsafe conditions, such as throw rugs on the floor over which a person could trip and fall, frayed electrical cords, too many items plugged into one extension cord, or broken and uneven stairs. Frequently, these conditions have existed for many years and thus everyone has forgotten how dangerous they can be.

ROLE DIFFERENTIATION

Each role has a specific and different goal so the choice of role is important. Thus, if the goal is intervention to change the functional status or behavior of an individual, then the role most likely will be that of behavior–changer. If the goal is to provide information and to educate, then the role is likely to be consultant–educator. The goal of the broker–advocate is to link a service to a person needing a service. The goal of the research–evaluator is to enhance practice and/or professional education. Caretakers and caregivers substitute their own knowledge and skill or someone else's knowledge and skill to compensate for loss or unavailable

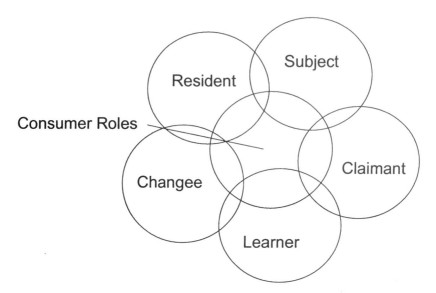

Figure 20.2. Consumer roles in the therapy process.

knowledge and skill of a particular client or consumer. Selecting the correct role is important to providing the right service. Matching the role and the goal is particularly important when more than one role and goal is being provided to the same person.

COUNSELOR–MENTOR

In professional practice, a counselor or mentor can provide assistance and guidance based on experience and accumulated knowledge and skills that a younger colleague has not yet acquired or a fellow professional has not needed in other situations. The counselor role involves listening, assisting, exploring options, and clarifying values, needs, and possible solutions. The mentor guides the younger or less experienced colleague using knowledge and skills that apply to specific topics and situations. The difference between the two roles is one of degree. Counseling is often more general in nature and wide-ranging in focus. Mentoring is usually focused on a particular objective such as helping the person prepare a manuscript for publication.

CONSUMER ROLES

In addition to the helper roles, Thomas suggests there are five client or consumer roles: changee, learner, claimant, subject, and resident (Figure 20.2). These roles complement the helper roles. Changee is the complement of the clinician–

behavior changer. Learner complements the consultant–educator. Claimant complements the broker–advocate role. Subject complements the research–evaluator and resident the caretaker–caregiver role. Thus, correspondence between the role(s) of the helper and the role(s) of the consumer should be cultivated and maintained for maximum results. Where multiple roles are involved—usually because of multiple goals—the helper may need to clarify with the consumer what role is assumed so confusion does not occur. As Thomas states, "not only should the client role be congruent with that of the helping person, both types of role need to be consistent with the desired change objective."

References

1. Thomas EJ. Designing Interventions for the Helping Professions. Beverly Hills: Sage, 1984.
2. Fischer J. Effective Case Work Practice: An Eclectic Approach. New York: McGraw-Hill, 1978.
3. Foster M. Process of practice. In: Turner A, Foster M, Johnson S. Occupational Therapy and Physical Dysfunction: Principles, Skills and Practice. 4th ed. New York: Churchill Livingstone, 1996:91.

CHAPTER 21

Clinical Reasoning

Clinical reasoning can be described as the types of inquiry or thinking that a therapist does to understand clients and their problems in doing routine occupations (1). Fleming suggests that therapists use three types of clinical reasoning in relation to working with clients: interactive reasoning, pattern recognition, and procedural reasoning. A visual example is provided in Figure 21.1. Interactive reasoning is used when the therapist wants to get to know and understand the client better as a person including feelings, preferences, interests, goals, lifestyle, coping skills, and adaptive responses. Interactive reasoning is usually based on talking directly with the person, family, and significant others. The interview is the most widely used method of obtaining information, but observation and written questionnaires may provide additional information. Although the data are valuable as factual information, therapists often view the information from a phenomenologic perspective to try to understand the client's perspective in terms of what is meaningful to the client as an individual.

Pattern recognition is a type of problem solving based on the ability of the therapist to observe and interpret cues. Cues are aspects of the situation the therapist observes and interprets as potentially significant to understanding the client's problems. Basically, "pattern recognition is the ability to observe a phenomenon, identify significant characteristics (cues), determine whether there is a relation among the cues, and compare the present observation to a previously learned category or type." Learning to use pattern recognition effectively is a major element in professional education. Each profession has a different set of pattern recognition skills although overlap occurs between closely associated professions. Pattern recognition skills usually improve with practice and modeling. Experienced practitioners may recognize a pattern in a few seconds whereas the student will struggle for several minutes to recognize the same pattern.

Procedural reasoning is used to link the client's problems to the intervention process—that is, to apply the tools and procedures of occupational therapy to the issues or problems identified through interactive reasoning and pattern recognition. Procedural reasoning is the process needed to create a plan of intervention, implement the plan, and determine when to end or revise implementation. Each profession has a different method for engaging procedural reasoning. Western medicine uses the sequence of etiology, diagnosis, treatment, and prognosis. Occupa-

Interactive reasoning

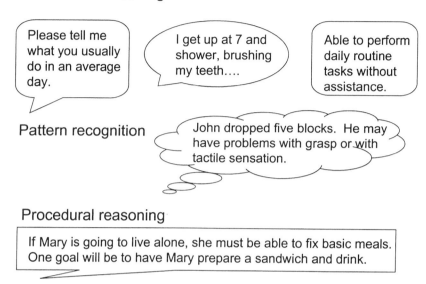

Figure 21.1. Three types of clinical reasoning according to Fleming.

tional therapists use the sequence of assessment (problem identification), analysis (occupational therapy diagnosis), planning (goal setting), program implementation, and intervention (treatment) and reassessment (determining results).

The division of clinical reasoning into three parts is most useful at the initial learning stage so that each part can be practiced and learned. Experienced therapists, however, probably collapse the first two types, interactive and pattern recognition, into one, called diagnostic reasoning (2). Rogers and Holm suggest the sequence for diagnostic reasoning includes a four-stage model of hypothetical reasoning: cue acquisition, hypothesis generation, cue interpretation, and hypothesis evaluation. Cue acquisition entails compiling the data garnered from the client, by using such sources as reading the client's chart, referral to occupational therapy, interviews, observation, and informal and formal testing. Cues, in singles or clusters, provide data concerning the source and types of dysfunction (problems), which in turn lead to the generation of one or more diagnostic hypotheses. Diagnostic hypotheses are tentative explanations of the source and types of dysfunction. In occupational therapy the diagnostic hypotheses may be called tentative occupational therapy diagnoses. The tentative occupational therapy diagnoses may be based on the occupational therapist's previous experience with clients who had similar problems, on interpretation based a particular theoretical view or practice model, or on a protocol (recipe or standard operative procedure) prepared by the facility or research project. Clinical or practice guidelines are examples of such protocols.

The diagnostic hypotheses provide the explanation for the third stage: cue interpretation. Cue interpretation is based on the relevance of the cues to the hypotheses being considered. Cues themselves can be divided into three groups: those indicative of normal function, those indicative of dysfunction based on one or more diagnostic hypotheses, and those that do not fit either categories and must be discarded or reorganized to create additional hypotheses. The skill in selecting tentative occupational therapy diagnoses determines whether the cue interpretation is correct, inaccurate, or misleading.

Correct interpretation of the cues is likely to result in success when the evidence (data, hypotheses, and cues) are reviewed during hypothesis evaluation. For each proposed occupational therapy diagnosis, the evidence is rechecked before proceeding to the planning and implementation stages. The evidence is analyzed to determine whether it better supports or refutes one hypothesis over another. The hypothesis with the preponderance of evidence is usually selected as the basis for planning and intervention. Evidence that does not fit the prevailing hypothesis must also be considered to determine if important information has been overlooked and an alternate hypothesis should be explored. A correct hypothesis is more likely to result in successful planning and intervention. Although it may save time if the occupational therapist quickly arrives at a hypothesis, effective intervention is more often related to arriving at the correct hypothesis than to arriving at a fast hypothesis.

Five other modes of clinical reasoning have also been identified in the occupational therapy literature (3,4). Mattingly and Fleming define theoretical reasoning as concerned "with what one can reliably predict will hold true in any specific case, or with what will give useful insight into a broad range of [a] particular situation." Theory is a useful guide to analyzing client problems, developing hypotheses, organizing a plan of intervention, and implementing the strategies, but the theory is not always sufficient to control or predict outcome for a given individual. Occupational therapists must be able to compare the client to the theory to see if a good fit exists between the client and the theoretical concepts and recommendations. Because a theory ought to work does not mean it will work. Clients are individuals and individuals do not always follow the expected course. Experienced occupational therapists weigh the pros and cons before initiating an intervention strategy based on a particular theory, monitor the results, and make changes when the results do not match the expectations proposed by the theory.

Mattingly and Fleming suggest that practical reasoning is similar to clinical reasoning except that practical reasoning is applied to everyday situations but not necessarily to professional situations such as working with clients. Practical reasoning involves "deliberation about what an appropriate action is in this particular case, with this particular person, at this particular time" (3, p. 10). One must know how to act, what course of action to take, and what is "good" in a particular case. What is "good" may have numerous working definitions in a multicultural society such as the United States.

The concept of "good" could also be explored using ethical reasoning. Hagedorn states that therapists can evaluate "proposed interventions in relation to the moral and ethical basis of practice, and with regard to any medicolegal consideration." There are ethical guidelines that therapists must follow. Such guidelines, together with the ability to apply the guidelines to the therapeutic process, are especially important when clients are vulnerable and may be unable to fully express personal needs or desires. Ethical reasoning requires that the occupational therapists think about what is "good" and "best" for the client: not what will achieve the most billable units for the accounting office or be easiest for the occupational therapist to do within a busy schedule.

Hagedorn also discusses predictive reasoning. She states that "during predictive reasoning the therapist weighs probabilities and possibilities and attempts to predict the effects of options for intervention and to gain a picture of probable outcomes in the case in relation to various imagined scenarios." Predictive reasoning could be considered a subcategory of hypotheses evaluation focusing on the outcomes of various occupational therapy diagnoses to determine which outcomes might be most desirable for the client.

Finally, Mattingly and Fleming discuss narrative reasoning. Narrative reasoning is the use of "stories to help frame practical decision about what to do" (3, p. 239). Storytelling can help place events within a temporal context which is particularly useful in reviewing historical information. By telling the story, the important cues often can be identified and actions can then be planned.

In summary, clinical reasoning is a specialized cognitive process that uses thinking and sometimes talking (narrative) to facilitate effective problem solving and decision making. Clinical reasoning relates to data collection, data analysis, and action plan development. There are several types and/or subtypes of clinical reasoning.

References

1. Fleming MH. Aspects of clinical reasoning in occupational therapy. In: Hopkins HL, Smith HD. Willard and Spackman's Occupational Therapy. Philadelphia: Lippincott, 1993:867–881.
2. Rogers JC, Holm MB. Occupational therapy diagnostic reasoning: a component of clinical reasoning. Am J Occup Ther 1991;45(11):1045–1053.
3. Mattingly C, Fleming MH. Clinical Reasoning: Forms of Inquiry in Therapeutic Practice. Philadelphia: FA Davis, 1994.
4. Hagedorn R. Foundations for Practice in Occupational Therapy. 2nd ed. New York: Churchill Livingstone, 1997:52.

CHAPTER 22

Assessment and Diagnosis

Assessment is part of the evaluation process but requires special skills. The evaluation process is discussed in the section on practice. Assessment in occupational therapy is the systematic collecting of data and information to determine the client's level of and ability to function or perform. Function and performance can be assessed in the occupations of self-care, self-maintenance, work and productivity, and play or leisure or in the occupational performance skills, which include sensorimotor, cognitive, and psychosocial. Analysis of the function is used to determine the following:

- Client's current level of growth and development within the life cycle
- Client's current level of function and performance of occupations and skills necessary to do daily tasks, perform in a productive setting, and enjoy play or leisure activities
- Client's need for and potential to benefit from intervention by occupational therapy services
- Information that would be useful for differential diagnosis
- Information necessary to make an occupational therapy diagnosis
- Information and data necessary to establish objectives and goals for an individualized plan
- Information and data necessary to develop strategies for an intervention program
- Information that will be useful in collaborative planning with other professionals
- Information and data for reassessment and/or termination

Occupational therapy practitioners need to understand that assessment is connected to planning and intervention. Assessment should provide the basis for planning and implementation. Figures 22.1 and 22.2 make the connection by illustrating the relationship. Assessment provides the data, and evaluation provides the analysis of the data to be applied in developing the objectives and goals in the intervention (treatment) plan. In turn, the intervention should be directly related to the intervention plan. There should be an obvious connection between what was assessed and what intervention strategies are used. The connection should be clear to the practitioner, the client and his or her family, and the reimbursement agency.

An assessor has several methods that can be used to collect data and informa-

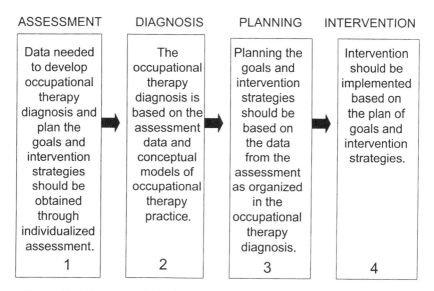

Figure 22.1. Assessment is the basis for diagnosis, planning, and implementation.

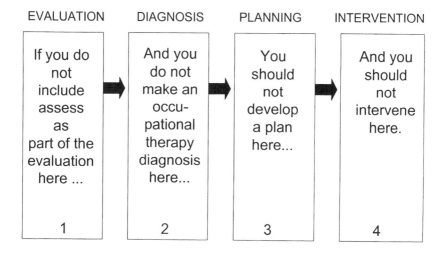

Figure 22.2. No assessment, no diagnosis, no plan, no intervention.

tion. These methods can be summarized as 1) interviewing; 2) observing; and 3) testing. Interviewing involves asking the person a series of questions and recording the answers. Interviews may be conducted verbally with the interviewer and person being interviewed sitting face-to-face, or an interview can be completed through the use of a questionnaire. Interviews are useful in collecting information directly from the individual that might be time-consuming to gather from other sources. Also, the person can be asked opinion-type questions as well as factual questions. For example, the interviewer can ask if the person likes living in a given community while asking for the person's address.

The disadvantages of interviewing are that the quality of the data depends on the willingness and ability of the interviewee to provide accurate information. A person may lie, forget, get confused, simply not know the answer, or not be willing to share the information. Older people sometimes answer questions about skills on the basis of what they used to be able to do or used to do frequently rather than their current status. The gap between what people think they can do and what they actually can do is always a problem in the interview format. Therefore, some practitioners prefer to combine interviewing with a demonstration or simulation. For example, if the person says "I take a bath everyday," have the person simulate taking a bath by getting in and out of an empty tub. If the person is unable to or has difficulty getting out of the tub, the person is probably not taking a bath in the tub but may be taking a sponge bath at the sink.

Observation is a method of gathering information based on the assessor's ability to see, hear, and feel what a person does in a given situation. The situation may be natural and unstructured or it may be contrived and structured. In the unstructured situation, the person does whatever would be done naturally and the observer watches, listens, or touches and then records the findings. Unstructured observation is useful for observing how a person works or plays in a given naturally occurring environment such as a home, office, playground, or neighborhood. A structured situation is prepared in advance by the observer. Only selected objects, such as toys or tools, are available. The observer knows in advance what skills will be required to use the toys or tools. When the person being assessed is introduced to the structured environment, the observer can focus attention directly on the person's performance since the environment is already preset.

Observation can provide an excellent source of real-life situation information. The practitioner can observe directly what actions the person does well and which ones cause problems. In a kitchen, for example, the person may be able to peel and mash the potatoes without difficulty but to carry the pan from the sink across 8 feet of open space to the stove may present a problem. The disadvantages are the limited observation skills of the assessor and limited opportunity to observer. Observation in a clinic environment is helpful in assessing function but the best place to observe is at the client's home. Clinics do not routinely have carpeted floors, narrow corridors, stairs without railings, and pets sitting in the doorways. In other words, homes have different situations to consider than an average occupational therapy clinic does.

Testing is the method most accepted for collecting data. This method involves an administrative procedure and a recording format that is routinely followed each time the test is administered. Tests may be informal nonstandardized or standardized. Informal testing is done by using a small part of a standardized or nonstandardized test to get an indication of whether more in-depth assessment should be done in a given area.

Nonstandardized tests may be developed by any therapist who wishes to use a routine checklist for clients with similar diagnosis. They are most useful when comparison to others is not important and not practical. For example, assessment of a prosthetic arm is important to the individual but comparing its function to a normal arm is unrealistic. Comparison to other persons with prosthetic arms may not be practical because each prosthetic arm must be adjusted to the individual. The important factor is how well the individual can use the arm.

Standardized tests are used when the client's achievement needs to be compared to the achievements of others to determine the degree of difference or similarity because the degree is critical to performance in society. Typing or keyboarding 20 words per minute is not sufficient in the job market that expects 50 to 60 words per minute. Taking 1 hour to get dressed may not be fast enough to allow a person to get up at 6:45 a.m., get to breakfast at 7:15 a.m. and to work by 8:00 a.m. Standardized tests can help determine if a person can function at an average level, above the average, or below.

Testing is useful when the test permits collection of information needed to determine levels of function. However, tests are not useful if the information is needed, but no test is available to record the data suitably. Some assessors like to use tests because of their recognized reliability in pinpointing certain information. However, if the information adds nothing to the decision-making process regarding need for intervention, differential diagnosis, selection of objectives, or collaborative planning, there is little reason to administer the test. In other words, there should be a reason for administering the test other than the fact that the test exists.

Selecting the right test can be a task in itself. Occupational therapy practitioners and researches have created more than 325 instruments, which have been identified by the authors. In addition, there are at least that many developed by persons other than occupational therapy personnel and used by practitioners. Some criteria can be helpful. Table 22.1 lists some of the considerations when selecting an assessment instrument.

Another approach to selecting a test is to use a classification system such as proposed in Table 22.2. Most of the groupings are self-explanatory. Test type includes battery, which means a test that includes multiple tests. Some of these tests may be single tests in their own right but have been grouped to provide more information and data than single test items could have provided. A checklist provides

Table 22.1. Test Analysis Form

I. **Reference Data**
   A. Title (full name of test):
   B. Alternate title (abbreviations, nicknames):
   C. Author (full names of all test developers from original and revisions):
   D. Publisher or Source (name, address, phone number, copyright):
   E. Publication dates (original and all revisions of manuals and test booklets):
   F. Population addressed (age, sex, race, culture, disability):
   G. Description of test and subtests materials (number of test items etc.):
   H. Purpose/application (screening, comprehensive, diagnosis):
   I. Theoretical base (frame of reference, conceptual model):

II. **Practical Considerations**
   A. Costs (current cost and format of materials):
   B. Time limits (time for subparts and total):
   C. Type/Format (checklist, interview, etc.):
   D. Alternate forms (number and type):
   E. Administration format (individual, group):
   F. Scores obtained (areas covered):
   G. Scoring procedures (total of numbers, graphic representation):
   H. Score interpretation (norms, proficiency, predictive):
   I. Equipment needed (included in test, other items needed):

III. **Technical Considerations**
   A. Dissemination of information:
      1. Availability of a manual:
      2. Presumption of validity by test title:
      3. Required qualifications:
   B. Validity
      1. Validity for each recommended use:
      2. Type of validity reported:
      3. Time elapsing between test administration and measurement of the criterion:
      4. Possibility of criterion contamination:
      5. Statistical procedures used to describe validity:
   C. Reliability
      1. Reliability for each recommended use:
      2. Means and standard deviations:
   D. Administration and scoring
      1. Clarity and completeness of instructions:
      2. Clarity and completeness of scoring directions:
      3. Safeguards against clerical errors in scoring:
   E. Scales and norms
      1. Types of norms provided:
         a. Scale scores
         b. Percentile ranks
         c. Stanines
         d. Grade equivalents
         e. Normal curve equivalents
         f. Anticipated achievement

continued

Table 22.1. Test Analysis Form

      g. Objective peformance index
      h. Standard error of measurement
      i. Grade mean equivalents
    2. Difficulty level of items:
    3. Comparability between old and revised norms:
    4. Description of the population used to select the norm group:
    5. Methods used to select the norm group from the population:
  F. Comments about fairness to persons of different ethnicity:
IV. **References or Bibliography**
  A. List of reference sources with citation information:
  B. Additional source information for further study:

Adapted from: Sax G. Principles of Educational and Psychological Measurement and Evaluation. 3rd ed. Belmont, CA: Wadsworth,1989:336–341.

---

a list of items that the person checks or ticks off. The checklist is used to indicate the presence or absence of a list of characteristics, factors, and/or behaviors. Checklists are frequently presented in tabular format for ease of recording answers. Most people have had experience with checklists.

A *coding system* translates qualitative information into categorical and numerical (quantitative) scores. This type of measurement instrument is concerned with degree of intensity of responses, including frequency of occurrence. A visual analogue is an example of a coding system. An *index* is a composite (often a ratio) of values or scores that describe a condition or variable that usually cannot be observed or measured directly. Many tests of functional assessment are actually indexes. The scoring is somewhat arbitrary relative to the amount of assistance needed and the value of performing one item over the next. *Projective techniques* provide a standardized method of eliciting responses to ambiguous stimuli. The stimuli may consist of pictures, phrases, or tasks that are loosely structured or defined and that allow respondents to reply as they wish. The technique is called "projective" because when asked to described the ambiguous stimuli, the respondent is believed to "project' feelings or thoughts onto the stimuli.

A *questionnaire* is a form or document that asks respondents to answer the questions presented. Questionnaires may be completed by the individual or in a group setting. A *rating scale* calls for opinions, judgments, or evaluations by a rater or a respondent. Responses are indicated by checking or circling words, phrases, or numbers. A *vignette* is a measurement using a scenario designed to assess a person's reactions to either hypothetical or actual situations. After reading a particular vignette (story, case study), respondents may be asked questions about the vignette, e.g., their attitudes toward the story characters, solutions to conflicts or problems depicted, or their possible reactions were they in the situation. Finally, there is a type of test called *test*. A test presents questions to assess or evaluate per-

Table 22.2.   Classification of Assessments in Occupational Therapy

1. Age
   1.1 Newborn 0–6 months
   1.2 Infant 0–2 years
   1.3 Preschool 2–5 years
   1.4 Child 6–12 years
   1.5 Adolescent 13–18 years
   1.6 Adult 19–64 years
   1.7 Aged (Geriatric) 65–80
   1.8 Elderly 80+
2. Areas of Practice
   2.1 Geriatrics
   2.2 Mental health
   2.3 Pediatric
   2.4 Physical disabilities
3. Occupational Areas
   3.1 Functional assessment
      3.1.1 BADL (self-care)
      3.1.2 IADL (community, homemaking, kitchen skills)
   3.2 Work/productivity
   3.3 Leisure skills
   3.4 Play skills
   3.5 School and academic skills
4. Occupational Components
   4.1 Sensorimotor
      4.1.1   Coordination
      4.1.2   Dexterity
      4.1.3   Fine motor skills
      4.1.4   Functional communication
      4.1.5   Gross motor skills
      4.1.6   Oral-motor
      4.1.7   Physiologic
         4.1.7.1   Breathing rate
         4.1.7.2   Endurance
         4.1.7.3   Exertion
         4.1.7.4   Heart rate
         4.1.7.5   Pain
      4.1.8   Preacademic skills
      4.1.9   Range of motion (joint)
         4.1.9.1   Functional
         4.1.9.2   Measures in degrees
      4.1.10 Sensory system
         4.1.10.1 Auditory
         4.1.10.2 Gustatory
         4.1.10.3 Kinesthetic
         4.1.10.4 Proprioception
         4.1.10.5 Tactile/touch
         4.1.10.6 Vestibular
         4.1.10.7 Vestibular

continued

Table 22.2. Classification of Assessments in Occupational Therapy

        4.1.11   Strength testing
        4.1.11.1 Grip of hand
        4.1.11.2 Individual muscles
        4.1.11.3 Muscle groups
        4.1.11.3 Pinch
    4.2 Cognitive
        4.2.1   Attention span and concentration
        4.2.2   General knowledge
        4.2.3   Generalization
        4.2.4   Judgment
        4.2.5   Level of arousal
        4.2.6   Memory
        4.2.7   Metacognition
        4.2.8   Problem solving
        4.2.9   Synthesis
        4.2.10   Transfer of training
    4.3 Psychosocial
        4.3.1   Dyad relationships
        4.3.2   Group skills
        4.3.3   Roles
        4.3.4   Self-concept/self-awareness
        4.3.5   Self-efficacy
        4.3.6   Sense of mastery, competence, achievement
        4.3.7   Stress
5. Technology
    5.1   Accessability—physical
    5.2   Communication system
    5.3   Environmental controls
    5.4   Prosthetic/orthotic checkout
    5.5   Mobility system
    5.6   Seating system
6. Test Mechanics
    6.1   Paper and pencil
    6.2   Object—singular
    6.3   Objects—multiple
7. Test Type
    7.1   Battery (contains multiple tests)
    7.2   Checklist
    7.3   Coding system
    7.4   Index
    7.5   Interview form
    7.6   Observation recording form
    7.7   Projective test
    7.8   Questionnaire
    7.9   Rating scale
    7.10   Self-report
    7.11   Test
    7.12   Vingette

continued

Table 22.2.   Classification of Assessments in Occupational Therapy

8. Purpose of Test
    8.1   Descriptive
    8.2   Evaluative
    8.3   Predictive
9. Time to Administer
    9.1   1–10 minutes
    9.2   11–20 min
    9.3   21–30 min
    9.4   31–60 min
    9.5   61–90 min
    9.6   91–120 min
    9.7   121+
10. Time to Score
    10.1   1–10 minutes
    10.2   11–20 min
    10.3   21–30 min
    10.4   31–60 min
    10.5   61+
11. Time to Learn to Administer
    11.1   1–30 min
    11.2   31–60 min
    11.3   1–2 hours
    11.4   3–5 hrs
    11.5   6–10 hrs
    11.6   11+
12. Ease of Administration
    12.1   Easy
    12.2   Difficult
13. Named Disability
    13.1   Alzheimer's disease
    13.2   Arthritis
    13.3   Cerebral palsy
    13.4   Cerebrovascular accident (stroke)
    13.5   Dysphagia/swallowing
    13.6   Mental retardation
    13.7   Neurological impairment
    13.8   Psychiatric
    13.9   Substance abuse
    13.10   Tumor/brain injury/head injury
14. Theoretical Background
    14.1   Occupational adaptation
    14.2   Occupational behavior
    14.3   Developmental
    14.4   Model of human occupation
    14.5   Motor control
    14.6   Sensory integration

continued

Table 22.2.   Classification of Assessments in Occupational Therapy

15. Ownership
    15.1 Commercial/proprietary
    15.2 Unpublished/nonproprietary
    15.3 Unrestricted
16. Price
    16.1 Original purchase price
    16.2 Replacement costs

formance, ability, knowledge, and/or behavior. Examples of tests are range of motion and muscle strength.

To summarize, assessments that occupational therapy practitioners administer and score may meet the objectives of assessing function and performance of skills; determine current levels of growth and development; determine if intervention is needed; contribute to differential diagnosis and occupational therapy diagnosis; provide information and data for program planning, intervention, and reassessment; and assist in collaborative planning with other disciplines. There are three major types of assessment: interview, observation, and tests. Tests include standardized and nonstandardized as well as several different types. Selecting a good assessment instrument is important. Guidelines are useful in evaluating which test to use.

OCCUPATIONAL THERAPY DIAGNOSIS

Occupational therapy practitioners have talked about occupational therapy diagnosis but have done little. The earliest reference to an occupational diagnosis appeared in Barton's article "Inoculation of the Bacillus of Work," presented at the founding meeting in 1917 (1). He stated that he makes an "occupational" diagnosis to discover latent interests. The most consistent literature about occupational therapy diagnosis is by Rogers and Holm who said that no classification system exists (2). Occupational therapy practitioners in the past may have been reluctant to use the term diagnosis because of its use in medicine but nursing has been using the term nursing diagnosis since 1973. The organization that maintains their diagnostic categories is called the North American Nursing Diagnosis Association (NANDA). With nursing at the lead, there should be no reluctance on the part of occupational therapy practitioners to also talk about diagnosis in connection with occupational therapy.

The word diagnosis comes from 'dia' meaning through or complete and 'gnosis' meaning knowledge. Complete knowledge includes the ability to distinguish, determine, differentiate and discriminate which are the terms most often associated with diagnosis (3, 4). Medical diagnosis can be described as the complete knowledge to distinguish disease or disorder according to the pathological frame of reference which physicians, by virtue of their education and experience, are able and licensed to treat. Nursing diagnosis can be described as the complete knowledge to distinguish health problems that nurses, by virtue of their education and experience, are able and licensed to treat (5, p. 1299). Occupational performance diagnosis can be described as the complete knowledge to distinguish occupational role and performance task problems and functional levels that occupational therapists, by virtue of their education and experience, are able and licensed to treat or manage. The term occupational performance diagnosis provides occupational therapy with an accurate description of a critical phase in the process of occupational therapy that links assessment to planning and intervention. The diagnostic process provides a sound, logical basis for decisions used in planning and intervention for a particular client at a particular time. The classification system organizes the possible occupational performance diagnoses into one list. Table 22.3 seen at the end of this chapter is a proposed classification system of occupational therapy diagnoses. The following information explains its development.

Components of a Diagnosis

According to King, diagnosis has three components (6). First, a preexisting series of categories or classes provides the frame of reference for the diagnosis. A classification system together with background knowledge of the categories or classes contained within the system provides an information base on which to analyze and derive a diagnosis. Therefore, a classification of occupation together with background knowledge of the types of occupational performance and dysfunction provides the basis on which to derive an occupational performance diagnosis. Second, there is the particular person to be diagnosed. The person is the source of information or data to be gathered. In occupational therapy, that information can include data about occupational roles, performance areas, and socioenvironmental expectations or situations. Data may be gathered or obtained through observation, interview, or tests, which provide cues to actual or potential problems that can be stated in a diagnostic hypothesis to be verified or discarded. Third, the deliberate or logical reasoning process results in a decision as to which object or problem belongs to *this* category rather than *that* one, differential diagnosis. Logical reasoning, also known as clinical reasoning, requires thought processes that 1) can collect and cluster data into recognized patterns, 2) have knowledge and understanding of probability, 3) form a judgment based on individual and collective knowledge and experience, and 4) have the ability to use the problem-solving or decision-making process. Overall, the purpose of diagnosis in occupational therapy is to classify the problem(s) to which intervention through occupational therapy can be applied and a prognosis or outcome concerning occupational performance can be predicted and measured. The Occupational Performance Diagnosis Classification System provides a framework for the identification of patient/client problems that can be remediated, potential problems that can be prevented, or functional performance that should be maintained through occupational therapy intervention and management. Criteria attached to each occupational performance diagnostic item can be used to establish the parameters that support the achievement of these goals and outcomes.

Defining Occupational Performance Diagnosis

An occupational performance diagnosis is a statement of the person's occupational role or performance task dysfunction or potential for dysfunction. The dysfunction is the problem that is causing, or may cause, the person difficulty in occupational performance and that brings the client to seek or be referred to occupational therapy. In contrast, an occupational performance goal or outcome is a statement of the expected change in the person's ability and skill in performing an occupational role and/or performance task. This change should occur during and as a result of occupational therapy intervention. The change is the expected outcome and should be stated in objective, measurable terms. When the change in the targeted direction occurs, the occupational therapy intervention process has been successful. In summary, the diagnosis defines the problem and the goal or outcome describes the direction and means to solve the problem and remove or decrease the dysfunction.

Occupational Performance Diagnosis Framework

Following King's model the first step in occupational performance diagnosis is the development of a classification system or taxonomy of conditions or problem statements that occupational therapists can assess, analyze, and diagnose, and that can be treated or managed through occupational therapy intervention and management. The frame of reference for the occupational performance diagnose classification system is based on a hierarchical model of functional abilities developed by Kemp and Mitchell (7). Kemp and Mitchell proposed a six-level model of functional abilities, which are labeled organ system, physical substrates, activities of daily living, instrumental activities of daily living, skilled performance, and social roles.

The model used to organize the Uniform Terminology for Occupational Therapy was explored as a frame of reference for organizing the occupational performance diagnoses (8). However, the occupational and performance areas do not lead to a hierarchy that can be used to develop priorities for organizing treatment goals and objectives. Also the Uniform Terminology focuses on what occurs or is seen in occupational therapy practice but does not define the actual problems that occupational therapists can diagnosis and manage. The purpose of the occupational performance diagnosis classification system is to define and outline the problems occupational therapists can identify and bring about positive change through the use of methods, techniques, and modalities that will improve or increase occupational performance and decrease or eliminate dysfunction. Therefore, the classification system is described in terms of the condition or problem in occupational roles or performance tasks.

Criteria for a Diagnosis

Campbell spelled out the criteria for a nursing diagnosis (9). Based on Campbell, the criteria for occupational performance diagnosis are as follows: 1) the diagnosis describes a human occupational role or performance task; 2) a professional occupational therapist can legally diagnose, prescribe, and implement the intervention and management program designed for the problem or problems in occupational performance; 3) the diagnosis occurs repeatedly in a significant number of clients so as to be recognizable by several occupational therapists; 4) one or more problems exist in human occupational roles or performance tasks; 5) the supporting data for the diagnosis can be obtained and analyzed by the professional occupational therapist using knowledge of occupational roles or performance tasks; and 6) the diagnostic problem is not a specific disease identified as such in the standard medical classification system but may be related to a health problem addressed in a nursing diagnosis.

Creating a Classification System

To identify the possible occupational performance problems, 42 models of occupational therapy theory and practice were reviewed for the problems that each model was developed to address. The problems were then organized into the occupational performance diagnostic framework (See Table 22.3). Labels or names and definitions were developed according to the concept in the originating model but reworded to meet the phraseology used to describe the problems in the occupational performance diagnosis outline. Key words are unable, altered, impaired, and high-risk. Unable to perform means the person cannot perform any of the steps required for the task or can perform so few steps as to make the performance of the role or task impractical in terms of energy expended, time consumed, satisfaction gained, or safety of the individual and significant others. A person with dressing apraxia is unable to dress himself or herself. Impaired means the person experiences difficulty performing one or more tasks within a designated skill. A person with dressing dyspraxia has difficulty performing the steps needed to dress. The difficulty might be caused by problems in coordination, sequencing, spatial organization, or memory of the steps that would be determined during the assessment process. Altered means one or more tasks must be performed in a manner different than is customary for the society or culture in which the person usually lives. A person who needs extended or enlarged handles to perform some steps within the dressing task uses an altered approach to dressing as defined by the norms in most cultures. High-risk means a person has a condition or situation that is known to frequently result in difficulty performing steps in a task. Problems in dressing occur frequently in persons with dementia or following a stroke. Therefore, these medical diagnoses would prompt the occupational therapist to consider persons with such labels as high-risk for dressing apraxia or dyspraxia. A step is a unit of sensory motor, cognitive, or psychosocial behavior, which when combined with other steps in a designated sequence, results in the performance of a task. A task consists of a series of sequential steps that lead to performance of the activity. Examples of steps are putting on, taking off, zipping, buttoning, putting the left arm through a sleeve, and tying a tie. An occupational role requires the performance of a group of tasks and behaviors which society condones and expects of individuals and that a person agrees to perform.

Each definition in the classification system must meet several criteria to be useful as a diagnosis. The definition must be clear, concise, and descriptive of an occupational performance problem or condition. Second, the definition must be meaningful and assist in differentiating the specific diagnosis from other diagnoses. Third, the definition must describe a documented occupational role dysfunction or a difficulty or potential deficiency in performing one or more performance tasks to meet the frame of reference used in the particular classification system.

Benefits of a Classification System

One benefit of the occupational performance diagnostic classification system is a list on which to build a taxonomy of the problems occupational therapists state in various publications that they can assess, analyze, diagnose, and provide intervention or management strategies to improve occupational performance. The list serves as a guide for the conceptual organization of problems by providing a label and definition. To each label (problem), a set of defining characteristics can be attached, a summary of the assessment tools used to identify each problem can be listed, effective intervention or management strategies can be described, and outcomes can be established and evaluated. In addition, the classification system provides a guide to determine which tasks or performance areas need additional research to support the claims made for precision and accuracy of the diagnosis and the effectiveness and efficiency of the intervention or management strategies. Linking practice and research provides increasing evidence that occupational therapy is serious about meeting the criteria to become a recognized profession.

A third benefit is that professionals can concentrate on those diagnoses for which research has shown that occupational therapists are most successful in improving performance or preventing dysfunctional performance. The list produced thus far is very long. Not all diagnoses included may be within the scope of services occupational therapists will want to provide or will be accepted by clients and third-party payers as services needed to regain or maintain health. Occupational therapists may decide to concentrate their resources on selected problems or prioritize the list of problems that will receive the most attention in practice or research.

A fourth benefit is improved communication to the public, clients/patients, third-party payers, and other health care professionals who frequently have difficulty understanding what occupational therapy is and what occupational therapists do. Occupational therapists have not been systematic about creating a comprehensive list of what they can do or what they can do better than others and for which occupational therapists can be held accountable in quality assurance reviews.

A fifth benefit is a system that can be used across various specialized areas of practice within occupational therapy. The classification system should be useful to all areas of practice because all problems addressed by occupational therapists can be included. Thus, the classification system can accommodate the diversity and variety of occupational roles and task performance.

A sixth benefit is the potential to increase the credibility and respectability of occupational therapy as a discipline within the social system of professionalism. A discipline is evaluated in part on its body of knowledge, scientific orderliness and translation into a unique practice arena that fills a distinct social need (9, p. 9).

Finally, the classification system may help organize occupational therapy educational curricula by providing a guideline of content to be included and a checklist to determine if the content has been covered. Continuing education or inservices may be developed to educate practitioners on content that has been recently added or is updated as practice, research, or changing healthcare needs has mandated.

Challenges

The challenge is to develop a useful classification system. The draft system may be too long, may not be inclusive enough, may contain vague or incomplete definitions, or may be more useful if organized within a different framework. Further analysis of the literature concerning occupational therapy and continuing research will be required to determine which diagnoses should be kept and which should be changed or discarded.

What work remains to be done? First, each diagnosis must be reviewed for clarity of the problem described in the definition. Some problems may need to be divided or subdivided to provide more accurate descriptions of problems known to cause occupational performance dysfunction. Second, each problem must be expanded to include the assessment instrument or instruments used to substantiate the diagnosis and differentiate the diagnosis from similar or related problems. Next, the intervention strategy or strategies along with the media, methods, techniques, and approaches used by occupational therapists to remediate or prevent the problem must be defined in the diagnosis. If intervention strategies are not found in the occupational therapy literature, then strategies must be developed or the problem removed from the list. Fourth, the classification system must be examined for missing diagnoses that need to be added or that might be combined because they are similar. In addition, some diagnoses may need to have assessment instruments or intervention strategies revised and reevaluated to improve effectiveness or efficiency in remediating or preventing the problem.

The classification system must also be reviewed with clients, reimbursement sources, and other healthcare professionals to determine whether the occupational performance diagnoses are understandable by persons or groups other than occupational therapists. Such review may enable changes to be made in marketing occupational therapy services, documenting occupational therapy services for billing purposes and criteria for referral, or consulting with occupational therapy personnel.

Occupational therapists do not always act alone to correct problems that affect occupational roles or task performance. Many problems causing occupational dysfunction present issues that may be defined as illness, lack of education, illegal, unsafe, or harmful. Carpenito refers to problems with overlapping concerns as collaborative problems (10). In such cases, occupational therapists must work in collaborative arrangements to correct the presenting problems. Each profession provides a perspective using the knowledge base of that profession. The occupational therapist uses the knowledge of occupational performance. Carpenito defines collaborative problems as "complications that professionals monitor to detect onset or changes in status" (10). Maintaining skin integrity and preventing skin breakdown is an example. Skin integrity is a prerequisite to performing most occupational roles and tasks and is a problem which will interfere with health, education, and personal safety.

Table 22.3. Occupational Therapy Diagnosis

ORGAN SYSTEMS: prerequisites include organ system integrity, nutrition, movement, and health

> Activity deficit: a state in which an individual does not perform a minimum number of daily activities to maintain basic physiological and psychological health
>
> Activity imbalance: a state in which an individual performs certain daily living activities to the exclusion or near exclusion of other important daily activities, including rest and sleep
>
> Activity intolerance: a state in which an individual has insufficient physiological or psychological energy to endure or complete required or desired daily activities***
>
> Activity intolerance, potential: a state in which an individual is at risk of having insufficient physiological or psychological energy to endure or complete required or desired daily activities***
>
> Fatigue: an overwhelming, sustained sense of exhaustion and decreased capacity for physical and mental work*

continued

Table 22.3. Occupational Therapy Diagnosis

Impairment: a state in which an individual experiences loss and/or abnormality of mental, emotional, physiological, or anatomical structure or function****

Incontinence, partial total: a state in which an individual experiences a continuous and unpredictable loss of urine*

Intellectual impairment: individual lacks cognitive skills that permit a person to learn and remember a variety of information and knowledge

Shortness of breath: a state in which an individual experiences difficulty getting enough air into his or her lungs

Skin/soft tissue breakdown/redness/soreness/decubiti: a state in which the individual's skin and/or soft tissue is adversely altered*

Skin/soft tissue, potential for breakdown/redness/soreness/decubiti: situation exists or apparently will exist in the foreseeable future for the skin and/or soft tissue to become adversely altered

PHYSICAL SUBSTRATES: prerequisites include organ system integrity plus desire, perseverance, motivation, and sensory ability

Sensory Motor Substrates: Sensory and Perceptual Systems

Sensory awareness/sensory registration, deficit/impaired (specify sensory system/systems or disuse syndrome): a state in which an individual lacks awareness or experiences diminished registration of sensory input

Sensory processing/sensory sensitivity, deficit/impaired (specify sensory modality or system such as blindness, low vision, deafness, hard of hearing, deaf-blind, hypersensitivity, hyposensitivity, phantom pain, chronic pain, tactile defensiveness): a state in which an individual overresponds or underresponds to sensory input, real or imaged

Sensory discrimination, deficit/impaired (specify sensory modality): a state in which an individual experiences inability or difficulty in differentiating one kind of sensory stimulus from another

> Auditory deficit/impaired: a state in which an individual is unable to or experiences difficulty receiving, processing, and organizing or interpreting sounds, including deafness, hard of hearing, hearing loss, localizing sounds, and discriminating background sounds based on previous knowledge or experience
>
> Gustatory deficit/impaired: a state in which an individual is unable to or experiences difficulty receiving, processing, and organizing or interpreting or discriminating between different tastes based on previous knowledge or experience
>
> Olfactory deficit/impaired: a state in which an individual is unable to or experiences difficulty receiving, processing, and organizing or interpreting or discriminating between different odors based on previous knowledge or experience
>
> Proprioceptive deficit/impaired: a state in which an individual is unable to or experiences difficulty receiving, processing, and organizing or interpreting or discriminating between body postures or movement positions proprioceptive input and based on previous knowledge/experience
>
> Tactile deficit/impaired: a state in which an individual is unable to or experiences difficulty receiving, processing, and organizing or interpreting

continued

Table 22.3.   Occupational Therapy Diagnosis

tactile input including light touch, pressure, vibration, and two-point stimuli through skin contact/receptors based on previous knowledge or experience

Vestibular deficit/impaired: a state in which an individual is unable to or experiences difficulty receiving, processing and organizing or interpreting vestibular input from the inner ear receptors regarding position of the head and body during movement through space (linear, curvilinear, or circular acceleration and deceleration)

Visual deficit/impaired: a state in which an individual is unable to or experiences difficulty in receiving, processing, organizing or interpreting visual input through the eyes, including blindness, homonomous hemianopsia, low vision, unilateral neglect

Perceptual deficit/impaired (specify perceptual disorder): an individual is unable to or experiences difficulty in perceiving and organizing information received through the sensory systems

Agraphesthesia: inability or difficulty in identifying symbols written on the skin

Astereognosis: inability or difficulty in identifying objects through the sense of touch

Body scheme, deficit/impaired: a state in which an individual is unable to or experiences difficulty in acquiring an internal perceptual awareness of the body and the relationship of body parts to each other

Color blindness: inability to perceive or difficulty in perceiving and differentiating one color, shade, or hue from another

Depth perception, lack of: inability to perceive or difficulty in perceiving the relative distance between objects, figures, or landmarks and one's self

Dyskinesthesia: a state in which an individual experiences difficulty in perceiving the excursion and direction of joint movement

Right-left discrimination, deficit/impaired: inability to perceive or difficulty in perceiving and differentiating between one side of the body from the other

Topographical orientation, deficit/impaired: inability to perceive or difficulty in perceiving and thus determining the locating of objects and settings and the route to the location

Visual closure, deficit/impaired: inability to perceive complete forms or objects based on an incomplete presentation

Visual discrimination, deficit/impaired: inability to perceive or difficulty in perceiving objects in the environment visually by their unique visual characteristics

Visual figure–ground deficit/impaired: inability to perceive or difficulty in perceiving and differentiating between objects or figures in the foreground and those in the background

Visual form/perceptual constancy/consistency, deficit/impaired: inability to perceive or difficulty in perceiving objects possessing invariant properties such as shape, position, and size regardless of the variability of presentation in the environment

Visual spatial relations, deficit/impaired: inability to perceive or difficulty in perceiving the relationship of figures and objects to one's self or in relation to other forms or objects

continued

Table 22.3. Occupational Therapy Diagnosis

Sensory integrative dysfunction: a state in which an individual experiences inability or difficulty in receiving, selecting, combining, integrating, and coordinating sensory information at the subcortical level for use in adaptive behavior and responses

Sensory Motor Substrates: Neuromuscular Systems (reflexes, joints, and muscles)

Ataxia: see Postural control

Endurance: see Physical endurance

Grip/hand strength, weakness: a state in which an individual demonstrates deviations in norms from his or her age group or occupation for grip or hand strength

Hand grasp patterns (functions), impaired: a state in which the individual experiences impaired ability in using different hand and finger grasp patterns to perform a variety of activities

Joint range of motion, deficit/loss of/limited: a state in which an individual demonstrates limited ability to move a joint through a range of motions consistent with accepted norms for his or her age group

Joint range of motion, potential for loss/limitation/contractures/deformity/immobility: situation exists or apparently will exist in the foreseeable future for loss of joint range of motion and/or joint deformity that is preventable

Joint stability, impaired: a state in which an individual experiences lack of joint stability and muscle cocontraction when resistance or body weight is applied

Muscle-joint synergies, reflexive: a state in which an individual is unable to initiate or maintain movement of muscles or joints without the synergy pattern dominating, controlling, or limiting the intended movement

Muscle power/strength, atrophy/paralysis: a state in which an individual demonstrates total or near total loss of ability to demonstrate muscle power within the norms for his or her age group or occupation

Muscle power/strength, dystrophy/weakness: a state in which an individual demonstrates impaired ability to demonstrate muscle power within the norms for his or her age group or occupation

Muscle power/strength, potential for loss: situation exists or apparently will exist in the foreseeable future in which the individual will lose muscle power/strength unless preventative measures are adopted and followed

Muscle tone, abnormal (specify hypertonicity, hypotonicity, athetosis, spasticity, imbalance, tremor, dystonia): a state in which an individual demonstrates muscle tone that deviates from the norm and interferes with movement

Physical endurance/fitness, low: a state in which an individual demonstrated deviations in norms from his or her age group or occupation in physical endurance or fitness

Pinch/finger strength, weakness: a state in which an individual demonstrates deviations in norms from his or her age group in pinch or finger strength

Postural control/stability (ataxia/loss of balance/disequilibrium), lack of: a state in which an individual is unable to or experiences impaired ability to maintain the upright position in sitting, standing, and walking

Postural integration/proximal stability, lack of: a state in which an individual is unable to maintain postural background control when engaged in voluntary movements or activities

continued

Table 22.3.   Occupational Therapy Diagnosis

Range of motion: see Joint range of motion
Reflex/reaction maturation and integration, delayed but no abnormality: a state in which the individual demonstrates deviations in norms from his or her age group in the maturation and integration of reflexes or reactions
Reflex/reaction response, abnormal: a state in which the individual demonstrates abnormal response to stimuli that elicit reflexes or reactions
Strength: see Muscle power/strength
Synergies: see Muscle-joint synergies
Tone: see Muscle tone

Sensory Motor Substrates: Motor Coordination and Dexterity

Akinesia: see Dyskinesia
Apraxia: see Dyspraxia
Bilateral integration, lack of: a state in which the individual is unable to or experiences impaired ability to use the two sides of the body together as a unit for movement in same direction at the same time or movements that require reciprocal action
Bilateral (parallel) movement, deficit: a state in which an individual is unable to perform the same movement pattern at the same time with two extremities
Change of dominance/handedness: a state in which an individual must change the preferred side of the body to the non preferred in order to perform some activities such as handwriting
Dyskinesia/akinesia/bradykinesia: a state in which an individual experiences impaired or slowed ability to initiate a voluntary movement or sequence of voluntary movements
Dysphagia: see Oral-motor incoordination
Dyspraxia/apraxia/motor planning deficit: a state in which an individual is unable to or experiences impaired ability to motor plan movements of the joints and muscles

> Constructional dyspraxia: a state in which an individual has an impaired ability to organize or combine details and component parts which must be perceived in relation to each other as a synthesis#
> Ideational apraxia: a state in which an individual has a disruption in the sequential organization of the gestures required to cary out a complex performance, owing to the disintegration or inadequacy of the plan of action#
> Motor apraxia: a state in which an individual is unable to perform skilled, purposeful movements

Fine motor incoordination, manipulation deficit, lack of dexterity: a state in which an individual experiences impaired ability to perform coordinated movement of fingers and hand
Gross motor incoordination (dyskinesia, dysdiadochokinesia): a state in which an individual experiences impaired ability to perform coordinated movements of the large joints and muscle groups
Gross motor skill, developmental delay: a state in which an individual demonstrates deviations in norms from his or her age group in the development of gross motor skills

continued

Table 22.3. Occupational Therapy Diagnosis

Gross motor skill, altered/impaired: a state in which an individual experiences impaired ability to perform gross motor skills

Laterality/dominance, deficit or lack of: a state in which an individual is unable to or experiences impaired ability to select and use a preferred side of the body as the lead or dominant side; relates to eyes, hands/arms, and feet/legs

Midline crossing, difficulty in: a state in which an individual is unable to or experiences impaired ability to place parts of the body such as arms or legs across the midline (center) of the body

Ocular control, deficit or impaired: a state in which an individual is unable to or experiences difficulty in controlling or coordinating the eyes (includes amblyopia, diplopia, squint, or strabismus)

Oral-motor incoordination (swallowing, impaired; chewing, undifferentiated): a state in which an individual is unable to chew or swallow or experiences impaired ability to chew or swallow

Reciprocal (opposite) movement, deficit: a state in which an individual is unable to alternate movement of, move in opposite directions, two extremities at the same time

Visual-motor (eye-hand, eye-foot) incoordination: a state in which an individual is unable to or experiences impaired ability using visual input to guide the direction and speed of movement of the hand or foot

Cognitive Substrates

Arousal level, low/not maintained, lethargy: a state in which an individual is unable to maintain a level of consciousness so as to permit performance of daily living skills; person is not alert and does not respond quickly to stimuli

Coma: see Arousal level

Confused or disoriented: a state in which an individual has difficulty responding correctly or is unable to respond correctly to questions regarding or locating one's self in relation to time, place, person, date, and destination

Disoriented or disorientation: see Confused or disoriented

Memory loss, deficit or impaired, temporary: a state in which an individual is temporarily unable to or has difficulty remembering information or knowledge previously learned or known

Memory loss, deficit or impaired, permanent: a state in which an individual is permanently unable to remember information and knowledge previously learned

Recall: see Recognition and recall

Recognition/recall deficit or impaired: a state in which an individual is unable to or has difficulty recognizing or recalling information or knowledge previously learned or known

Sequencing (of time and/or task activity), deficit or impaired: a state in which an individual is unable to or inaccurately states the relation of events or performs a series of tasks according to an established time sequence or schedule of activities

Stupor: see Arousal level

Psychosocial Substrates

Dynamic a states: term is used to specify those aspects of an individual that change or respond to environmental influences (includes needs, emotions, interests, motivation, and values)

continued

Table 22.3. Occupational Therapy Diagnosis

Anger, hostility: individual feels he or she is mistreated and is mad at various persons, situations, or events

Anxiety: individual has a subjective feeling of apprehension and tension manifested by physiological arousal and varying patterns of behavior; the source of anxiety is nonspecific or unknown to the individual*

Apathy, depression: individual feels he or she has no energy to give to any activity and no activity is worth performing

Depression: see Apathy

Depressive reaction to illness: individual feels overwhelmed by an illness and may grieve for loss of health and ability to perform activities

Fear: individual feels a sense of threat or danger to self arising from an identifiable source that the person validates

Grieving: individual perceives the loss or anticipates the loss of an object (person, job, possessions) that is significant or important to the person

Hopelessness: individual feels that alternatives and personal choices are limited or nonexistent, and therefore is unable to mobilize energy on his or her own behalf

Hostility: see Anger

Interests/motivators, lack of: individual is unable to identify mental or physical activities that create pleasure and maintain his or her attention

Initiative, lack of (unmotivated): individual is unable to engage in a physical or mental activity at an appropriate time

Mania: individual feels his or her energy is unlimited and any and everything can be accomplished without regard for time or cost

Mood/affect, altered (specify whether constricted, blunt, or flat): inability or difficulty in expressing emotion consistent with the situation, circumstances, and cultural background

Motivation: see Initiative

Needs, basic: individual is unable to meet or satisfy basic needs for maintenance of life and personal safety

Negative emotions: a person responds to most or all situation(s) with one or more of the following: dissatisfaction, fear or anxiety, dislike, hatred, anger, or depression

Object relations, deficit or impaired: a person is unable to or experiences difficulty in investing emotions and psychic energy in objects (human beings including the self, abstract concepts, or nonhuman things) that have the potential for satisfying needs

Termination, lack of (perseveration): individual is unable to stop an activity at an appropriate time

Violence, potential for self directed or directed at others: individual expresses behaviors that can be physically harmful either to the self or others*

Intrapsychic dynamics: refers to the phenomena of conscious and unconscious, psychodynamics and defense mechanisms

Conflict resolution, unresolved: discordance between opposing desires and between desires and prohibitions which the individual experiences difficulty resolving

Defense mechanisms, inappropriate: overuse of defense mechanisms (denial, introjection, projection, repression) to avoid dealing with various life situations

continued

Table 22.3. Occupational Therapy Diagnosis

Denial, ineffective: individual consciously or unconsciously disavows
knowledge or meaning of an event to reduce anxiety or fear, to the
detriment of his or her health*
Ego strength, inadequate: individual lacks physical energy
Emotional immaturity: individual does not demonstrate ability to response
to situations with the emotional maturity or control consistent with age
and cultural situation

ACTIVITIES OF DAILY LIVING (self-maintenance or self-care): Prerequisites
include physical substrates plus memory and help from others if needed)

Bathing/hygiene, deficit: a state in which the individual is unable to perform
independently bathing or hygiene activities due to lack of knowledge and/or
opportunity to practice or implement the required skills
Bathing/hygiene, altered/impaired: a state in which the individual experiences
impaired ability to perform or complete any or all bathing or hygiene activities
for him or herself owing to changes in skill performance components*
Dressing/grooming, deficit: a state in which the individual is unable to perform
independently dressing or grooming activities as a result of lack of knowledge
and/or opportunity to practice or implement the required skills
Dressing/grooming, altered/impaired: a state in which the individual
experiences impaired ability to perform or complete any or all dressing or
grooming activities for him or herself*
Feeding/eating, deficit: a state in which the individual is unable to perform
independently feeding or eating activities owing to lack of knowledge and/or
opportunity to practice or implement the required skills
Feeding/eating, altered/impaired: a state in which the individual experiences
impaired ability to perform or complete any or all feeding or eating activities
for him or herself*
Physical mobility or ambulation, deficit: a state in which the individual is
unable to move independently owing to a lack the knowledge or opportunity
to practice required skills
Physical mobility or ambulation, altered/impaired/lost: a state in which the
individual experiences a limitation of ability for independent physical
movement*
Rest and sleep disturbance: a state in which disruption of rest or sleep time
causes discomfort or interferes with an individual's desired lifestyle*
Sexual dysfunction: a state in which problems with sexual function exist*
Sexuality patterns, altered/impaired: a state in which an individual expresses
concern regarding his or her sexuality*
Toileting, (bowel and bladder) deficit: a state in which the individual is unable
to perform independently toileting activities becuase of lack of knowledge
and/or opportunity to practice or implement the required skills
Toileting, (bowel and bladder) altered/impaired: a state in which the individual
experiences impaired ability to perform or complete any or all toileting
activities for himself or herself*
Transfers, deficit: a state in which the individual is unable to perform transfers
from bed to chair, chair to tub, etc., owing to lack of knowledge and/or the
required skills

continued

Table 22.3.   Occupational Therapy Diagnosis

Transfers, altered/impaired: a state in which the individual experiences impaired ability to perform or complete any or all transfer activities independently

Potential for loss (specify): situation exists or apparently will exist within the foreseeable future when the individual will loose the ability to perform independently one or more self-care skills

INSTRUMENTAL ACTIVITIES OF DAILY LIVING: prerequisites include ADL requirements plus basic cognition, gross skills, purpose, interest, social interaction

Appointments, deficit: a state in which the individual lacks the knowledge or opportunity to practice required skills needed to contact the doctor or other healthcare professional and set a appointment to get together with the professional for some purpose and some specified time

Appointments, scheduling: a state in which the individual experiences impaired ability to perform or complete any or all appointment scheduling tasks

Functional communication, deficit: a state in which the individual is unable to use language, verbal or nonverbal skills, to communicate basic needs and wishes owing to the lack of knowledge or opportunity to practice required skills

Functional communication, altered/impaired (aphasia, disarticulation): a state in which the individual experiences impaired ability to perform or complete language, verbal or nonverbal skills necessary to communicate basic needs and wishes

Functional limitation: a state in which an individual is restricted or lacks the ability to perform an action or activity in the manner or within the range considered normal that results from impairment**** (limitation should be specified)

Health maintenance/prevention, deficit: the lack of knowledge or opportunity to practice required skills in maintaining health and preventing disease, disorders, or discomfort

Health maintenance/prevention, altered/impaired: the inability to identify, manage, and/or seek out help to maintain health*

Home management: cleaning living quarters, deficit: a state in which the individual is unable to maintain the living quarters in a clean and orderly condition resulting from lack of knowledge or opportunity to practice required skills

Home management (cleaning living quarters, altered/impaired): a state in which the individual experiences impaired ability to keep the living quarters in a clean and orderly condition

Home management (clothing care, deficit): a state in which the individual is unable to maintain clothing clean, pressed, and mended owing to lack of knowledge or opportunity to practice required skills Also includes the selection and purchase on clothing appropriate for daily activities performed by the individual

Home management (clothing care, altered/impaired): a state in which the individual experiences impaired ability to perform or complete skills necessary to keep clothing in good condition (clean, pressed, and mended)

continued

Table 22.3. Occupational Therapy Diagnosis

Home management (household maintenance/repair, deficit): a state in which an individual is unable to keep a home in good condition and repair owing to lack of knowledge or opportunity to practice required skills

Home management (household maintenance/repair, altered/impaired): a state in which an individual experiences impaired ability to keep a home in good condition and repair

Home management (meal preparation and cleanup, deficit): a state in which the individual is unable to prepare meals and cleanup afterwards owing to lack of knowledge or opportunity to practice required skills

Home management (meal preparation and cleanup, altered/impaired): a state in which the individual experiences impairment in the ability to prepare meals and cleanup afterward

Home management (money management, deficit): a state in which the individual is unable to develop and stay within a budget, maintain a checking account, and pay for goods and services with cash or check, resulting from lack of knowledge or opportunity to practice required skills

Home management (money management, altered/impaired): a state in which the individual experiences impaired ability to develop and stay within a budget, maintain a checking account, and pay for goods and services with cash or checks

Home management (safety procedures, deficit): a state in which an individual is unable to keep a home safe from hazards (fire, poison, structural weakness, or deficits which can cause injury, flooding, insect invasion, electrocution, theft), owing to lack of knowledge or opportunity to practice required skills

Home management (safety procedures, altered/impaired): a state in which an individual experiences impaired ability to maintain a safe living environment

Home management (shopping/purchasing goods and services, deficit): a state in which the individual is unable to shop for or purchase goods and services because of lack of knowledge or opportunity to practice required skills

Home management (shopping/purchasing goods and services, altered/impaired): a state in which the individual experiences impaired ability to shop for or purchase goods and services

Medication schedule, deficit: a state in which the individual is unable to take medications according to the prescribed schedule or take the correct amount as a result of lack of knowledge and/or the required skills

Medication schedule, altered/impaired: a state in which the individual experiences impaired ability to perform or complete any or all skills required to take medications according to the prescribed schedule or take the correct amount

Telephone use, deficit: a state in which the individual is unable to use the telephone to call out or answer an incoming call owing to lack of knowledge and/or the required skills; includes looking up a number in the telephone book and dialing emergency numbers

Telephone use, altered/impaired: a state in which the individual experiences impaired ability to perform or complete any or all telephone use tasks

Transportation/powered mobility (private or public) skills/performance, deficit: a state in which an individual is unable to use public (such as catching a bus) or private (such as driving a car) transportation owing to lack of knowledge or opportunity to practice required skills

continued

Table 22.3. Occupational Therapy Diagnosis

Transportation/powered mobility (private or public) altered/impaired: a state in which an individual experiences impaired ability to use public or private transportation

SKILLED PERFORMANCE: prerequisites include IADL requirements plus intelligence, advanced skills, and positive personality

Sensory Motor Skills

Accuracy performance standard, deficit or impaired: a state in which an individual is unable to or has difficulty performing to a standard or expected level of correctness, trueness, precision, or exactness

Orthotic/prosthetic use/tolerance: a state in which an individual needs to learn to use, tolerate for an extended time, and maintain in good condition an orthotic or prosthetic device

Precision, deficit or impaired: a state in which an individual is unable to or has difficulty performing a movement so that the result is exactly what was intended; see also Accuracy

Speed/velocity, deficit or impaired: a state in which an individual is unable to achieve or maintain the rate of movement considered necessary to perform a task with efficiency (timeliness) and effectiveness (desire result or accuracy)

Timing, deficit or impaired: a state in which an individual is unable to start, stop, or maintain a movement within the proper sequence or context

Cognitive Skills (thinking, thought processes, memory, intelligence and a state of consciousness)

Abstract reasoning, deficit or impaired: a state in which an individual shows inability to think using abstract concepts; person can use only concrete concepts

Amnesia: a state in which an individual has a temporary or permanent memory deficit

Association, deficit or impaired: a state in which an individual is unable to or has difficulty connecting the significance of events in one situation with those of another situation

Attention disorder: see Inattentive/distractible

Attention span, short/lack of: a state in which an individual has difficulty focusing and maintaining attention on one activity for a time period consistent with norms for his or her age-group

Categorization, deficit or impaired: a state in which an individual is unable to or inaccurately groups like or related ideas or objects together

Concept formation, deficit or impaired: a state in which an individual is unable to or inaccurately organizes ideas or objects together by specific attitudes

Dementia: a state in which a person has loss of cognitive functioning which was previously acquired

Distractible: see Inattentive

Generalization of learning/transfer of training deficit/impaired: a state in which an individual is unable to or has impaired ability to use knowledge or information learned in one situation and apply the knowledge or information is another situation which is the same or similar and requires the same or similar response

Impersistence: a state in which an individual has difficulty sustaining action when attention is needed

continued

Table 22.3. Occupational Therapy Diagnosis

Impulsivity: a state in which an individual acts without attention to consequences of the actions

Inattention/distractibility: a state in which an individual has difficulty focusing and maintaining attention, i.e., concentrating on one activity to the exclusion of other stimuli in the environment

Insight, deficit or impaired (lack of): inability to understand or evaluate one's own mental processes, reactions, abilities, or self-knowledge

Integration of learning, deficit or impaired: a state in which the individual is unable to or has impaired ability to incorporate previously acquire concepts and behavior into variety of new situations

Judgment (of safety), deficit or impaired: a state in which an individual is unable to or has impaired ability to determine whether a situation is potentially harmful or dangerous to self or others

Knowledge/educational, deficit: an individual's lack of information or inability to state or explain information or demonstrate a required skill related to disease management procedures; it is also the inability to explain or use self-care practices recommended to restore health or maintain wellness; it may appear as a cognitive or psychomotor deficit or a combination of the two***

Noncompliance: the a state in which an individual who has expressed the desire and intent to adhere to a therapeutic recommendation does not adhere to the recommendation***

Perseveration: a state in which the individual had difficulty with set shifting or changing focus of attention and therefore continues to perform with the same response pattern

Problem solving/decision making, deficit or impaired: a state in which an individual is unable to or has impaired ability defining a problem, listing alternative solutions, and selecting the best solution for a given situation

Synthesis of learning, deficit or impaired: a state in which the individual is unable to or has impaired ability to restructure previously learned concepts and behavior into new patterns

Thought process, altered (paranoid, suspicious, phobic): individual experiences a disruption in cognitive operations and activities

Time management, deficit or impaired: a state in which an individual is unable to plan a schedule of activities that contributes to a balanced lifestyle

Time management, deficit or impaired (disorganized or imbalanced): a state in which an individual is unable to organize his or her activities (spends too much time in certain activities to the exclusion or minimization of others) into a balanced lifestyle that promotes satisfaction and health

Vigilance, deficit or impaired: see Attention span

*Psychosocial Skills (psychological aspects, emotions, feelings, self-awareness)**

Concept of human and nonhuman environment

Concept of others, negative: a state in which a person does not perceive people or humans as basically trustworthy, as willing to share and provide assistance, and as not deliberately seeking to inflict pain or harm on the individual

Concept of world in general, negative: a state in which a person perceives the nonself environment as hostile, harmful, and "out to get" the individual

continued

Table 22.3. Occupational Therapy Diagnosis

Reality testing: evaluating the actual environment (physical, economic interpersonal, attitudes, emotions) objectively

Reality, misinterpretation (hallucinations, delusions, obsessions, phobias, preoccupations): a state in which an individual's response to information from the internal or external environment is distorted or incorrect

Self-concept: how a person views one's self as a person, one's sense of self, one's knowledge about oneself, one's beliefs in regard to the self, and the value or worth ascribed to the self

Body image disturbance: individual experiences a disruption in the perception of boundary, physical self, or real self

Identity crisis: see Personal identity disturbance

Personal identity disturbance: individual is uncertain about components of self (who he or she is or wants to become as a person) especially in relation to making choices regarding vocation, social relations, and lifestyle

Self-centered/egocentric: individual is concerned only with his or her own feelings, thoughts, actions, behaviors, skills, or abilities

Self-concept disturbance: a state in which an individual has negative self-evaluation or feelings about self or capabilities, which may be directly or indirectly expressed*

Self-concept (self-esteem, self-image, self-worth), chronic low: a state in which an individual has a long-standing negative self-evaluation or feelings about self or self capabilities*

Self-concept (self-esteem, self-image, self-worth), situation low: a state in which the individual has negative self-evaluations or feelings about self that develop in response to a loss or change in an individual who previously had a positive self evaluation*

Self-evaluation, deficit or impaired: lack of knowledge and understanding of one's assets and limitations based on feedback from the environment

Sexual identity disturbance: a state in which an individual is unclear about or unaware of feelings about, and interactions with others as a sexual being

Self-discipline: refers to an individual's capacity to manage him or herself in the conduct of daily life activities

Adaptive behavior, deficit/impaired: difficulty or inability in meeting the standards of personal independence and social responsibility expected of a individual based on age and cultural group

Adjustment, impaired: inability to change or modify lifestyle or behavior consistent with changes in health status or disability

Coping/stress management, ineffective, individual: individual is unable to use effectively adaptive behaviors and problem-solving abilities to meet life's demands and roles

Coping/stress management, posttrauma response: individual experiences a intense, sustained emotional response to a traumatic experience or natural or man-made disaster*

Dealing or managing with adversity, success, failure, frustration or anxiety: see Coping/stress management

continued

Table 22.3.   Occupational Therapy Diagnosis

Lack of self control: see Locus of control or Self-responsibility

Locus of control, lack or loss of (powerlessness): a state in which an individual feels that he or she is not in control of what happens to oneself or ones environment: that he or she is a victim of others actions or circumstances

Self responsibility and direction, deficit or impaired: a state in which a person does not recognize or does not act independently to satisfy personal needs, establish person goals, or select a preferred life style

Volition (will), deficit or impaired: a state in which a person is unable to or experiences difficulty in making a deliberate, conscious choice of a course of action, or in exercising the power to choose and control one's own actions

Self-efficacy/self-mastery, lack of: an individual does not feel a sense of confidence and competence in his or her ability to respond to environmental needs, demands, and constraints

Self-expression, lack of: individual is unable to use a variety of styles and skills to express thoughts, feelings, and needs

Values, lack of clarity/commitment: individual is unable to clarify which ideas or beliefs are intrinsically important to him or her

Psychosocial Skills (social roles and relationships)

Dyadic interaction, deficit/impaired: individual is unable to maintain a mutually satisfying relationship with one other person

Group interaction, deficit/impaired: individual is unable to maintain a mutually satisfying relationship with a group of people

Interpersonal relationships, deficit/impaired: individual is unable to maintain a variety of satisfying relationships with individuals and groups from different areas of his or her life situations

Role behavior/performance, deficit (irresponsible): individual is unable to or unwilling to take responsibility for his or her failure to perform behaviors associated with one or more roles

Role behavior/performance, altered/impaired: individual experiences impaired ability to perform behaviors associated with one or more roles

Role conflict, individual: a state in which an individual finds some roles conflict or compete with other roles and the individual is unable to work out or experiences difficulty in working out a satisfactory compromise

Role conflict, social: individual feels that society expects him or her to perform behaviors that appear to the person to be oppositional

Role identity confusion: a state in which an individual is unclear about what roles he or she should have assumed or acquired

Structured social interaction, deficit or impaired: individual is unable to participate appropriately in social situations which require cooperation, compromise, and negotiation

Structured social interplay, deficit or impaired: individual is unable to participate appropriately in social situations that require assertiveness and/or competition

Social isolation/withdrawal: individual selects to withdraw or becomes isolated from social situations

continued

Table 22.3. Occupational Therapy Diagnosis

Socialization or social conversation, deficit or impaired: individual is unable to or experiences impaired ability to initiate or maintain a social conversation
Social support, deficit: individual feels he or she lacks or really does lack support for his or her activities from family or friends

SOCIAL ROLES (productivity or work occupations): prerequisites include skilled performance requirements plus social skills, opportunity, and attitude

Caregiver/parenting skills/performance deficit: a state in which an individual is unable to perform caregiving/parenting skills due to lack of knowledge or opportunity to practice required skills
Caregiver/parenting, altered/impaired: a state in which the individual experiences impaired ability to perform caregiving/parenting skills
Disability: a state in which an individual experiences an inability or limitation in performing socially defined activities and roles expected of individuals with a social and physical environment****
Educational (student) skills/performance deficit: a state in which an individual is unable to perform student behaviors and skills owing to lack of knowledge or opportunity to practice required skills
Educational (student) skills/performance, altered/impaired: a state in which an individual experiences impaired ability to perform student behaviors and skills
Job acquisition, altered/impaired: a state in which an individual experiences impaired ability to get a job
Job acquisition skills/performance deficit: a state in which an individual is unable to perform tasks needed to get a job due to lack of knowledge or opportunity to practice/implement required skills
Leisure skills/performance/recreation, deficit: a state in which the individual is unable in engage in leisure activities due to lack of knowledge or opportunity to practice or implement required skills
Leisure skills/performance/recreation, altered/impaired: a state in which the individual experiences impaired ability to engage in or perform leisure activities
Leisure skills/performance/recreation, potential for decrease or loss: situation exists or apparently will exist in the foreseeable future when the individual will lose the ability to engage in play or leisure activities
Play/leisure skills, lack of exploration: a state in which the individual is unable to engage in explorative play skills due to lack of knowledge or opportunity to practice or implement required skills
Play skills, developmentally delayed: a state in which the individual demonstrates deviations in norms from his or her age group in the development and performance of play skills
Play skills, altered/impaired: a state in which the individual experiences impaired ability to perform or engage in play skills
Productivity/work skills/performance, potential for loss (specify): situation exists or apparently will exist within the foreseeable future when the individual will loose the ability to perform one or more productive skills
Retirement planning skills/performance, deficit: a state in which an individual is unable to plan for retirement due to lack of knowledge or opportunity to practice or implement required skills

continued

Table 22.3. Occupational Therapy Diagnosis

Retirement planning, altered/impaired: a state in which an individual experiences impaired ability to plan for retirement

Vocational exploration skills/performance deficit: a state in which an individual is unable to perform or explore career opportunities owing to lack of knowledge or opportunity to practice required skills

Vocational exploration, altered/impaired: a state in which an individual experiences impaired ability to explore career opportunities

Volunteering skills/performance, deficit: a state in which an individual is unable to seek and perform volunteer activities owing to lack of knowledge or opportunity to practice or implement required skills

Volunteering, altered/impaired: a state in which an individual experiences impaired ability to seek or perform volunteer activities

Work/job skills/performance, deficit: a state in which an individual is unable to perform work or job tasks and skills owing to lack of knowledge and/or opportunity to practice or implement required skills

Work/job skills/performance, altered/impaired: a state in which an individual experiences impaired ability to perform work or job tasks and skills

ENVIRONMENTAL (SOCIOCULTURAL) PROBLEMS

Community, lack of access: individual is unable to find a community that is accessible or can be modified to accommodate his or her limitations

Community, unsafe/potential for injury: individual is unable to find a community that is free of unsafe conditions and potentials for injury

Family coping/stress management, ineffective: behavior of one or more family members incapacitates the family to adapt effectively to the existing health challenge***

Family process, altered: family that normally functions effectively experiences a dysfunction***

Home/living quarters, lack of access: individual or family is unable to find suitable housing that the individual or family can afford and is accessible to all members

Home/living quarters, unsafe/potential for injury: individual or family is unable to maintain housing in a condition that is free of unsafe conditions and potentials for injury

Workplace, lack of access: individual is unable to find employment in a setting that is accessible or can be modified to accommodate his or her limitations

Workplace, unsafe/potential for injury: individual is unable to find employment in a setting that is free of unsafe conditions and potentials for injury

*Definition from: Uniform terminology for occupational therapy. 2nd ed. Am J Occup Ther 1989;43(12):808–815.
** Categories based on Performance Components in: Mosey AC. Psychosocial Components of Occupational Therapy. New York: Raven Press, 1986:42, Table 3–1.
*** Categories and/or definitions from: Carpenito LJ. Nursing Diagnosis: Application to Clinical Practice. 4th ed. Philadelphia: Lippincott, 1992.
****Categories and/or definitions from: Institute of Medicine: Disability in America. Washington, DC: National Academy Press, 1991:79.
Categories and/or definitions from: Van Duesen J, Brunt D. Assessment in Occupational Therapy and Physical Therapy. Philadelphia: Saunders, 1996.

References

1. Barton GE. Inoculation of the bacillus of work. Mod Hosp 1917;8:399–403.
2. Rogers JC, Holm MB. Diagnostic reasoning: the process of problem identification. In: Christiansen C, Baum C. Occupational Therapy: Enabling Function and Well-Being. Thorofare, NJ: Slack Inc.,1997:137–156.
3. Dorland WAN. Dorland's Illustrated Medical Dictionary. 27th ed. Philadelphia: Saunders, 1988.
4. Stedman T. Stedman's Medical Dictionary, Illustrated. Baltimore: Williams & Wilkins, 1990.
5. Gordon M. Nursing diagnoses and the diagnostic process. Am J Nurs 1976;76(8): 1298–1300.
6. King LS. What is a diagnosis? JAMA 1967;202(8):154–157.
7. Kemp BJ, Mitchell JM. Functional assessment in geriatric mental health. In: Birren JE, Sloane RB, Cohen GD. Handbook of Mental Health and Aging. 2nd ed. San Diego: Academic Press, 1992.
8. American Occupational Therapy Association: Uniform terminology for occupational therapy. 2nd ed. Am J Occup Ther 1989;43(12):808–815.
9. Campbell C. Nursing Diagnosis and Intervention in Nursing Practice. 2nd ed. New York: John Wiley & Sons, 1984:7.
10. Carpenito LJ. Nursing Diagnosis: Application to Clinical Practice. 5th ed. Philadelphia: Lippincott, 1993.

CHAPTER 23

Planning and Intervention

Program planning is the process of organizing information so that the problems in function are delineated, goals are specified, principles of intervention are identified, and activities are selected. The process of planning is designed to permit a comprehensive approach to bring the client and the occupational therapist together. The client has strengths and weaknesses that were found in the assessments. The occupational therapist has knowledge of intervention principles and activities that may help the client solve or overcome any problems. Together, the client and occupational therapist can set goals and objectives to correct the problems.

A good plan allows an overview of the intervention process at a glance. Several formats may be used to outline the plan. The outline in Figure 23.1 will serve as an example. First, the problems are listed down the left column. Listing problems according to occupational areas and performance components enables the therapist to note strengths and weaknesses quickly. The client's strengths should be those areas and components that have few problems while weaknesses have more problems. Listing also permits the opportunity to recognize interrelations of problems. A child with sensory integration problems may have social conduct problems as well. The latter frequently are coping behaviors. Correcting the sensory integration problems reduces the need for coping behaviors. As a result, social conduct problems improve without direct intervention. Knowledge and observation of interrelated problems can help the therapist set intervention priorities.

Time and energy dictate that a limited number of problems, usually two to four, can be worked on during the initial intervention sessions. Thus, the therapist must have a means of selecting which problems will be alleviated first. One guideline is to select the most basic or underlying problem. The example of the child with sensory integration problems illustrates this guideline. Intervention would be directed at the sensory integration problems while the social conduct problems are monitored to see if improvement occurs as sensory integration problems improve.

Another guideline for selecting the initial problems for intervention is to ask the client which problems are most annoying or are of most concern. Most persons over the age of 2 or 3 years can answer the question. Alleviating an annoying problem enhances the therapist–client relationship and may set the stage for better cooperation between the therapist and client to attack problems that are complex or difficult to overcome.

Problems	Goals	Principles	Strategies
Based on analysis of formative assessment, what are the problems?	Based on expected outcomes, what results can be achieved?	Based on the rationale for intervention, why can the goal be achieved?	Based on the intervention principle, how can the goal achieved?
Self-maintenance	Prevent . . .	Feeding skills can . . .	Select:
Productivity	Develop . . .	Computer skills	Medium or media
Leisure	Increase . . .	can . . .	Modality or modali-
ties			
Sensorimotor	Improve . . .	Bowling skills can . . .	Teaching method(s)
Cognitive	Restore . . .	Movement can . . .	Therapeutic
Psychosocial	Aid adjustment . . .		Range of motion
approaches: normal			
	Provide	can . . .	or specialized
	adaptive . . .	Muscle strength	
	Maintain . . .	can . . .	
	Reestablish . . .	Physical tolerance	
	Do not use:	can . . .	
	Get rid of	Developmental task	
	Decrease	can . . .	
	Diminish	Sensory function	
	Habilitate	can . . .	
	Make better	Reality testing can . . .	

Figure 23.1. Intervention plan.

A third guideline is to select first those problems that most annoy staff or family and take up excessive staff time. For example, a person may need to be fed by the staff because the individual cannot hold onto the silverware due to arthritis. Feeding someone beyond the age of 2 or 3 years is time-consuming and not especially enjoyable. If the person could eat without assistance by slipping the fork into a cuff around the hand, both time and energy can be spent on other tasks. Staff and family as well as the client usually appreciate assistance in solving such problems and will, as a result, cooperate more in approaching other problems.

The fourth guideline is to select initially those problems that seem to have an easy solution. Enlarging handles, substituting Velcro for buttons, and placing nonskid strips in the bathtub are easy solutions to particular problems. The impact on both therapist and client is that progress is being made. Again, better cooperation may be achieved when results of intervention can be seen quickly.

After the problems are listed, goals need to be established to determine when intervention can be discontinued and the direction such intervention should take. Goals should be based on the therapist's best estimate of what competencies are needed at what level and what can be accomplished in the intervention setting. Overestimating potential serves only to frustrate both the therapist and the client. Underestimating robs the client of accomplishing a better skill level. Goals, however, can be revised and should be whenever information is available to warrant a change.

Goals are written in terms of change statements that indicate the direction and type of change expected. There are several key words that commonly appear in goal statements. The direction may be to prevent something from happening that would be detrimental to health. Examples include preventing contractures, loss of muscle strength, and disorientation. In some cases, the direction is consistent with development or learning of skills. Examples include developing play skills or improving group interaction. Another direction may be to increase, improve, or restore the amount or degree of a skill. Examples include increasing or improving muscle strength, range of motion, balance, coordination, attention span, reality orientation, or social skills.

Some clients will need to adjust or adapt to certain conditions. These may include adjusting or adapting to using a prosthesis, a wheelchair, or eating devices. Finally, some clients will need to maintain a skill level. Examples include maintaining muscle strength, range of motion, or autonomy.

These three skill categories are the primary ones used in describing competency goals. Competency goals can be stated to decrease the level of a performance skill. However, decreasing performance is rarely successful without increasing or substituting another skill. A person may hit others, break objects, throw food, scream, or run away. All of these behaviors may prompt a request to decrease the behavior. However, behavior serves the purpose of communicating and doing. To decrease a behavior without offering a constructive alternative behavior leaves the person using his or her own devices. The new self-generated behavior may be no more socially acceptable than the original behavior that was eliminated by intervention. Therefore, the therapist should always attempt to increase an acceptable behavior when decreasing an unacceptable one.

Goals represent the final outcome of performance to be achieved in terms of type of performance or level of performance in a specific time period. The final outcome is most often the result of accomplishing a series of steps between the starting and end point. Such steps must be recognized. For example, to dress oneself requires putting on several garments. Each garment to be put on requires a slightly different approach. Thus, dressing requires a complex set of skills. These skills are taught most easily by teaching a person to put on one garment at a time. A goal, therefore, must be analyzed in terms of the steps needed to achieve it. Some therapists prefer to list the steps as well as the competency. This approach allows progress to be checked off as it occurs.

To this point, the emphasis has been focused on short-term and not long-term goals. Long-term goals are not listed as a ride on the intervention plan for occupational therapy but on a comprehensive plan developed by the planning team.

Each team member should be aware of the long-term goals to be reached by the client so that short-term goals can be coordinated toward the long-term goals.

Principles and assumptions explain why the therapist feels that intervention will be successful. In other words, principles and assumptions are the rationale for intervening. Actually, principles and assumptions are the same except that a principle has scientific proof that it works as described whereas an assumption seems logical based on available knowledge but has not been proven. In effect, principles should not change much over time. Once a principle has been learned, it is sound knowledge. On the other hand, assumptions may or may not change, depending on whether research proves assumptions true or false. If true, an assumption becomes a principle. If false, an assumption should be abandoned.

The following examples may clarify the terms. A principle in therapy is that progressive resistive exercise will increase muscle strength; that is, requiring an individual to lift more weight against gravity will increase the amount of weight a muscle group can lift, thereby, increasing the strength of that muscle group. This principle of progressive resistive exercise is the rationale for weight lifting. Muscles become stronger and can do more work when they are required to lift increasingly heavier weights.

An example of an assumption is the old medical treatment of bloodletting for various diseases. The assumption was that draining "bad" blood permitted "good" blood to take its place. This assumption was false for two reasons, based on scientific research. First, diseases are not caused by "bad" blood but by organisms invading the body. Second, loss of blood can be fatal in itself because blood is needed to carry oxygen and nutrients to the cells and carry away wastes. Therefore, the assumption that bloodletting is a cure for disease is false, and the treatment should be abandoned.

On the intervention plan, each goal should be followed by a principle or assumption. Whether the statement is a principle or an assumption depends on the state of knowledge in relation to the goal. As the previous example illustrated, progressive resistive exercise has been proven to increase muscle strength. Therefore, if the goal is to increase muscle strength in the shoulder and arm muscles, the principle would be progressive resistive exercise. However, if the goal is to teach a child to walk, there is no principle. Studies have not proven which method of teaching a child to walk is best. Two assumptions have been popular. One says a child should crawl and creep before walking is encouraged because activity on hands and knees organizes the brain. Another assumption states that practice in standing balance is needed because walking is a progression of losing and regaining balance on the alternately extended legs. Whichever assumption is used, the therapist must realize that new information may soon invalidate or support that assumption. Changing rationales and explanations are inevitable as knowledge increases.

The example of teaching walking further illustrates the interdependence of problems and the need for therapists to recognize the complex problems. Many occupational therapists would feel that walking is a problem for physical therapy, not occupational therapy. What rationale physical therapy uses is of no concern to occupational therapy. This thinking is short-sighted. Activity in the lower extremities affects the upper extremities and hands. Moving on hands and knees gives direct stimulation to the hands, wrists, elbows, and shoulders. Standing may appear not to involve the upper extremities, but, in fact, the upper extremities are involved actively in balancing and counterbalancing the upper torso against the lower extremities and lower torso. This activity will have some effect on purposeful movement of the upper extremities for such tasks as writing, throwing a ball, or putting on a T-shirt. Whether the effect is positive or negative must be determined by the team members in terms of which goals are receiving immediate attention and which are the long-term goals.

In summary, the importance of stating principles and assumptions is to provide a rationale for intervention and to permit analysis of the effects of setting certain goals on others.

INTERVENTION STRATEGIES

The last section of the intervention plan is the strategies to be used to implement the plan. Strategies should be selected that 1) will accomplish the goal, 2) are acceptable to the client, 3) are available to the therapist, and 4) are efficient in terms of time, energy, and money. All factors are important to consider because there is usually more than one strategy that can be used to implement each goal. More important, one strategy may implement more than one goal. Intervention strategies include three interrelated subsystems as shown in Figure 23.2. These are 1) techniques,

Techniques	Media and Modalties		Methods and Approaches	
Normal or Adapted Techniques	Media or Agent Types	Modality Groups	Teaching Methods	Therapeutic Approaches
A. Normal techniques	A. Inanimate	A.	Functional activities	A. Demonstration and perfor-
A. Normal developmental			B. Self-care activities	
B. Adapted individual mance techniques	1. sequencing arts and	Creative	B.	Exploration and sequencing
B. Normal activity		C. Work-related activities	discovery	
C. Adapted environmental techniques	crafts	D. Leisure/avocational activities	C. Explanation and	C. Tasks analysis discussion D.
(see Table 23.4)	2. Manual arts and	E. Homemaking activities		
Graded activities	crafts		D. Role playing/ simulation	E. Adapted acitivity F. Activity groups
	3. Games and sports		E.	Problem solving and
G. Normal environment	4. Education		decision making	H. Adapted environ-
ment	and learn-		F.	Audiovisual aids
I. One on one	ing tasks		G. Practice and repetition	J. Consulting
	5. Toys			K. Adapted therapy equipment
	6. Computer		H. Behavioral management	
	B. Animate		I. Patient education	
	1. Self			
	2. Dyad			

Figure 23.2. Intervention strategies.

2) media or modalities; and 3) teaching methods or therapeutic approaches. At least one item from each of the three subsystems must be selected to complete an intervention plan. Techniques relate to the performance area or areas to be addressed in the intervention plan. In other words, techniques designate which performance will be stressed. Media or modalities organize what will be used to implement the techniques. Teaching methods or therapeutic approaches outline how the therapist will attempt to assist the client to achieve the goal or goals. Although the subsystems are interrelated, they will be described separately for the purpose of illustration.

Techniques

Three primary guidelines exist for selecting techniques in occupational therapy based on potential outcome. The first guideline is based on the outcome of normal performance. The goal is to enable the person to gain or regain performance of occupations/activities in the normal mode. In other words, the person will do tasks just like everybody else does them.

The second guideline is based on changing the individual's method of performing some occupations. This method is adopted only when normal performance is impossible or impractical. Examples might include amputation, paralysis, or injury of an arm. The individual cannot be expected to perform occupations with one arm in the same manner as previously performed with two. Therefore, some modification, substitution, or compensation will be necessary on the part of the individual to get the occupations performed. Some techniques, such as biofeedback and splinting, are external to the individual, but their presence is considered temporary and their function is to assist the individual to adapt or change. A list of adapted individual techniques is provided in Table 23.1 at the end of this chapter.

The third outcome is based on changing the external environment. This outcome is used only when individual performance, normal or adapted, is insufficient or impractical. In other words, adapting the environment is done only when the first two alternatives fail. Examples might include amputation, paralysis, or injury to a large part of the body, such as spinal cord injuries, or arthritis. The person needs adaptation beyond that which the individual can do. The situation probably will be a permanent arrangement. Wheelchairs, ramps, tenodesis splints, braille, and modified handles on utensils are all examples of physical environmental adaptations designed to substitute or compensate for an individual's inability to perform occupations normally or adapted. Moving to a new apartment away from family is an example of a physical change that may provide a much needed psychological change. Regardless of the rationale, the purpose of the environmental adaptations or modifications is to enable the individual to perform the occupation or occupations required of the individual to function in society and to achieve self-satisfaction. Figure 23.3 underlines the criteria for determining whether a technique should be considered. A list of adapted environmental techniques is provided in Table 23.2 at the end of this chapter.

Normal Techniques	Adapted Individual Techniques	Adapted Environmental Techniques
Technique is used to teach normal individual	Technique is not taught to normal individual	Technique is considered more or less permanent
Task is performed in the same manner as performed by normal the individual	Technique is considered a temporary measure	Talk will be performed for a long time in manner prescribed
Equipment is used regularly used as is by normal person	Task is performed in a manner different from the way normal persons perform it	Equipment will be for a long time
Supplies are used regularly needed by normal individual	Equipment is not used regularly by normal individuals	Supplies will be for a long time
Concept of prevention is applicable to normal individual	Supplies are not used regularly by normal individuals	Need to prevent specific problems will be present for a long time
	Concept of prevention is not needed by normal	Is a more or less permanent

Figure 23.3. Criteria for categorization.

Figure 23.4 shows the techniques used in occupational therapy divided into three subsections. Techniques should be selected from column one before column two or three. Likewise, techniques in column two should be selected before three. If techniques are selected from column three, the therapist should be sure that techniques from column one or two are not possible. Techniques in column three may include a high price tag, such as an electric wheelchair. If the person does not need an electric wheelchair, the expense is not justified. Also, the therapist should be aware that clients may resist using "all that fancy" adapted equipment even when it is justified to achieve independent functioning. Helping a client gain "gadget tolerance" may be just as important as teaching the person to use the gadgets.

Media and Modalities

A medium is an agent or activity through which something is accomplished. A good or useful medium facilitates the accomplishment. Conversely, a poor or useless medium hinders. Selection of a medium, therefore, should be thought out in relation to the goal or objective to be achieved and in relation to the person who is trying to achieve the goal.

Media abound in occupational therapy. This abundance is both a help and a hindrance. The help is the wide variety of choices usually available to accomplish a particular goal or objective. The hindrance is the wide knowledge and skill needed by the occupational therapist to make the best use of the media available. It is easy for the occupational therapist to select a few media and use them repeatedly. The media may provide the processes needed to accomplish the goal, but the media may be of no interest to the client. Thus, there is a poor fit between the medium, the goal, and the client. An example might be asking an older woman to sand a board with both hands using a bilateral sander to encourage movement of the shoulders to increase range of motion. If the woman has not had experience with sanding or thinks of sanding wood as a man's activity, she may not think much of the activity and participate as little as possible in the therapy. The same goal could be achieved by shelving dishes or getting can goods off shelves of various heights, which probably would relate to the woman's life experience.

Of course, it is possible to select a medium that cannot provide processes necessary to reach a goal but which the client enjoys doing. The client may enjoy watching the afternoon soap operas on television, but watching the TV will not increase range of motion in her shoulder. The point is, however, the media should be selected both for the potential of the medium to facilitate attainment of the goal or objective and for its intrinsic interest to the client.

To gain knowledge of media, students are required to practice skills in many activities—the more, the better. Creative use of media can make a big difference in how well the clients achieve goals. Occupational therapy differs from many medical fields because it depends on the client's active participation in the process, through the medium, rather than passive participation in which the medium, such as heat or sound, is applied. The more knowledge the occupational therapist has about activity, the wider range of choices the therapist can offer the client to attract one's interest in the process and participation in achievement of the goal or objective of therapy.

In Figure 23.2 and Table 23.3, the media have been divided into inanimate and animate. The classification is simply one of convenience. A creative occupational therapist should be able to think of several other ways to classify media so that one or more goals will be of interest to one or more clients. In Figure 23.4, the modalities have been divided into occupational groups because occupation is a central concept to the practice of occupational therapy. The modalities can also be divided by the occupational roles that a person wants or needs to fulfill. This approach permits the scope of occupations to be tailored to the individual client so that specific performance skills can be assessed and taught as needed.

Teaching Methods and Approaches

Teaching or instructing is an essential aspect in the therapeutic process. It is the means occupational therapists use to communicate what goal or objective is to be accomplished through the use of what medium. Frequently, the medium is

Examples of Normal Techniques	Examples of Adapted Individual Techniques	Examples of Adapted Environmental Techniques
Self maintenance	Daily living class	Self-help aids
Self-care training	Work hardening	Adapted housing
Self-mobility training	Leisure counseling	Mobility aids
Productivity	One-handed techniques	Transportation aid
Homemaking training	Bilateral techniques	Electronic assisted
Child care training	Reciprocal techniques	living
Play skills	Orthotic techniques	Accessibility
Task skills	Biofeedback	Adapted workstation
Work performance skills	Facilitation/inhibition	Adapted sports
training	techniques	Adapted social activities
Work simplication	Sensory integrative	Prosthetic training
techniques	techniques	Orthotic training—long
Leisure	Sensory substitution	term
Develop avocational	Pressure garments	Sensory aids
interests	Sensory awareness	Therapeutic
Plan and use leisure time	training	horsemanship
Sensimotor		
Motor skills	Computer-assisted	Communication
boards/	therapy	devices
Coordination and	Cognitive retraining	Changing attitudes
dexterity training and		
Muscle-strengthening	Stress management	social customs
activities	Reminiscence training	
Muscle tone control	Remotivation training	
Physical endurance	Reality orientation	
activities	Support groups	
Physical skills		
development		
Range of motion activities		
Reflex training		
Positioning		
Joint protection		
Sensory skills		
Auditory perception		
training		
Proprioceptive/		
kinesthetic training		
Sensorimotor training		
Sensory stimulation		
training		
Tactile perception training		
Vestibualr system training		
Visual perception training		
Cognitive skills		
Attention training		
Cognitive schema training		
Communication techniques		
Comprehension training		
Concept formation training		
Integration of learning		
Judgment training		
Memory and retention		
Problem-solving		
Time organization training		
Activity configuration		
Psychosocial		
Intrapersonal skills		
Autonomy		
Develop coping skills		
Decrease/substitute defense mechanisms		
Increase motivation		
Relaxation techniques		
Object relations techniques		
Incease self-control		
Improve self-concept		
Reality testing		
Synthesis		
Interpersonal skills		
Dyadic interaction skills		

Figure 23.4. Examples of techniques used in occupational therapy.

adapted slightly or significantly to better fit the goal or objective. For example, checkers played with cone-shaped pieces is still checkers, but the hand grip used is altered from the usual finger and thumb grip to a full hand grip. If the client knows how to play checkers, the only instruction needed is to inform the client that the pieces are different for a purpose. The purpose is to practice opening and closing the hand. If the client does not know how to play checkers, the teaching process will be more involved. Teaching checkers is more complicated because a person must understand rules, comprehend taking turns, and have the visual perceptual skills to see diagonal as well as vertical and horizontal patterns.

Occupational therapists work frequently with people for whom learning or relearning is difficult. Clients with brain damage, head injuries, mental retardation, learning disabilities, or Alzheimer's disease are just a few. Occupational therapists must know several methods of teaching the same task or activity so that when one method does not help a person learn to perform the task, another method can be tried until one is successful.

Students are asked to practice a variety of teaching methods and therapeutic approaches during their education and training—the more practice, the better. Learning to find the right teaching method or approach requires practice and experience (Table 23.4).

Tables 23.5 and 23.6 at the end of the chapter are representative of the teaching methods and therapeutic approaches used in occupational therapy but are not necessarily exhaustive. Students and practicing occupational therapists should always be looking for better methods of teaching and instructing clients.

Summary

Each aspect of planning has been presented separately for ease of explanation. In implementing and managing a person's intervention plan, the techniques, media and modalities, and teaching methods and therapeutic approaches may be used in a variety of combinations. The combination chosen depends, in part, on the problem to be addressed, the patient/client's choice, and on the protocol (standard plan) used to manage patients/clients in a given facility. Some teaching methods, for example, lend themselves to use with some techniques more than others. For instance, it is difficult to explain to someone how to walk or knit. Demonstration of the normal sequence is much easier. Also, some people learn more easily through one method than another. One person may like the challenge of learning through exploration, whereas another may prefer the guidance offered by explanation and discussion.

MANAGEMENT OF THE INTERVENTION PROGRAM

Management of the intervention program includes five items: 1) scheduling the therapy sessions and coordinating the schedule with other services; 2) obtaining the necessary equipment and supplies; 3) setting up or preparing for the therapy session; 4) conducting the therapy session; and 5) cleaning up.

Scheduling

Scheduling is the process of deciding how often and when to see the client for therapy. Factors that may affect the decision are the nature of the problem; status of the client, such as inpatient or outpatient; preferences and reactions of the client; total number of clients the therapist already has scheduled; and the number of other services in which the client is involved. In other words, scheduling often must be negotiated between the client, other professionals, and occupational therapy. The client's problems may respond best to twice-daily therapy sessions, but physical therapy, speech pathology, respiratory therapy, social work, and daily nursing care must be scheduled also. The hours are limited, and the client's health condition requires rest. If the client has too many activities scheduled, the therapist may be treating a sleeping individual. As students already know, it is difficult to pay attention when one is asleep. Drug therapy is another factor that may influence the response to therapy. Certain drugs have side effects that cause drowsiness, but others may be necessary to reduce pain before therapy begins.

Inpatient schedules are usually more frequent than outpatient. Inpatients may be scheduled twice a day to maximize the time available during hospitalization. On the other hand, outpatients may be seen only once a week or once every 2 weeks because the client must travel long distances or because little change can be expected between sessions.

The therapist must keep in mind the total number of treatment sessions that can be given in a day's time and still leave time for recording and reporting. A heavy schedule increases the need to record progress frequently. Otherwise, the therapist is likely to forget important details.

In summary, scheduling is more than filling up time slots on a piece of paper. Scheduling requires consideration of the client, the client's health conditions and problems, the client's location in or out of the hospital, the therapist's schedule, and the schedules of other professional who must see the person.

Equipment and Supplies

Equipment and supplies must be obtained to conduct the therapy session. Few things are more frustrating to both therapist and client than getting ready for a therapy session only to discover that equipment or supplies are not to be found. It is hard to assess a client when the assessment test has gone into hiding. It is difficult to work on self-feeding when the utensils have disappeared. Another problem arises when two clients are scheduled at the same time, need the same piece of equipment, only one piece is available, and sharing is out of the question.

A third problem is not having the equipment or supplies at all. Certain therapy techniques are very dependent on having the right equipment. Table 23.7 lists some examples of techniques and the equipment associated with those techniques.

The list is a sample and is not intended to be complete. Therapists may use other types of equipment.

A fourth problem is size. Obviously, children may need smaller sizes than adults. Chairs, tables, splints, and eating utensils are some items for which size is important.

Preparation Time

Therapists can reduce the frustration and aggravation of discovering the client is waiting but the equipment is not available by planning ahead. Preparation or set-up time often is necessary to prepare for a therapy session. In a small clinic or private practice, preparation is the therapist's responsibility. In a large clinic, an aide may be available to organize the equipment and supplies needed for a therapy session. Either way, the therapist must do the planning. The aide must be told what is needed (see Table 23.7).

Preparation time can be reduced by designating a specific space for equipment and supplies and always putting items in their place. The logic is self-explanatory but the follow-through may be lacking. A disorganized clinic or therapy area is a disaster waiting to happen. Probably more tempers may have been lost over misplaced equipment than for any other reason. Therapists who are otherwise very cooperative and considerate of their fellow therapists suddenly turn their smile upside down when equipment has "sprouted legs." A little organization will reduce the hassles for everyone.

CONDUCTING THE THERAPY SESSION

When the equipment and supplies are assembled, the therapy session can begin, provided that the client arrives and is ready to work. Occasionally, the therapist may find that the client is in no condition to proceed with the activities planned for that session. An alternative plan of activities may avoid a wasted therapy session.

CLEANING UP

After the therapy session is over, cleanup begins. Cleaning up is not most practitioner's favorite activity. Frankly, cleaning up is a chore. In a large clinic, therapists may avoid cleaning up by assigning the responsibility to an aide. A clever practitioner may also discover a way to integrate cleanup activities into the therapy session so the client assists in putting things away. Picking up objects increases hand skills. Putting objects on shelves increases shoulder and elbow range of motion. Putting objects where they are normally stored requires following directions. In other words, cleanup can be a part of the therapy program. Nevertheless, if there is no aide and cleanup is not integrated into the client's program, the practitioner will be doing the cleaning and putting away. A word to the wise; do it now! Therapy areas have a way of becoming a jumble and a jungle in short order.

SUMMARY

Intervention and management require organization and attention to details. Time schedules, equipment, and supplies are examples of the details that may need attention. Coordination and cooperation with other services and therapists frequently are necessary. One client cannot be everywhere at once. Decisions must be made as to which service the client attends at what time. Equally important are the client's time and money. Therapy is expensive even if insurance is available. When the client has to wait while the details of schedules, equipment, and supplies are worked out, money is being wasted. Preparation and cleanup may not be glamorous, but they are practical.

Table 23.1. Adapted Individual Techniques

A. **Problems in Self-care Performance**—the person needs assistance to modify or to adapt the method of performing some self-care activities.

   Daily living class—person needs to learn how to apply makeup to minimize variations in skin color after facial surgery for cancer or facial injuries.

   Examples: A group of persons who have had facial surgery meet to discuss the use of makeup and try out different makeup routines.

B. **Problems in Productive Performance**—the person needs assistance to modify or to adapt the method of performing some work-related activities.

   Work hardening—person needs to increase physical endurance, without excessive fatigue and injury, and improve general productivity, with acceptable quality control, to a level acceptable to the employer

   Examples: Person practices lifting items using the legs instead of the back, gradually increasing the weight of the lifts. Person practices assembling door locks according to a specific set of instructions until the acceptable rate of assembly and quality is obtained.

C. **Problems in Leisure Performance**—the person needs assistance to modify or to adapt the method of performing some leisure-related activities.

   Leisure counseling—person who has had a heart attack or has arthritis needs assistance in determining what sports activities can be done safely within physical limitations

   Examples: Person with history of heart disease learns to monitor heart rate and to stop activity when the maximum heart rate is obtained. Person with arthritis learns which sports activities produce less joint trauma, such as swimming.

D. **Musculoskeletal Dysfunction**—the person needs assistance to modify or to adapt the method of performing some motor activities.

   One-handed techniques—person is unable to use one hand or arm because of disease or injury. The disability may be temporary as with a fracture or permanent as sometimes happens in hemiplegia.

   Examples: The person must learn to button buttons, tie shoe laces, put on and take off clothes with one hand. The person may also have to switch dominance if the disability is on the dominant side. Therefore, the person may have to learn to write, throw, and catch a ball, and turn the key in the lock with the nondominant hand.

   Bilateral techniques—person may benefit from using both hands, arms, feet, or legs at the same time and in the same direction to perform a task to encourage ipsilateral input and feedback.

   Examples: Using a sanding block with handles, both hands are placed on the handles and sanding proceeds bilaterally. Use of a hand pump to blow up various inflatable balls, tires, or mats.

   Reciprocal techniques—person may benefit from using both hands, arms, feet, or legs at the same time but in opposite directions to perform a task to encourage ipsilateral input and feedback.

   Example: Using a bicycle jigsaw in which power is generated from the cycling to operate the blade.

   Orthotic techniques—person needs a splint or sling to prevent further deformity, reduce the risk of additional injury, or alleviate pain.

continued

Table 23.1.   Adapted Individual Techniques

Examples: A resting splint may be used to keep the wrist and hand in a functional position and to avoid stretching the extensor tendons at the wrist. A sling may be used to maintain the shoulder joint.

Biofeedback—person can benefit from additional information (feedback) to isolate muscle contraction and learn or relearn movement patterns.

Examples: A person with a peripheral nerve injury to the radial nerve may benefit from biofeedback to isolate muscle contraction in the wrist extensors. A person with hemiplegia may benefit from biofeedback to isolate muscle contraction in the anterior tibialis muscle to pick up the foot and avoid foot drag.

E. *Sensorimotor Dysfunction*—person needs assistance to modify or to adapt the method of performing some sensorimotor activities.

Facilitation/inhibition techniques—person can benefit from controlled and selected sensory stimulation used to provoke or reduce muscle contraction.

Examples: Ice placed briefly in the palm of hand helps promote extension and tonic response in the upper extremity. An orthokinetic cuff is applied to the upper arm to decrease spasticity and increase range of motion.

Sensory integrative techniques—person can benefit from selected sensory stimulation from the vestibular, tactile, and proprioceptive systems used to promote adaptive responses to environmental demands.

Examples: Child rides a scooter board down a ramp to stimulate gravity and motion receptors, activate reflexes in the neck, body, and legs, and provide feedback from the neck and eye muscles. Child is rolled up in a soft blanket to get touch and pressure sensations that calm the nervous system.

F. *Sensory Dysfunction*—person needs assistance to modify or to adapt methods of performing some sensory activities.

Sensory substitution techniques—person can benefit from learning to rely on another sensory system to provide information previously sought from the original sensory system.

Examples: A person who is losing sight due to degeneration of the retina learns to use hearing and touch to orient to the environment and locate objects. A person who has lost hearing learns to use a computer and modem to transmit information over the telephone.

Sensory awareness training—person can benefit from an organized program designed to counteract the effects of sensory deprivation, which occurred from disuse, malfunction, or retreat from the environment.

Examples: Person with chronic schizophrenia is added to a group that is directed in simple exercises to all body muscles and joints to stimulate body awareness. A person with Alzheimer's disease is provided with selected sensory simulation to activate vision, hearing, touch, smell, and taste to increase awareness and response to the external environment.

Pressure garments—person will benefit from pressure applied to the skin surface to promote smooth healing of the skin surfaces.

Example: A person who received burns to hands and face wears pressure gloves and mask to aid healing and avoid keloids (raised scars) from forming.

G. *Cognitive Dysfunction*—person needs assistance to modify or to adapt methods of performing some cognitive activities.

continued

Table 23.1. Adapted Individual Techniques

Computer-assisted therapy—person can benefit from consistent feedback, repetitive but versatile programs, and infinite patience, which the computer can provide.
Examples: Person with a head injury is using a computer program designed to increase auditory memory of a series of numbers as in a telephone number, and lists of words as in a grocery list. Person who is mentally retarded is using a computer program designed to teach safety while walking on the sidewalk and crossing the street.

Cognitive retraining—person can benefit from specific techniques designed to facilitate the performance of functions and skills, such as arousal, perception, discrimination, orientation, problem-solving, recall, and memory.
Examples: Person is assisted to write a schedule of the day's activities on a 3 × 5 card that will be put in the shirt pocket for easy reference. A person who recently was in a coma attempts to recognize familiar voices on a tape and match them to photographs.

Stress management—person can benefit from learning specific skills to cope successfully with events and situations that produce frustration and loss of control.
Examples: Person practices planning ahead for dinner party so that food will be prepared in a sequence that permits all items to be ready at about the time the guests arrive. A person role plays how to respond to questions asked in a job interview.

H. *Psychosocial Dysfunction*—person needs assistance to modify or to adapt methods of performing some psychosocial activities.

Reminiscence training—person can benefit from reviewing life events and memories as part of the final stage of life.
Examples: Older person records events that happened during the Depression years. Older person organizes a scrapbook of clippings and photographs that have been collected over the years.

Remotivation training—person with chronic depression can benefit from an emphasis on paying attention to daily happenings and current events.
Examples: Discussion for the day might be about what kind of activities a homemaker does. Some slides are shown of old advertisements and the group talks about how products and prices have changed over the years.

Reality orientation—person with mental confusion can benefit from a group experience that focuses on orientation to time, place, and/or person.
Examples: Group completes a bulletin board that includes year, day, date, next meal, weather, and next holiday. Each member has a cardboard clock that must be set to correspond to the questions posed by the leaders, such as "When do we eat breakfast?".

Support group—person and family members want to know how other families handle the problems of dealing with a person who has had a serious illness or injury and is now at home.
Examples: A group of patients/clients who have had a stroke and their families meet once a month in the occupational therapy clinic to discuss problems and to try out new methods of dealing with problems that occur now that the person is at home. A group of parents who have children with cerebral palsy meet to discuss and get information on raising a handicapped child, including rights to education, use of respite care, and job opportunities for the handicapped.

Table 23.2.   Adapted Environmental Techniques

A. *Problems in Self-maintenance*—person is unable to modify or to adapt performance to function satisfactorily and requires external, environmental adaptive techniques.

Self-help aids—equipment designed to compensate for problems in grasp, strength, range of motion, reach, balance, and safety.

Examples: A person with arthritis, which makes grasping utensils difficult, may use an enlarged handle that fits over the regular handle. A person in a wheelchair may use an extended handle with grippers to reach items overhead or on the floor.

Adapted housing—adjustments are made during the building or remodeling of an existing structure to permit the person to move about the structure and to use the facilities provided.

Examples: A person in a wheelchair may need a ramp instead of stairs and a wider door to permit entry and exit from the housing unit. A very short person may need kitchen, bathroom, and utility cabinets built lower to permit access to the sinks and overhead storage.

Mobility aids—equipment designed to compensate for a person's ability to walk with ease and safety.

Examples: A person with a spinal cord injury uses a wheelchair to move from place to place. A child with spina bifida may use a tricycle that can be pedalled with the hands instead of the feet.

Transportation aids—equipment and vehicles that have been modified or adapted to permit persons to drive and ride with ease and safety.

Examples: A van is adapted by removing the driver's seat so that a person in a wheelchair can get close to the steering wheel and controls. A bus is adapted by adding a hydraulic lift and ramp, which permits a person in a wheelchair to roll the chair onto the ramp and be lifted up to the floor level of the bus.

Electronic assisted living—equipment designed to perform functions within easy access of the individual that would normally be placed elsewhere.

Examples: A master control switch for lights is placed on a collar around the person's neck, which can be operated by shrugging the shoulder and lateral flexion of the neck. The telephone can be answered by turning on a switch with the teeth.

B. *Productivity*—person is unable to adapt or modify performance of productive activities satisfactorily and requires external, environmental adaptive techniques.

Accessibility—equipment and facilities are designed to permit a person with limited sensory acuity, strength, or mobility to move about the facilities without special assistance from others.

Examples: An elevator is available to go from floor to floor; it has braille signs for floor numbers, makes a sound when the doors are opening and closing, and has a timer that can be adjusted to keep the doors open longer for persons who move slowly. Doors can be opened electronically to permit entrance and exit by those with weak grasp, such as a bilateral amputee, and inadequate strength, such as an older individual.

Adapted workstation—site of work is modified to fit the needs of the individual worker.

continued

Table 23.2.   Adapted Environmental Techniques

Examples: A person in a wheelchair may need a higher desk to permit the wheelchair to fit under it. A person who is blind needs frequently used items within easy reach to avoid groping about for things.

C. **Problems in Leisure Performance**—person is unable to adapt or to modify performance of leisure activities to function satisfactorily and requires external, environmental adaptations.

Adapted sports—games that have equipment and rules already modified to permit persons with handicaps to participate.

Examples: Wheelchair basketball, in which all team members, whether able bodied or handicapped, must play from a wheelchair. Bowling ramp in which the ball is placed and then released toward the pins.

Adapted social activities—events that have been modified to permit persons with handicaps to participate.

Examples: Wheelchair square dancing, in which the sets or squares are formed by persons in wheelchairs. Musical instruments that have been modified for use by persons with various handicaps.

D. **Problems in Motor Performance**—person is unable to adapt or to modify motor performance to function satisfactorily and requires external, environmental adaptations.

Prosthetic training—assisting a person to learn to use an artificial device designed to substitute for a missing or amputated limb of part of limb.

Examples: A person with an artificial arm and hand is given practice in opening, closing, reaching, lifting, moving, placing, dialing, typing, writing, pushing, and pulling to enable the person to use the prosthesis effectively and efficiently in performing motor activities.

Orthotic training (long-term)—assisting a person to learn to use an orthotic device that will be needed for more than a few weeks or months.

Example: A person who has C5–6 spinal cord injury probably will need a tenodesis splint to facilitate hand grasp for writing, eating, and handling smaller objects.

E. **Problems in Sensory Performance**—person is unable to adapt or to modify sensory performance to function satisfactorily and requires external, environmental adaptations.

Sensory aids—use of special glasses and hearing aids for persons with low vision and profound loss of hearing.

Examples: Person with loss of peripheral vision (tunnel) learns to use the focal (sharp) vision and glasses to scan the horizon. Person with profound loss of hearing learns to use the hearing aid to listen for low sounds and correlate their meaning to the environment.

Therapeutic horsemanship—use of horseriding to stimulate vestibular, kinesthetic, and proprioceptive receptors to increase awareness of and response to motion and movement.

Examples: A child with cerebral palsy feels what coordinated, smooth movement is like. A person with a head injury practices balancing on a changing surface and keeping the head upright.

F. **Problems in Cognitive Performance**—person is unable to adapt or to modify cognitive performance to function satisfactorily and requires external, environmental adaptations.

continued

Table 23.2. Adapted Environmental Techniques

Communication boards—devices on which letters of the alphabet, words or pictures have been attached to permit nonverbal language communication. *Examples:* A person with expressive aphasia (unable to speak) points to letters on the board to spell out words to talk with friends. A person with cerebral palsy who cannot speak clearly, uses an electronic board that scrolls the board until stopped on the desired picture or word.

G. *Problems in Psychosocial Performance*—person is unable to participate in social activities because of discrimination.

Community awareness program—programs are sponsored by the facility on various topics to inform the community and subsections of the community about the abilities and assets of persons with physical or mental problems.

Community awareness publications—publications are written and published by the facility on various topics to inform the community and subsections of the community about the abilities and assets of person with physical or mental problems.

Table 23.3. Media or Agent Types

A. *Inanimate Media*

Creative arts and crafts—products that result from the translation of mental imagery to a recognizable form.

Examples: painting, drawing, sculpture, writing, dancing, writing music, cooking, baking.

Manual arts and crafts—products that result from the skillful alteration of selected materials through such processes as assembly, molding, stamping, carving, pounding, folding, cutting, pasting, gluing, weaving, sewing, knotting, braiding, knitting, crocheting, and chemical reactions, including melting, dyeing, etching, inking, and fusing together.

Examples: woodworking, ceramics, leather, metal working, jewelry, origami, macrame, loom weaving, needlecrafts, basketry, enameling, batik, printing.

Games and sports—use of rules to organize play and control equipment.

Examples: Board games, table games, card games, dart games, ball games, water sports, snow and ice sports, track sports.

Educational and learning tasks—associated with learning to read, write, spell, using numbers, paying attention, following directions.

Examples: Reading street signs, advertisements, application forms, newspapers, magazines and books; writing letters, signing one's name, filling out forms, writing short stories; adding, subtracting, multiplying, and dividing; concentrating on a task, auditory discrimination, auditory memory, sequencing, verbal memory; visual discrimination, visual memory.

Toys—objects associated with children's play.

Examples: construction and building toys, musical toys, occupational toys, concept toys, manipulative toys, developmental toys, windup toys, electrical toys, dolls.

Computer—an electronic device that operates on mathematical and symbolic logic.

Examples: Computer games, computer-assisted learning, telecommunications, word processing, calculations, data storage and retrieval.

B. *Animate*

Self—use of the therapist as a therapeutic medium.

Examples: verbal communication, gestures, attitudes expressed verbally and nonverbally, knowledge and information giver, caregiver.

Dyad—usually the therapist and client/patient functioning as a unit.

Examples: friend, advisor, counselor, role model, confidante.

Group—several clients meet together with a therapist for a specific therapeutic purpose, which all share in common.

Examples: task oriented group, development group, thematic group, topical group, instrumental group.

Animals—use of domesticated animals as adjunct therapists.

Examples: teach responsibility for care, promote conversation and socialization, provide sensory stimulation, establish relationships.

Plants and nature—use of plants and nature as adjuncts to therapy.

Examples: teach responsibility for care, promote conversation and socialization, provide sensory stimulation.

Table 23.4. Modalities Agent Group

A. *Functional Activities*
1. Grasp and release movements
2. Eye-hand coordinated movements
3. Reaching and fetching movements
4. Holding and carrying movements
5. Lifting and placing movements
6. Opening and closing movements

B. *Self-care Activities*
1. Learning how to care for one's physical body, including grooming, oral hygiene, bathing, and toilet hygiene
2. Learning how to clothe oneself
3. Understanding nutrition and proper eating habits
4. Learning communication skills
5. Learning how to move safely from place to place
6. Learning appropriate sexual expression

C. *Word-related Activities*
1. Learning about work
2. Identifying with a worker
3. Developing a self-concept as a worker
4. Developing basic word habits including responsibility, punctuality, and quality control
5. Learning to get along with peers
6. Learning to handle and adjust to authority

D. *Leisure/Avocational Activities*
1. Learning to follow the rules
2. Learning to function as a team player
3. Learning how to win and lose
4. Learning how to set a goal and work toward it

E. *Homemaking Activities*
1. Planning and preparing meals
2. Shopping for groceries and other staples
3. Scrubbing, vacuuming, and dusting
4. Making and changing beds
5. Washing, drying, sorting, and putting clothes away
6. Home safety—locks, electricity, throw rugs
7. Organizing closets and drawers

Table 23.5.   Teaching Methods

A teaching method is a means of presenting the task to the individual or group. Teaching methods as used in occupational therapy are described briefly. Most can be implemented in a one-to-one situation between the therapist and the person seeking help or in a group situation.

A. *Demonstration and Performance*

The most basic type of demonstration is imitation. The therapist does something and the person attempts to do the same thing. For example, the therapist places a peg in a hole, then the person tries to place a peg in a hole. Demonstration becomes more complex when several movements are demonstrated by the therapist before the person is permitted to try to copy the actions.

Demonstration can be separated from performance, but the therapist cannot be assured that the person can perform the movement to complete an activity unless performance is required. Since occupational therapy is concerned with the ability to do, not just observe, performance is an integral part of the demonstration.

B. *Exploration and Discovery*

Exploration and discovery are used frequently in children's play. Various activities are arranged, such as on a playground, and the child is permitted to select the activity of choice and try it without specific adult guidance. The child learns by exploring the object(s) and discovering what can be done with them. Adults can use exploration and discovery also. Art materials, for example, provide opportunities to try a variety of approaches. Oil paints can be used differently than water paints. Pastels produce a different effect than felt tip pens.

Exploration and discovery encourage maximum involvement of the individual in the activity or task. The disadvantage is that the therapist has less control and structure over the individual's performance.

C. *Explanation and Discussion*

Some learning tasks can be acquired, in part, by explaining verbally about the task and discussing the various activities involved in the task. Explanation and discussion are useful for planning an activity or task in advance, or in reviewing what happened after an activity or task has been completed. For instance, a person is getting ready to apply for a job. The therapist can explain to the person how to go about applying for a job and discuss misconceptions the person may have. After the interview, the therapist can discuss with the individual how the interview went and explain aspects the person may have misunderstood. The disadvantage is that performance may not be observed. An individual can say one thing and do something else.

D. *Role-playing and Simulation*

Another approach to the job interview would be role playing or simulation. In role playing, the therapist may assume the role of job interviewer while the individual plays the interviewee. The interviewer (therapist) asks the same questions that are likely to be asked by an actual job interviewer. The interviewee tries to answer the questions as they would be answered in a real interview. The advantage of the technique is the opportunity to try out behavior before actually doing the behavior. Changes or adaptations can be

continued

Table 23.5.   Teaching Methods

made before the person fails an interview. A disadvantage is that the therapist can never be sure that the person will act the same way in an actual interview as was performed in the role playing.

Simulation is similar to role playing except that objects are involved rather than human behavior alone. Specific jobs are simulated to permit analysis of performance and practice before doing the real job. Perhaps the most familiar job simulator is the driving simulator used in driving education courses, which permits the person to experience driving behaviors of watching the road, steering, accelerating, and braking before actually driving a car on the road. Again, however, the therapist or driving instructor cannot be sure the simulated learning will be transferred to the real situation.

E. *Problem Solving*

Problem-solving in therapy is a process of teaching an individual to examine a problem situation by carefully defining the problem, outlining a variety of possible solutions, and then selecting the solution that appears to have the best chance of solving the problem. The solution is tried and, if necessary, an alternative solution or variation of the solution is tried for even better results. The problem-solving approach is useful in solving life situations, like selecting a living place away from home or finding a way to enable a person with hand dysfunction to hold a pencil. In the case of the living place, the therapist can help define the problem by identifying the individual's needs, such as cost, distance from school or work, type of housing, furnished or unfurnished, special needs for wide doors, handrails, and no stairs. Then the therapist might accompany the individual to visit some possible accommodations.

Holding a pencil may be solved by enlarging the size of pencil, changing the grip from finger prehension to palm or spherical grasp or eliminating prehension by slipping a bar around the hand. Another solution may be to switch from handwriting to a typewriter.

The limitation of problem-solving is that the process can be time-consuming, requires several trial and error attempts, and needs the full cooperation of the individual. The advantage is that the individual can learn to solve future problems based on the approach. Future time and frustration can be reduced.

F. *Audiovisual Aids*

Audiovisual materials can be useful teaching and learning aids because they provide the opportunity to teach a person the same thing in repetition using the exact teaching style.

Such materials may be used when the therapist is not present, such as evenings and weekends. Examples of such teaching aids might be a movie on wheelchair safety, a video tape of meat preparation using one hand, or a series of slides and a tape illustrating architectural barriers and ways to eliminate barriers in the home.

The advantage of audiovisual aids is that the material may be repeated numerous times without the therapist becoming irritated at the amount of time required to do the task. A disadvantage is the limited opportunity to vary the presentation style to meet individual needs.

continued

Table 23.5. Teaching Methods

G. *Repetition and Practice*

The major purposes of repetition and practice are to increase speed and accuracy. Behavior that is fast but results in many errors is ineffective. Likewise, behavior that is slow but accurate may be ineffective. Most behaviors have an approximate time allotment and error rate that is considered acceptable. Exceeding either the time or number of errors may be considered unacceptable. A person who can type only ten words a minute probably would not be hired as a typist or word processor. The same would be true if the person made ten errors per minute.

Ideally, speed and accuracy should improve together since one without the other is of limited use. The problem for the therapist is to find the best method to achieve the twin goals. The first step is to make sure the person has a mental picture or cognitive map of the desired performance. With motor tasks, one good demonstration usually is better than a thousand words. Second, the person must understand why the repetition and practice are necessary and want to put the effort into learning or relearning the task. Performance does not necessarily improve because repetition and practice have occurred. If practice made perfect, most adults would have beautiful handwriting. Most adults do not write well because the motivation to do so is not present. The third step is to decide on a schedule. Learning and performance are dependent on an alert nervous system. Fatigue and central nervous system depressor drugs decrease both learning and performance. The therapist must observe the person carefully. If speed and accuracy are improving, then repetition and practice should continue. When either is decreasing, the session should be terminated. There is little gain in slowing down and repeating errors.

H. *Behavioral Management*

Behavioral management is based on the concept of focusing on one or more specific behaviors separate from a cause-effect relationship. In other words, behavioral management is not concerned with what may or may not have contributed to the development of the behavior; only that the behavior exists. Some programs of behavioral management target behaviors that are seen as inappropriate or undesirable, such as head banging, hitting people, wearing dirty clothes, eating with fingers, failure to do an assigned task, or saying swear words. Other programs are designed to promote a desired behavior, such as saying "thank you," buttoning a shirt, or wearing a splint. First, the behavior is selected and operationally defined so that the program managers agree on examples of the behavior. Then, a target performance is described, such as no head banging for a 2-hour period when awake or no hitting in an 8-hour time period. Third, a reward is established, such as points, tokens, or an event, to encourage the desired behavior, and, finally, the program is implemented. Behavioral management is a powerful learning method. Thus, it can be used and misused. Misuse occurs when the individual focus is sacrificed for the convenience of an institution. If a person loses privileges for hitting others but can be spanked (a form of hitting) for various other rule infractions, the effectiveness of the behavioral management program is suspect. Another misuse is the failure to determine whether the person can control the behavior. Trying to toilet train a 6-

continued

Table 23.5.   Teaching Methods

month-old child clearly will not succeed because the child cannot control the sphincter. The desired behavior must be available to the person. A person must be able to say and use words other than swear words or the program will fail since total silence is not the objective. Finally, if the person whose behavior is targeted does not want to change the behavior, he or she may sabotage the program by appearing to cooperate but not really changing a behavior pattern at all except in the specific situation. Many behavioral management programs have appeared to be successful in the hospital only to disappear when the client goes home. Therefore, behavioral management programs must be carefully thought out and checked to determine if any carry over occurs to other situations. Getting a person to wear a splint in the hospital is nice but it is better if the client wears the splint at home too. If the splint spends most of its time on the back seat of the car, the behavioral management program has not been successful.

I. *Patient Education*

Patient/client education is an important part of most intervention programs but is often neglected. If, however, the person is expected to gain or regain independent function, that person must learn how to live with continuing problems brought on by the illness or injury and how to prevent additional problems if possible. Some learning does take place during regular intervention sessions but such learning should not be the sole means of acquiring information. Patient/client education means a formal, organized, systematic approach to imparting knowledge and information. The focus is on the individual receiving services but the learning sessions may include the spouse, children, parents, or other family members who are part of the living arrangement.

When should patient/client education begin? Usually, the acute phase of an illness or injury is not a good time. The person and family are not ready physically or emotionally. Even if there is no "acute phase" in the medical sense, a person who has been recently diagnosed may not be ready to deal with the long-term problems right away. Convalescence is a good time for patient/client education. Since many patients/clients are sent home to convalesce, educational sessions may begin after hospitalization. The primary objectives usually are: (*a*) to teach the person and family about the nature of the disease or injury, including etiology, prognosis, and treatment; (*b*) to provide instruction in self-care procedures; (*c*) to suggest ways to prevent additional or recurrent health problems; and (*d*) to inform the person and family of other community services that might be useful.

Patient/client education is important especially for persons with long-term conditions. The individual's willingness to learn and take responsibility for maintaining personal health is critical. Failure to take medication, refusing to wear a corrective splint, and "forgetting" to practice or exercise decrease the chances of the individual avoiding additional health problems. Patients/clients are more likely to follow through with a home program if that program has been carefully explained and the steps have been demonstrated by and practiced with the therapist. Written instructions, even with drawings or pictures, are difficult to follow when the objective is murky. Therapists must take responsibility for providing good instruction at the level the person or family can understand.

Table 23.6. Therapeutic Approaches

A therapeutic approach is a means of organizing tasks or activities into a series of steps based on a system of logic.

A. *Normal Developmental Sequencing*

Activities or tasks are selected according to the normal progression of skill acquisition in the average child or adult. The specific activity or task is chosen because it is the next item in sequence that the person cannot do. For example, if the child can stand with support, the next activity is standing without support, and the next task is walking.

Using the developmental sequence is helpful in program planning and implementation because the sequence is provided automatically on a developmental chart. The disadvantage is that, for handicapped persons, the developmental sequence may increase problems rather than reduce them. A child with spastic muscles who spends time learning to creep and crawl may develop hip and knee contractions, which will interfere with standing. In walking, standing with hips and knees extended is very desirable.

B. *Normal Activity Sequencing*

Many activities have a logical sequence of steps that facilitates task performance. The steps are not necessarily invariant, but a sequence may require less total time of repetition of steps. For example, in dressing or putting on clothes, normally undergarments are put on first, then overgarments and, finally, outer garments, such as a coat. If slacks are put on before underpants, the slacks will have to be taken off. Once the underpants are on, the slacks must be put on again. Normal activity sequencing provides an easy therapeutic approach to follow for any task with which the therapist is familiar. However, the normal sequence may not be advantageous for a person with handicaps. A person with balance problems may do better to put on all items that dress the upper part of the body while sitting. Then items for the lower part of the body can be put on as a group, thus reducing the number of times the person must get up and sit down. The result is a safer, if not more efficient, approach.

C. *Task Analysis*

Task analysis permits the therapist and individual to examine in detail the steps or processes that compose an activity or task. Most activities or tasks are complex and require several steps and units of behavior to complete. Even such a basic skill as brushing one's teeth is complex. One must get a toothbrush using finger prehension. Next, the toothpaste must be secured while the cap is unscrewed. Then the tube must be held and squeezed over the toothbrush until the right amount of paste is on the brush. The cap must be replaced on the tube. The brush is brought to the mouth to brush upper and lower teeth both in front and in back. Motions involve up and down and sideways movements. Finally, some water must be poured into a cup and placed in the mouth to rinse out the mouth.

Task analysis allows an examination of each step in a sequence in terms of the requirements, which, in turn provides an opportunity to note which steps a person can and cannot perform. A major drawback is that performance does not occur normally in a step by step approach but rather as an integrated continuous flow of behavioral performance. Failure to provide practice in the whole sequence may result in a halting, awkward performance.

continued

Table 23.6. Therapeutic Approaches

D. Graded Activities

"Graded activities" is the term used to refer to the technique of categorizing tasks or toys into degrees of difficulty or complexity. Most activities can be classified according to how long a task takes to complete; how much equipment is needed; how much instruction is needed; how much skill is needed; how much space is needed to perform the activity; whether the activity can be done lying down, sitting, or standing; whether the activity creates a mess; and whether the materials are structured or free form. For example, making a link belt is usually a short-term project that requires very little equipment, has few instructions, requires little skill, can be done in a limited amount of space, such as in bed, does not create a large mess, and is fairly structured. In contrast, making, glazing, and firing a set of ceramic dishes probably would take several days, require several pieces of equipment, has many directions to be followed, requires a fair amount of skill if a potter's wheel is used, needs a lot of space, cannot be done in bed, creates a mess, and is a free form activity until the clay is fired.

The purpose of grading or categorizing activities is to permit the task to be selected within the client's functional ability but at the same time meet the client's needs. A link belt might be within the ability level of an 8-year-old child, a person confined to bed, or a person who has had little experience in using fine finger motions. Working on the potter's wheel, on the other hand, probably would be more suitable with a teenaged or older client who was able to sit or stand for several minutes and who had experience in using the hands to make projects. The needs of the client, however, would determine if either the link belt or potter's wheel would actually be selected of if another project or toy would be a better choice.

E. Adapted Activity

Activities may be adapted when the client cannot perform the task in the normal or usual manner. An activity may be adapted by modifying or changing the equipment used, omitting or condensing steps in the sequence, altering the environment, or altering the person's approach to the task.

Equipment can be changed by altering the tool. For example, a hand saw can be made two-handed, an embroidery hoop can be mounted on a stand that sits over the knee for one-handed work, a spoon handle can be lengthened or enlarged.

Steps can be omitted by using partially prepared materials, such as leather billfold kits, cake mixes, or ceramic molds. The environment can be altered by performing the activity in different locations, such as the client's room, the clinic, outdoors, the community center or home, of in a different position, such as placing an activity overhead, higher or lower than normal. Altering the person's approach can be accomplished by changing the client's position from sitting to lying down to standing or from one hand to two hands.

As with the graded activity approach, the adaptation must make the activity possible for the client to perform. Adaptations, however, are not useful unless the activity meets the client's needs.

F. Activity Group

An activity group involves the organizing of a number of clients into a group for a particular purpose or objective, which all members need to gain. There

continued

Table 23.6. Therapeutic Approaches

are three types of activity groups used most commonly in occupational therapy. The most basic is the parallel activity group in which each client is engaged in an individual activity. The therapist interacts with each client by observing the activity, answering questions, and commenting off the progress. Clients are not expected to interact or share supplies and equipment with each other, although some general conversation may occur about the weather, sports events, or local news.

The second type of activity group is called a project group. In the project group, some sharing of supplies and equipment is required and some interaction among clients is expected. The therapist encourages the sharing and interacting, both by structuring the activity setting before the group begins and by actions taken during the time the group is together.

In the third activity group, called a cooperative or egocentric-cooperative group, the amount of sharing and interacting is again increased. Usually only one activity or task is selected by the therapist or chosen by the group among alternatives offered by the therapist. Group members are expected to participate in the total activity or task. The therapist guides but does not control the actions of group members.

Activity groups are used to encourage social skills, such as talking and working in a group situation. Usually the group will have eight to twelve members. Groups offer the advantage of providing realistic situations where people interact and perform together. After the activity or task is completed, the group can critique the session and provide feedback for each other that can be useful. The overall effectiveness of activity groups, however, depends on the therapist's ability to organize and direct each member according to individual needs.

G. *Normal Environment*

Use of the normal environment at first glance may not seem to be a therapeutic or special approach. However, in some cases, it is practice in the normal environment that has not occurred because of fear or lack of opportunity. Use of the normal environment permits the client and therapist to assess whether a person can perform in the "real world" since the normal environment is, in fact, the real world.

Precautions in using the normal environment pertain to the recognition of the risks involved. For example, a person who is learning to drive only using hand controls needs to practice in a safe environment first before tackling the freeway traffic at rush hour. It is the therapist's responsibility to discuss the risks of performing in the normal environment with the client prior to actual practice.

H. *Adapted/Structured Environment*

An adapted or structured environment means that there is more structure or guidance and less risk involved for the client. The therapist plans the practice session in an environmental setting, such as the occupational therapy clinic where situations can be controlled to minimize the risk of failure or serious physical injury.

Use of an adapted environment is usually a first or initial approach before the client tries out new or released skills in the normal environment. The primary drawback of the adapted environment is overreliance on its security and protection. A hundred performances in an adapted environment are no

continued

Table 23.6.   Therapeutic Approaches

match for one performance in the normal environment. The therapist must learn when to start encouraging some clients to think about trying it "for real" and when to discourage the eager beaver.

I. *One-to-One*

In the one-to-one approach, the therapist works with one client at a time. This is a very intense relationship in which the therapist may assume the role of parent surrogate, advisor, friend, supervisor, or observer, depending on the program plan. As the plan changes, the role may change also. A one-to-one approach is very effective with clients who cannot function in a group situation because of skill deficiencies or fear of ridicule and failure. One limitation is the possibility that the client will become overly dependent on the therapist and not want to let go. Another limitation is the expense. One-to-one programs are costly and limit the number of clients that can be seen in a given time period.

J. *Consulting*

Consulting is the process of examining the problem and giving advice to a person as to how to solve the problem. To qualify as a direct service, consultation must be given to the individual, not to other professionals or community agencies. Consultation can provide ideas and possible answers to problems, but does not include trying out the suggested solutions. Because no tryout is required, the person may not use the advice. This is the major drawback to consultation. Advice is given but need not be accepted or used.

Table 23.7. Examples of Therapy Equipment List by Types and Categories

Functional Activities—Object Manipulation
Adapted needle-working tools
Adapted woodworking tools
Adapted leather tools
Cones, stacking
Coordination boards
Dexterity boards
Handles—enlarged, elongated
Peg boards
Reachers
Function Activities—Activities of Daily Living (ADLs)
ADL boards
Adapted utensils
Adapted grooming aids
Adapted dressing aids
Other self-help devices
Functional Activities—Transportation
Driving aids
Driving simulator or computer program
Modified or adapted vans
Modified or adapted buses
Range of Motion
Skateboard
Powder board
Herring track
Floor-type weaving loom
Floor-type manual printing press
Cuffs or mitts
Sanding blocks
Positioning
Corner chair
Benches
Bolsters or rolls
Easels
Hammocks
Positioning boards, prone
Tables
Trays
Progressive Resistive Exercise
Weights
Adapted weaving loom–rehabilitation loom
Adapted printing press with attachable weights
Sensory Integration
Barrels
Balls—large diameter
Crawlers

continued

Table 23.7. Examples of Therapy Equipment List by Types and Categories

Hammocks or nets
Scooter boards
Swings, platform
Vestibular board
Wedges
Sensorimotor
Mats
Slings
Splints
Powered toys
Vibrators
Cognitive Retraining
Computer games
Computer programs for cognitive tasks
Computer simulation programs
Developmental
Dolls with and without handicaps
Computer-adapted toys
Computer programs for developmental tasks
Toy lending library for handicapped children
Mobility
Adapted tricycles
Wheelchair adductor pads
Wheelchairs
Wheelchair cushions
Wheelchair footrests
Joy sticks
Communication
Language boards
Adapted typewriters
Adapted computers
Adapted tape recorders
Head operated controls
Homemaking—Kitchen
Adapted cooking aids
Adapted cleaning aids
Gravity Lessening Aids
Counterbalanced sling
Overhead sling
Rancho aid
Mobile arm supports
Muscle Reeducation
Biofeedback trainers
Group Activities
Parachutes
Earth ball
Trampoline

continued

Table 23.7. Examples of Therapy Equipment List by Types and Categories

Orthotics Equipment and Supplies
Splints
Slings
Cast cutter
Casting supplies
Plastic, metal, fabric supplies
Work Evaluation and Training Systems
BTE (Baltimore Therapeutic Equipment)
Valpar system
WEST system (West Evaluation Systems Technology)

The Practice Base

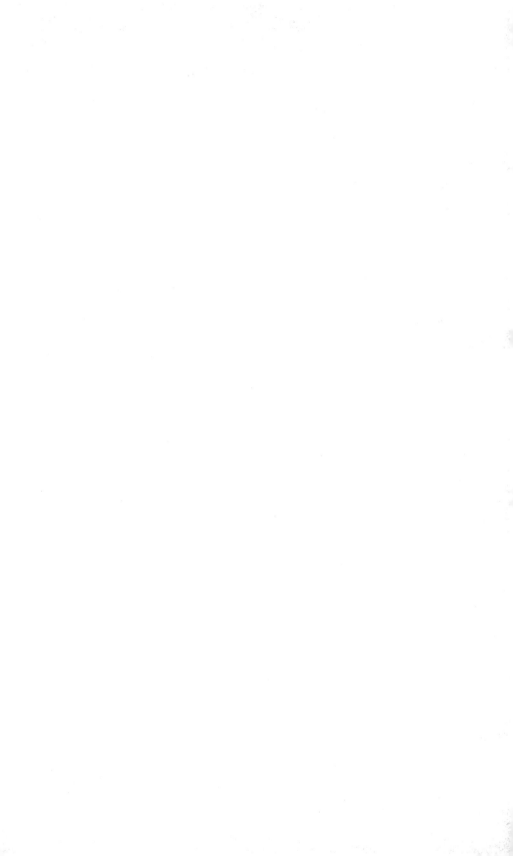

CHAPTER 24

Occupational Therapy Process Model

Occupational therapy was established on the concept of providing direct services to people; that is, the knowledge and skills of occupational therapy would be applied for the immediate benefit of the persons receiving occupational therapy. To apply occupational therapy knowledge and skills for maximum benefit, a process or series of stages should be followed. The process is based on a problem-solving approach and is graphically presented in the occupational therapy process model in Chapter 1 (see Fig. 1.1) and outlines in Table 24.1. The twelve stages can be identified as follows: 1) referral, 2) theoretical model, 3) screening evaluation, 4) comprehensive evaluation, 5) occupational therapy diagnosis, 6) practice model, 7) plan intervention, 8) implementation and management, 9) review, 10) revision, 11) discharge, and 12) follow-up. These steps form the direct service functions of occupational therapy, which are as follows:

1. To receive a referral, whatever its source
2. Select tentative conceptual model(s)
3. Complete screening evaluation
4. Complete comprehensive evaluation
5. Make occupational therapy diagnosis
6. Select practice model consistent with conceptual model
7. Plan intervention by setting goals and selecting media, modalities, and methods
8. Implement and manage intervention plan
9. Review the client and intervention plan
10. Revise the intervention plan, if needed
11. Discharge client when goals are achieved or progress has reached a plateau
12. Follow-up

   The occupational therapy process is outlined in Table 24.1 and is described in the following.

Table 24.1.   Occupational Therapy Process Model

REFERRAL STAGE

Process
Receive referral
Identify pertinent data from referral
Collect additional data, if needed
Summarize the referring data
Interpret data from referral
Action decision question
What does the referring agent or party expect from occupational therapy regarding this referral?
What information can occupational therapy provide?
Prioritize the answers

OCCUPATIONAL THERAPY CONCEPTUAL MODEL SELECTION STAGE

Process
Review possible occupational therapy conceptual models
Select a tentative theoretical model
Action decision questions
What theoretical model would most likely facilitate the collection and analysis of data needed to reply to the referring agent's questions?
What theoretical model would most likely permit an evaluation of the client's strengths, weaknesses, and potential to benefit from occupational therapy services?

SCREENING EVALUATION STAGE

Process
Select a screening instrument(s) consistent with the theoretical model
Collect the data by administering and scoring the instrument(s)
Interpret the data from the instrument(s)
Summarize the data (may require a written report)
Communicate the results to the referral source
Action decision questions
Can occupational therapy services be of benefit in resolving the problems of the referred client?
If yes, continue to the comprehensive evaluation stage
If no, write a report summarizing the assessments used, data analyzed, and the rationale for rejecting the potential client
If client is accepted, prioritize the problems that require additional information to clarify the goals and strategies for intervention

COMPREHENSIVE EVALUATION STAGE

Process
Review list of comprehensive assessment techniques consistent with the conceptual model
Select those assessment techniques based on the priorities established from the referal and screening stages
Administer the assessments in the order of priority

continued

Table 24.1. Occupational Therapy Process Model

Score the assessments
Interpret the assessments
Summarize the results of the assessments and other data
Determine if additional data is needed and how to obtain that data
Action decision questions
What are the problems manifested in the evaluation stage?
What strengths can be identified to assist in problem resolution?

OCCUPATIONAL THERAPY DIAGNOSIS STAGE

Process
List all the problems identified
Group the problems into categories suggested by the conceptual model
List and prioritize the problems and/or categories according to the conceptual model
Describe the findings to the client and also to the family and referral source if requested
Action decision questions
What groups or categories of similiar problems can be identified?
What occupational therapy diagnosis or diagnoses best fit the problems identified in the categories?

OCCUPATIONAL THERAPY PRACTICE MODEL SELECTION STAGE

Process
Review tentatively selected theoretical model
Considering the occupational therapy diagnosis, select the theoretical model that best addresses the diagnosis
Identify possible occupational therapy practice models based on the theorectical model
Select a tentative occupational therapy practice model
Action decision questions
What theoretical model best fits the categories of problems identified by this client?
What practice model is most likely to resolve these problems?

PLANNING STAGE

Process
Prioritize the list of categories and problems based on client (family, referral source) and therapist discussion
Develop a list of expected changes
Determine when these changes should be expected
Based on the practice model consider possible intervention strategies (media, modalities, and methods) to use in resolving the categories of problems (or individual problems) and achieve the goals
Select initial intervention strategies
Write goal statements incorporating the expected changes, timelines, and intervention strategies to be applied
Determine where, when, and for how long intervention sessions will be held

continued

Table 24.1. Occupational Therapy Process Model

Action decision questions
In what order will the problem categores be addressed?
What changes in the client are expected when the problem categories are resolved?
What will the client be able to do that he or she cannot or does not do now?
What intervention strategies will be applied?

IMPLEMENTATION STAGE

Process
Begin with first goal statement
Continue with goal list
Action decision questions
Are the items in the goal statements being implemented as planned?
If yes, continue plan and proceed to the review stage
If no, proceed to the revision stage

REVIEW STAGE

Process
Select an assessment methodology that can detect change in client performance which will measure the problem(s) being addressed in the goal statements.
Adminster and score the instrument, if necessary
Interpret the results
Summarize the results
Action decision questions
Are the goal statements being achieved?
If yes, continue intervention plan and strategies
If no, proceed to the revision stage

REVISION STAGE

Process
Determine what barriers are occurring
Explore what options are reducing the barriers
Determine if other categories of problems exist which did not appear in the original assessment or were not selected for intervention for whatever reason.
Determine if occupational therapy services are required to resolve the problems
Reformulate the goal statements based on the new information
Action decision questions
Can the goal statements be revised to increase the potential for problem resolution?
What changes are needed to achieve a more workable situation in which problems can be resolved and the goals can be accomplished?

DISCHARGE STAGE

Process
Collect data on the progress toward all goal statements
Administer, score, and interpret any instruments used

continued

Table 24.1.   Occupational Therapy Process Model

Intrepret and summarize the data
Document the status on goal statements at discharge
Discharge the client
Action decision questions
Have all goal statements been obtained?
Are the client, therapist, and referral source person, satisfied with the
  progress made?
If yes, proceed to the follow-up stage
If no, proceed to the revision stage

FOLLOW-UP STAGE

Process
Discuss with the client (family and referring source) the need for followup
  including check-up visits and referral to other resources/agencies
Arrange for follow-up visits, if needed
Make referrals, if needed
Document arrangements for follow-up visits
Document referrals in writing
Action decision questions
Does client need follow-up visits?
Should client be referred to other resources/agencies?

OCCUPATIONAL THERAPY PROCESS

Referral Stage

Technically, the source of referral can be from anyone including the consumer. An occupational therapy practitioner can refer a client as well as any other professional. A neighbor, friend, or family member can make a referral for occupational therapy services. In reality, however, there is often a chain of command that determines how and when referrals are made. Without the proper authorization, reimbursement is jeopardized or hours of credit for therapy may not be recognized. In addition, often a specific form must be used for the referral, which must be placed in the client's chart or permanent record. Even in private practice, referrals often must be recorded in a certain manner if reimbursement is involved. Clients who pay themselves may need a record of the referral and subsequent intervention to submit to their insurance company or to provide record of therapy expenses for tax deductions. In summary, referral sources vary depending on the worksite, but keeping a record of all referrals in a consistent manner is always a good idea.

The process involved in the referral stage includes receiving the referral, identifying pertinent data from the referral, collecting additional data if needed, summarizing the referral data, and interpreting the data from the referral in preparation for the screening. These five stages may take only a few minutes or several hours depending on the situation. Pertinent data includes the client's identifying information such as name, age, name of referral source, reason for referral, information justifying why the referral was made, and expected results from occupational therapy services. If any of the previous mentioned data is missing, it will need to be acquired. Additional data that may be useful are the results of assessments by other professionals, previous response to therapy, medications prescribed, educational level, work history, and family support. How much data is needed often depends on the reason for the referral. A referral to assess the sucking and swallowing reflexes of a newborn infant may not require much additional information. A referral to assist a 67-year-old person who had a stroke to return home may require additional data. Summarizing the referring data involves gathering the pertinent data together so it can be interpreted. Some referral sources state the goals to be achieved through occupational therapy quite clearly; others do not state any goals. Knowing the purpose of the referral clearly increases the possibility of assessing the client to obtain that data.

Two questions should guide the action in the referral stage. What does the referring source expect from occupational therapy regarding the referral? And what information can occupational therapy provide? If more than one answer would be expected, prioritize the answers so the information gained during the evaluation stage will be sure to be obtained.

Occupational Therapy Conceptual Model Selection

The second stage involves reviewing possible occupational therapy conceptual models that appear to address the expectations of the referral source. From the possibilities, select one or two if both are very similar. Selecting a tentative conceptual model is important because the model provides the guidance to determine which assessment instrument or instruments should be used to gather information. For example, is recovery from a stroke primarily a motor control problem or a cognitive reeducation problem? The answer to that question will determine what assessment data is needed from the screening and comprehensive evaluations.

Some occupational therapy practitioners may say they use an eclectic model. If they mean they use a combination of two models which can named and explained that is acceptable. More often the term "eclectic" is used because the practitioner does not identify what theoretical model or models are being used. The profession of occupational therapy cannot appear to be unknowing and occupational therapy practitioners should not appear to foster the idea. Also research methods require that concepts be defined so they can be measured. Defining eclecticism does not allow for very precise measurement. Therefore, occupational therapy practitioners need to know, describe, and define what they are doing.

Action decision questions are: What conceptual model would most likely facilitate the collection and analysis of data needed to repay to the referring agent's request? What conceptual model would most likely permit an evaluation of the client's strengths, weaknesses, and potential to benefit from occupational therapy services?

Screening Evaluation Stage

Screening evaluation has five substages: selecting a screening instrument(s) consistent with the theoretical model, collecting the data by administering the scoring instrument(s), recording any other data collected, interpreting the data, and summarizing the data.

Screening evaluation is basically the determination of an individual's function or performance in the parameters specified in the theoretical model. Many of the parameters may be measured by administering a screening instrument or instruments. Other important data may be obtained through structured interview and observation. For example, if the occupational therapy practitioner is using a model based on occupational performance, the therapist should assess those performance skills that are presently within or above normal limits and those that are not. Both areas of information are needed because most models of occupational performance are concerned both with maintaining and continuing normal performance throughout the life span and with correcting and upgrading those problems that are limiting performance. Deficient or inadequate performance skills frequently are easiest to recognize. Normal and above normal performance skill areas may be overlooked unless the assessment is complete. However, these normal areas of function may be most useful in the intervention program to assist in developing, restoring, compensating for, or maintaining skill in problem areas of occupational performance.

The primary purposes of an assessment are to gather, analyze, and interpret data. In gathering data, decisions must be made concerning what data are needed and which methods or tests are used to obtain it. When a therapist assesses a person, the model provides some indication of what information may be of value. For example, a 4-year-old child may be referred for an assessment of occupational and developmental skills before entering kindergarten. The conceptual model might be concerned with occupational role performance. For the child about to enter school, the role will be that of a student who needs the skills to perform the tasks expected in kindergarten. An initial data-gathering tool could be the Denver Developmental Screening Test, which evaluates gross motor, fine motor, language, and personal–social development. The results would indicate whether performance skills in each occupational area are within normal limits. Suppose the child's language development is advanced, but physical development is lagging. The higher level of language development could be an asset in an intervention program. The child probably would be able to understand a simple explanation of the intervention management procedures, which would assist the child to cooperate in sessions with the therapist. The primary problem will be in occupational areas that require motor skills as prerequisites to performance. Most self-maintenance activities require motor skills. Coloring, writing, and scissor cutting also require motor skills as do many childhood games and sports. This child may be seriously disabled in all occupational performance areas. How much of a disability will be determined in a comprehensive assessment?

Other sources of information important to the student role may be observed while administering the DDST such as ability to follow directions, attention span, and postural control while performing the items on the DDST. Assessment instruments that provide maximum data in minimum time are important to consider when time is short, which is usually the case for practitioners.

After the data have been gathered, the information should be recorded in a systematic and concise form. This step is necessary so that data can be used later as a reference base to see if change has occurred. Written records are essential. Memory is not accurate enough, especially over long periods of time.

In essence, screening evaluation requires learning how to locate pertinent data, identifying and administering appropriate tests, and summarizing the data for possible use in setting up an intervention program if one is needed. It should be stressed that an intervention program is not the inevitable outcome of screening evaluation. The evaluation may indicate that no program is needed. In the area of prevention, such as a wellness clinic, the assessment procedure may be the end of the contact when performance skills and occupational development are within normal limits. Also, an intervention program may not be indicated if occupational therapy has no intervention to offer that is likely to be effective. An assessment that indicates a program is not necessary or will be of little value is just as important as one that indicates a program will be needed. No individual can afford to pay for programs that are not needed, and no occupational therapist should afford the time.

Analysis of Initial Data

Analysis of the initial assessment may be the most important step in the occupational therapy process model. The basic questions are as follows: 1) Can the consumer or potential client benefit from occupational therapy service? and 2) Can occupational therapy service be provided?

Benefit implies that progress can be made toward promoting better occupational performance and adaptation or toward reducing the possibility of deterioration of occupational performance and adaptation. The benefit, furthermore, must be feasible, through an occupational therapy service program in this case. Thus, if no benefit through occupational therapy can be expected, no program of occupational therapy should be planned or implemented. Such an analysis is fairly understandable in concept but more difficult to determine in reality. Determining if benefit is possible and the degree of benefit expected is based on judgment, knowledge, experience, and research.

Once a decision about benefit is achieved, the next question can be just as difficult. Namely, can the occupational therapy services needed to benefit the consumer be made available? First, the occupational therapy program must be functioning; second, there must be space on a therapist's schedule; and third, the consumer must agree to accept the program being offered.

If there is a service program available and space is available in the program, the consumer has the option to accept or not to accept client status. However, if there is limited space in the program, what criteria will be used to decide which potential clients will receive service? Should those who need the most service or the least service be chosen first? There is no simple answer. Some therapists will say those who need the least service should be seen first because they will benefit quickly from service and be able to function independently again. Others will argue that those who need the most service should be seen first because any improvement in performance, especially in self-maintenance activities, will reduce the amount of care required by others. The savings in resources will be in money, time, and energy.

Another problem occurs if no occupational therapy service is available. Can other resources be used? Can occupational therapy service be started? These are questions the occupational therapy assessor must answer before recommending that a consumer be seen as a client in occupational therapy.

The action decision question is: Can occupational therapy services be of benefit in resolving the problems of the referred client? If yes, continue to the comprehensive evaluation stage. If no, write a report summarizing the assessment used, data analyzed, and the rational for rejecting the potential client. If the client is accepted, prioritize the problems that require additional information to clarify the goals and strategies for intervention.

Comprehensive Evaluation

Comprehensive evaluation begins when a decision is made by the occupational therapy practitioner that an intervention program of occupational therapy service can be useful to the person and that the service can and will be provided by the therapist and the facility. The decision may be made in cooperation with other professionals. Ultimately, however, the occupational therapy practitioner must make a final determination because accepting a person for occupational therapy services carries the obligation to perform such services to the best of the occupational therapy practitioner's ability.

A comprehensive evaluation builds on information obtained in the initial assessment phase. The occupational therapy practitioner reviews a list of comprehensive assessment techniques consistent with the theoretical model, selects those assessment techniques based on the priorities established from the referral and screening stages, administers the assessment, scores and interprets the assessment, and summarizes the results of the assessment and other data, determines if any additional data is needed and, if so, how to obtain that data. The information obtained is integrated with the information obtained from the initial assessment procedures to provide a comprehensive database. Analysis of the data should provide a list of problems or deficiencies and assets that will form the basis for program planning.

Assessment Process Using an Occupational Performance Model

Assessment using a model of occupational performance might include consideration of self-maintenance, productivity, and leisure occupations plus the performance components of sensorimotor, cognitive, and psychosocial skills.

The *self-maintenance* area of occupation is assessed in terms of what activities
are needed to maintain the individual's life support needs and the individual's abil-
ity/skill to perform these needs. Although each individual has a unique combination of self-maintenance needs, there are common areas, including eating, dressing, toileting, being mobile, communicating, and problem solving. These
self-maintenance needs must be performed. If the individual cannot perform the
skills needed to complete the activities, someone else must perform part or all of
the self-maintenance activities for the person. The more someone else must assist
in self-maintenance activities, the less independence an individual can achieve
in managing all occupational functions. In addition, the cost in terms of the resources of time and money are greater for a dependent person than for one who
is independent.

The *productive* area is assessed in terms of the skills a person has to provide goods
and services for others to use or from which they can derive benefit. Assessment includes the acquisition of basic work skills, such as being punctual, following directions, and using judgment, as well as the actual application of skills to a specific
work situation. Thus, for children, productivity is learning school work; for adults,
productivity is holding a job for pay or in lieu of paying someone else (homemaking). For older adults, productivity is volunteer work or holding a part-time job.

The *leisure* area can be assessed by examining the types of activities a person
does for individual enjoyment. Assessment of leisure skills indicates what activities the individual is able to perform and which ones actually are done with what
frequency and amount of time. It is important to emphasize that leisure activities
are for the enjoyment of the individual engaged in the activity. Activities of leisure
for one person may be productivity or work for another.

The *sensorimotor* component of performance is assessed to determine if the sensory, neuromuscular, and motor systems are able to perform the basic functions
and skills needed to perform occupational requirements. The senses need to function separately and in combination with each other. The sensory system is the primary means of gaining information from the outside world. The neuromuscular
and motor systems must be able to perform the basic movement skills a person
needs to complete the tasks required for occupational performance, such as getting food on the eating utensil and into the mouth or mounting a tire on an automobile or throwing a bowling ball.

The *cognitive* component of performance is assessed to determine if the person is
able to attend to a task long enough or well enough to learn to perform it and to solve
problems that arise in performing tasks. Memory is assessed to establish whether the
person can remember knowledge and skills over a short or long period of time.

The *psychosocial* component is assessed to determine if the person is able to relate effectively to a human and nonhuman environment. A person should be able to distinguish reality from fantasy and to cope with that reality. The person may use self-concept, self-control, and coping skills to relate to the environment. The person also must be able to relate to other humans whether in a dyad or group situation. Role behavior and social skills further refine psychosocial skills.

The action decision questions are: What are the problems manifested in the evaluation stage? What strengths can be identified to assist in problem resolution?

Occupational Therapy Diagnosis Stage

The purpose of the occupational therapy diagnosis stage is to organize the problems and strengths of the client from the perspective of occupational therapy. Occupational therapy is a unique discipline and it views problems in living from a unique perspective, which is occupation. Therefore, the problems in occupation, whether viewed from the vantage of performance, function, or adaptation, form the occupational therapy diagnosis. The substages in occupational therapy diagnosis are as follows: list all the problems identified from the evaluation stages, group the problems into categories suggested by the theoretical model, prioritize the categories according to the theoretical model, report the findings to the client and referral sources. Reports to family members and other professionals may also be necessary.

For example, if an occupational performance model is used, the list of problems might be grouped into roles related to self-care or self-maintenance, work or productivity, and play or leisure. In addition, the problems may be grouped into sensorimotor, cognitive, and psychosocial. Problems related to role performance are more likely to be understood by the client and family members. Problems phrased in the language of poor motor control, perceptual deficits, cognitive dysfunction, and loss of social skills may be more understandable to professionals. As many occupational therapy practitioners have discovered, the same problems may need to be stated in different words for different audiences.

The action decision questions are: What groups or categories of similar problems can be identified? What occupational therapy diagnosis or diagnoses best fit the problems identified in the groups or categories?

Practice Model Select Stage

The purpose of a practice model is to translate the concepts and interrelationships among concepts into action steps (methods, approaches, or techniques) that the occupational therapy practitioner can incorporate in the intervention program. Thus, the practice model must be consistent with the conceptual model. Although the original theoretical model is the most likely basis for selecting the practice model, a review of the occupational therapy diagnosis may suggest to the occupational therapy practitioner that another conceptual model would provide a better rationale for organizing the intervention program and a better choice of practice model. Therefore, the first substage is to review the tentatively selected conceptual model and by considering the occupational therapy diagnosis, select the conceptual model that best addresses the diagnosis. Next, identify possible occupational therapy practice models based on the theoretical model and finally select a tentative occupational therapy practice model.

The action decision questions are: What conceptual model best fits the categories of problems and occupational therapy diagnosis identified for this client? What practice model is most likely to resolve these problems?

Planning Stage

Program planning involves identifying goals and proposing or outlining a program of action from the practice model that indicates how the goals are to be accomplished. There are seven substages to be considered in the planning stage. First, the list of problems and categories must be prioritized based on discussions with the client, family, referral source, and other professionals in the facility. At the same time, a list must be made of expected change or goals along with time lines for when the changes are most likely to occur. Based on the practice model selected, the occupational therapy practitioner should consider possible intervention strategies (media, modalities, and methods) to use in resolving the categories of problems or individual problems to achieve the goals. Selection of media, modalities, and methods should be based on styles of learning, an activity analysis, the goals desired, what is available, and the interests of the person involved. Together with the clients and with others as appropriate, the selection of initial intervention strategies is made. All goal statements incorporating the expected changes, time lines, and intervention strategies should be written down. In addition, decisions should be made regarding the where, when, and for how long intervention sessions will be held.

In hospitals, nursing homes, and other institutions, there is often a staffing meeting to discuss new clients and reevaluate clients already being seen. In other settings, the occupational therapy practitioner may need to initiate a conference.

Determining goals is very important. Goals need to be obtainable. The word obtainable is stressed. Some goals may be desirable but are not realistic. Furthermore, goals are usually set down in a hierarchy; that is, some goals may be more important or should be accomplished before others. A strong note of caution is in order here. Too often, the decision regarding which goals should come first is made by the occupational therapy practitioner or team members without consulting the client and family members for whom the goals are set. The client may have a different list of priorities. Many plans have been ineffective because the client and family did not participate in the planning and did not have the same sense of direction for goal attainment that the occupational therapy practitioner had.

Finally, the plan must be in writing. This substage is overlooked most frequently by practicing occupational therapists. Students need to write detailed plans so they do not miss any of the steps and so that the supervising therapist can see how well they apply the problem-solving approach. Practitioners, however, need to outline their plan for record keeping, legal requirements for documentation, and for use by others if the original practitioner is absent or unable to continue the program.

The action decision questions are: In what order will the problem categories within the occupational therapy diagnosis or diagnoses be addressed? What changes in the client are expected when the problem categories are resolved? What will the client be able to do that he or she cannot or does not do now? What intervention strategies will be applied?

Setting Goals

After an assessment has been completed and the data have been analyzed, a plan of action may be outlined to enable a person to have normal occupational skills within the limits of the individual's ability. The outcome of the action plan may be to develop, improve, reestablish, or maintain occupational functions and performance. Developing a skill is desirable if the individual has never learned to perform a particular activity, such as a young child who has not learned to sit without support or a young adult who does not know how to participate in a social conversation.

Improving a skill is indicated when the person knows some aspects of the skill but not enough to make the skill functional or useful. For instance, a person may know how to type but may not have the speed and accuracy acceptable for employment. More practice and some instruction may improve the typing skill to a rate and quality desirable for employment as a typist.

Reestablishing a skill is helpful to a person who once was able to perform the skill but lost the ability due to long disuse, an accident, an injury, or a disease process. For example, a person who breaks a forearm may lose some range of motion because the cast limits the ability to move. Also, the skill in moving the forearm may be lost due to inactivity. Exercise and practice should enable the person to reestablish functional performance.

Maintaining skill performance is important to everyone. However, some people have more difficulty maintaining skills than others. Older people or those who are hospitalized for long periods of time are more likely to lose skills because of disuse. Disuse often leads to other problems in a cyclical pattern. An effective means of avoiding these problems is to maintain skills. For example, walking helps to maintain muscle tone, joint mobility, and cardiopulmonary output. Although gaining normal occupational roles (function) and performance skills is important, programs designed to avoid loss of occupational function and performance are equally important. Thus, occupational therapists attempt to prevent, remediate, or minimize dysfunctional performance. Prevention can occur in three ways. Programs can be designed to avoid situations that might lead to loss, such as assessing a child's skills periodically to minimize developmental delay. If some loss has occurred, the therapist can intervene to prevent additional loss, such as preventing contractures in an arthritic joint. A third type of prevention is to avoid a cycle of problems, such as might occur when a person loses a job.

Remediation is especially important in sequential skills. The remedial activity is designed to avoid the problem of falling farther and farther behind. For instance, the child who does not sit on schedule probably will not stand on schedule because both skills depend on balance and protective reflexes to avoid falling. If sitting can be facilitated, standing can be encouraged. Thus, remediation of the sitting problem reduced the sequential delay in standing.

Sometimes, the therapist cannot prevent or remediate the problem. A person with a spinal cord injury cannot walk. The loss of function has occurred. However, the therapist can help the person minimize the dysfunction that is a result of the loss. Learning to use a wheelchair and perform skills from the wheelchair will minimize the loss of function as a walking person.

In summary, the four goals of occupational therapy are directed toward promoting and maintaining health through functional performance of occupational skills. Occupational skills are assessed throughout the life span and in stages of the health-illness continuum. Thus, the therapist may plan and implement change in occupational performance for persons of all ages whose state of health is poor or good.

Program Implementation Stage

Program Intervention and Management

Program intervention involves setting up the program. Primarily, setting up involves checking to see that the necessary equipment and supplies are available, in working order, and in sufficient quantity. In addition, it may be necessary to "set the stage" of the proposed program environment to see if it is suitable for the proposed plan. Sanding a board may be a good activity for increasing range of motion, but doing so in bed may result in complaints from those responsible for maintaining good skin care.

There is only one step in the management process: to carry out the plan. Although the actual management is the heart of an occupational therapy program, it is dependent on the previous processes being completed correctly. Also, the occupational therapist must watch to be sure that all aspects of the intervention program are consistent with the goals set forth in the plan. For example, if a therapist is attempting to interact with a person only when the individual is "working" on assigned tasks and not when talking about various aches and pains, it is then inconsistent for the occupational therapist to talk about a painful sunburn acquired from a weekend at pool side.

Another point to consider is the time dimension. Sometimes inexperienced therapists forget to determine how much time will be needed for a given activity. The result is that too many activities are planned for one session, or a long-term project, such as a ratchet rug, is assigned to a person who will be seen for only a few sessions.

Action decision question is: Are the items in the goal statements being implemented as planned? If yes, continue plan and proceed to the review stage. If no, proceed to the revision stage.

Review or Reevaluation Stage

The next stage is to review or reevaluate. Review is the feedback link that acts as a check and balance on the previous processes. The substages are to select an assessment methodology that can detect change in client performance and which will measure the problem(s) being addressed in the goal statements, administer and score the assessment instrument, and interpret and summarize the results. However, the focus is on what has taken place since the initial assessment. In other words, what changes, if any, have occurred? Were the projected goals reached? Again, assessment should be in written form. One form would be a progress note used for reporting to appropriate persons, such as the physician, agency, parent, or person involved in the total management program.

What if there is no specific time schedule for a review or reevaluation? Actually, it begins as soon as any management program is begun. However, in reality, it is helpful to set up a schedule, such as once a week or once a month, so that conscious attention can be paid to the process and any changes in the plan can be recorded in writing.

Action decision question is: Are the goal statements being achieved? If yes, continue intervention plan and strategies. If no, proceed to revision stage.

Revision Stage

The revision stage is important if the review stage indicates that some goal is not being achieved. Revision involves five substages. First, determine what barriers are occurring. In other words, why is the goal or goals not being achieved? Second, explore options that are reducing the barriers. Third, determine if other categories of problems exist now that did not appear in the original assessment or were not selected for intervention for whatever reason. Fourth, determine if occupational therapy services are required to resolve the problems or if referral to other services may be in order. Fifth, reformulate the goals statements based on the new information.

The action statements are: Can the goal statements be revised to increase the potential for problem resolution? What changes are needed to achieve a more workable situation in which problems can be resolved and the goals accomplished?

Discharge Stage

If the review stage reveals that all goals have been reached and maximum change has occurred, the client is ready to be considered for discharge. Usually, the referral agent is notified that the client is being considered for discharge. In a facility using the team approach, the team agrees on a discharge date. When the discharge is agreed on, a final summary or discharge note is written that reviews the initial assessment, program plan, and progress and change and then makes any recommendations to other agencies or services in the community that might provide additional assistance to the client. For example, the Visiting Nurse Association might be helpful if nursing skills are still needed. A home health aide may be useful in organizing the home for awhile. Meals on Wheels service may be needed to ensure the person has at least one good meal a day. Community services should be used if available. Other professional services should also be recommended if needed. Speech pathology, vocational counseling, outpatient physical therapy, and occupational therapy are just a few of the professional services that may be useful to continue the progress started in the occupational therapy service program.

The failure to provide recommendations and discuss with the client how to implement the recommendations is a common failure in many service programs, including occupational therapy. Sometimes no recommendations are made, and sometimes no one checks to ensure the recommendations are understood by the client and feasible to carry out in the home and community environment. Architectural, social, and environmental barriers are most common in the home and community. Doors at home are too narrow for a wheelchair, the neighbors are afraid to speak to the former mental patient, and public transportation is inaccessible for the older person who no longer drives. These are the problems that confront the client after occupational therapy and other services have given their best service. The client may still find that the skills achieved are not good enough to meet the challenge of the home and community. Occupational therapy practitioners and other professionals must be reasonably certain that the gains achieved in the service program are not lost because no one investigated the home and community. The client should be discharged *to* the home and community, not just *from* the facility or therapist.

The action decision questions are: Have all goal statements been reached? Are the client, therapist, and referral agent satisfied with the progress made? If yes, proceed to follow-up stage. If no, proceed to the revision stage.

Follow-up Stage

In preparation for the follow-up stage the occupational therapy practitioner should discuss the need for follow-up including check-up visits and referral to other resources/agencies. Second, the occupational therapy practitioner can assist in the arrangements for follow-up visits, if needed. Third, the occupational therapy practitioner can make referrals, if needed. Fourth, the practitioner can make document arrangements for follow-up visits and, fifth, document referrals in writing.

Action decision questions are: Does the client need follow-up visits? Should the client be referred to other resources or agencies?

PHILOSOPHY AND THEORY

There is one remaining basic process to discuss—that of philosophy and theory. The actual development of a philosophy or theory is beyond the scope of this book. However, the important points to be considered are that a philosophy must be identified and that the other processes must be consistent with and build on it. Failure to integrate philosophy with the other processes leads to a breakdown in the management program.

It should be noted that philosophy and theory are useful in many settings. For the practicing therapist, it is important to identify the philosophy of the total institution and that of the occupational therapy program. These should be consistent. To illustrate, if a therapist evaluates a person using a projective test based on the psychoanalytic model, the therapist might learn many items of information about the person's defense mechanisms and inner conflicts. However, if the facility in which the therapist is working bases its management program on behavior modification principles, the therapist would have difficulty planning a program that would include only observable, measurable behavior. In addition, communication with other professionals involved in the overall management program would be incomplete because they would not be interested in learning about the unconscious conflicts.

A second use of philosophy and theory is to guide research, whether the research is a literary survey or a field experiment. A third use relates directly to education. In education, knowledge of the basic processes makes reliance on diagnoses or function–dysfunction models of organization unnecessary.

APPLICATION OF THE MODEL

The basic problem-solving process model can be applied to any area of occupational therapy. Psychosocial or physical dysfunction, young or old, group or individual, disability or diagnosis makes no difference. Setting and location also do not change the use of the approach. Regardless of the environment the therapist works in, whether a hospital, clinic, community healthcare center, or home program, the problem-solving approach is always applicable.

When the model is applied to the education of occupational therapy personnel, it can help organize the major types of information the student will need to practice the profession. In theory courses, the process model provides a consistent frame of reference in which to organize new material. The student can identify what must be learned in terms of theories used to plan management programs, to select evaluation tools, and to choose specialized media and techniques.

MEDIA AND THE BASIC PROCESSES

The planning process involved selection of media. Thus, remembering the major types of media used by occupational therapists is useful. Media have been identified and classified by several methods, but only one is presented here for simplification. The eight major media areas are as follows: 1) creative arts (arts and crafts), 2) manual skills, 3) educational tasks, 4) daily living tasks, 5) functional equipment, 6) avocational activities (recreation), 7) prevocational exploration and training (tasks), and 8) use of self. A ninth medium, exercise, is identified and accepted on a limited basis in occupational therapy. Exercise is an acceptable medium only when no activity or few activities are available for use, such as for finger extension. Some neuromuscular facilitation patterns also may be thought of primarily as exercise. With these possible exceptions, exercise is more appropriately considered as a medium for physical therapy.

The eight major media areas have one feature in common. They all require active participation by the individual in treatment. Active participation is a basic premise of occupational therapy. Activities are performed by and with the individual in treatment, not to the person. Even with an unconscious person, the occupational therapy practitioner is trying to promote an active response. The individual involved in occupational therapy is expected to do as much as possible without assistance, no matter how limited the initial responses may be. The role of the occupational therapy practitioner is to assist, not do the activity for, the individual.

In summary, the basic processes model is designed to provide a frame of reference for students, teachers, and therapists to use in organizing the information needed to practice occupational therapy. If theory courses are organized according to the framework, students will know the primary objectives of each course and should be able to see the interrelationships. The basic processes framework also should help students and therapists see the continuum between conceptual models and practice models.

CHAPTER 25

Service Programs

In Chapter 6, the outcomes or goals of occupational therapy were discussed. However, such outcomes or goals do not indicate which service program the client may need. Service programs in occupational therapy must be based on client needs. If the needs are met, the outcome or goal should be achieved. This chapter focuses on the types of client needs and the processes that can be organized into particular occupational therapy delivery programs to meet those needs. Client needs have been divided into five different types: prevention, development, remediation, environmental adjustment, and health maintenance.

PREVENTION

The client enters a prevention service when there is a perceived threat to health, even though the individual is functioning currently in the community with relative satisfaction. A common example of prevention is the use of immunization shots given to a child to prevent the youngster from getting childhood diseases. A prevention program is focused on keeping problems from happening (primary prevention), or if a problem has developed, to keep it from worsening (secondary prevention). Possible examples of primary prevention programs in occupational therapy include screening children to determine if problems in development are likely to occur, establishing a group of persons in their forties or fifties to discuss how to plan for retirement, or running a group for young adults on how to become good parents. Secondary prevention programs might include a discussion group with parents of disabled children regarding how to parent such a child to promote maximum development or a cardiac rehabilitation program that promotes changing life patterns to avoid cardiac stress, thus reducing the chance of a second or third heart attack.

A client completes the goal of a prevention program and exits when that person is able to avoid developmental regression, and biogenic, psychogenic, or sociogenic disorders to the extent that current knowledge and technology will permit. In other words, the client has been provided with the knowledge and skills to avoid certain health problems. A prevention program cannot assure that the client will use the knowledge and skills to advantage.

395

DEVELOPMENT

The developmental program is designed for an individual who has not developed or learned the skills and tasks appropriate to chronological age. Because development occurs throughout the life span, there is no upper age limit on a developmental program. Usually a person enters the developmental program because there is a known deficit in the person's developmental progression. Illustrations of developmental programs might be 1) a neonatal nursery of premature infants who need sensory stimulation to develop more normally; 2) a nursery school program, which stresses readiness skills that children with disabilities will need to enter school in the first grade; 3) a sheltered workshop designed to teach basic work skills to adults who are retarded; or 4) a creative and leisure program for older persons who did not learn recreational skills as children or young adults.

A person leaves a developmental program when he or she has gained skills appropriate to chronological age level and life tasks or to the nearest level personally attainable, given existing circumstances. The developmental program is designed to eliminate or reduce the developmental delay between average performance and individual performance. Sometimes the delay can be overcome. Other times, such as in some cases of mental disabilities, not enough is known to enable therapists to eliminate the delay, but it can be reduced. The reduction in delay may enable the person to acquire enough skills, however, to move from a total care institution to a group home. Increasing the developmental level usually increases the skills in independent functioning.

REMEDIATION AND ENVIRONMENTAL ADJUSTMENT

The remediation program accepts individuals who have lost skills owing to illness or trauma but can be expected to regain some skills or relearn some activities through a "specialized intervention" program. Remediation is the most recognized program in occupational therapy. Programs include helping persons with strokes, arthritis, or cancer regain functional skill levels. Other programs help those who have lost skills as a result of mental health problems regain their ability to perform occupational tasks. When the individual completes a remediation program, he or she has regained skills and relearned activities to his or her former level or close to that level. These skills should be performed without the use of adapted devices, splints, or other special equipment.

Environmental adjustment frequently is an alternative to the remediation program. The client requires an environmental adjustment when change and recovery within the individual have achieved a level of functioning that can be expected in the immediate or long-range future. Further improvement in function, however, can be expected if the external environment is changed to reduce barriers to performance. Examples of environmental change are the use of adapted devices, such as splints, braces, or wheelchairs; the elimination of stairs; the widening of doorways, or the provision of braille signs.

In reality, the remediation and environmental adjustment programs are used side by side. A client is encouraged to regain and relearn skills without special environmental assistance, but aids may be used to facilitate progress. However, if function is not possible or can be assisted by environmental aids, these are introduced, and use is maintained as long as needed. For example, a person who has had a stroke might need a splint to facilitate eating for a while until muscle strength and tone are improved. Then, splint use is discontinued. In this case, environmental adjustment is temporary. In contrast, a person with a spinal cord injury may need braces or a wheelchair for the rest of his or her life. Without the environmental adjustment, the person with a spinal cord injury is impaired seriously in developing any degree of independent functioning.

If environmental adjustment is successful, the client will continue to gain or learn skill performance to a level satisfactory for independent living. Some changes in the method of performance are inevitable. Mobility in a wheelchair cannot be the same as walking. Use of a splint to position the hand for writing will change the quality and speed of the handwriting.

HEALTH MAINTENANCE

Finally, occupational therapy can provide a health maintenance or supportive program. Usually, the client is able to perform many skills independently but must continue to perform these skills in order to maintain health. Many clients in health maintenance have a life-threatening disease, such as AIDS or cancer, or are older individuals; however, no age limit is imposed. The primary recipient of health maintenance is the individual whose life situation does not always demand that known skills be employed.

Older people or people living alone or in semiprotected environments, such as residential or nursing homes, may not use the skills available to them. Nonuse of skills may lead to disuse, atrophy, and forgetting. In some instances, the disuse may be because a skill appears to be needed less. Food preparation skills may be used less because the older person is not as hungry or lives alone. Loss of hunger and companionship can lead to skipping meals. Lack of nutrition leads to various health problems. If the individual can learn to prepare nutritious and appetizing meals with a minimum of effort and is reminded of the importance of nutrition to health, that individual can maintain health and independent living for a longer period of time.

In residential or nursing homes, skills can be lost because someone else is available to help do the activities. The staff may encourage dependency because the staff can do the activity faster. For example, they bathe and dress the people rather than encourage residents to bathe themselves because the tasks can be completed faster. The result is that residents lose their independence and cannot return to or be placed in a situation that requires independence in bathing and dressing.

The client has achieved a satisfactory level of health maintenance when he or she can maintain or increase skill performance in all occupational areas to the degree needed for independent living and self-satisfaction in the community. If independent living is not feasible, health maintenance is directed at maintaining as many skills as possible.

IMPACT AND INTEGRATION OF SERVICES

Another way of viewing the types of occupational therapy service programs is to view them graphically. The chart in Figure 25.1 shows the impact of services on a hypothetical health line. Without any services, it is assumed that the health line would decelerate or, at best, maintain a straight horizontal pattern. The vertical line indicates the point of intervention by occupational therapy. In the prevention program, a successful intervention should be reflected in a continuous or rising

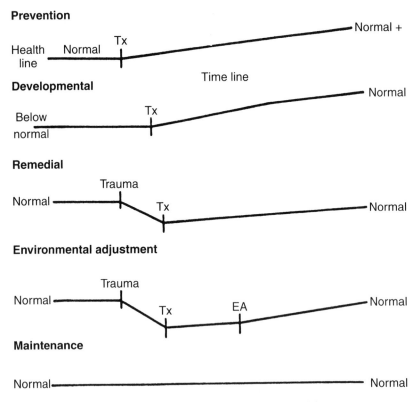

Figure 25.1. Health care programs in occupational therapy.

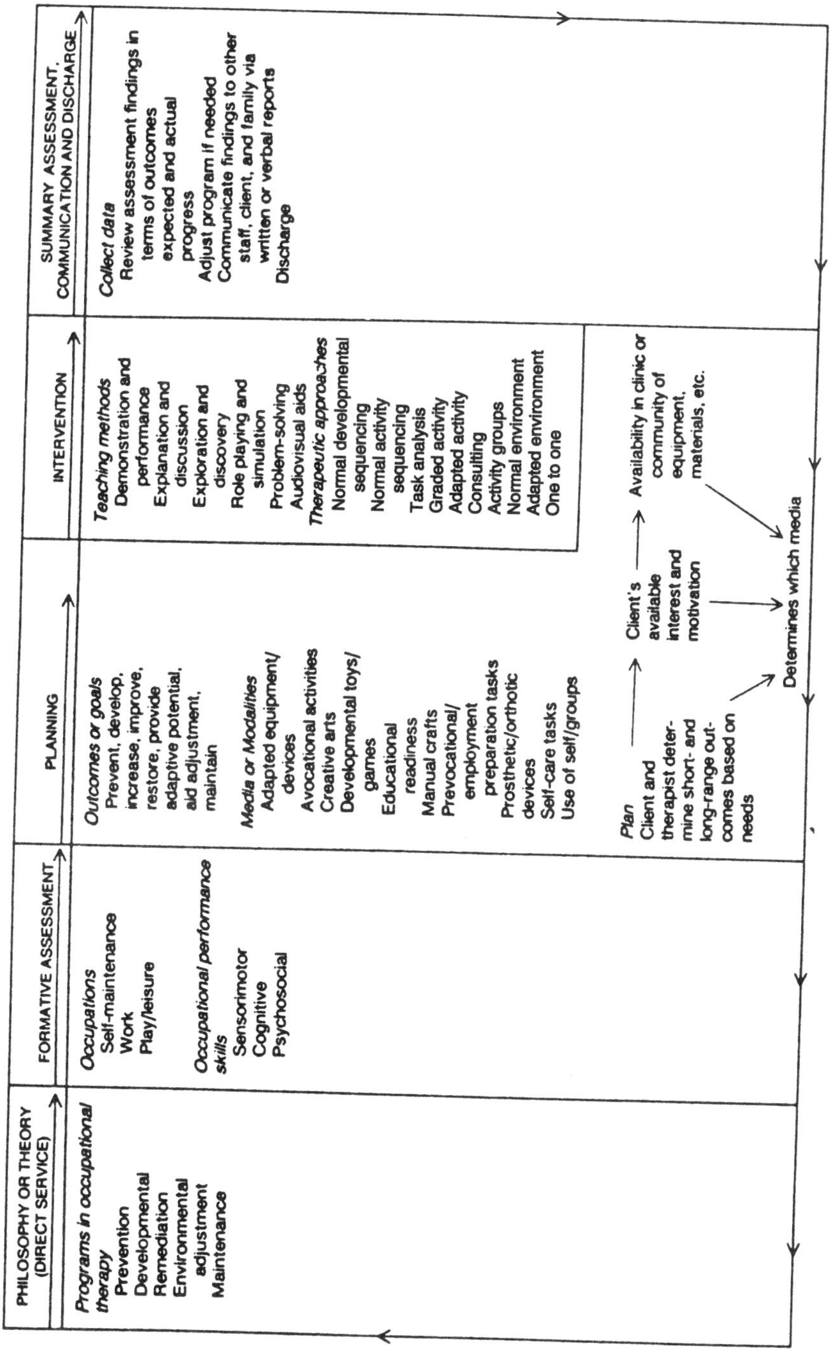

PHILOSOPHY OR THEORY (DIRECT SERVICE)	FORMATIVE ASSESSMENT	PLANNING	INTERVENTION	SUMMARY ASSESSMENT, COMMUNICATION AND DISCHARGE
Programs in occupational therapy	*Occupations*	*Outcomes or goals*	*Teaching methods*	*Collect data*
Prevention	Self-maintenance	Prevent, develop,	Demonstration and	Review assessment findings in
Developmental	Work	increase, improve,	performance	terms of outcomes
Remediation	Play/leisure	restore, provide	Explanation and	expected and actual
Environmental		adaptive potential,	discussion	progress
adjustment	*Occupational performance*	aid adjustment,	Exploration and	Adjust program if needed
Maintenance	*skills*	maintain	discovery	Communicate findings to other
	Sensorimotor		Role playing and	staff, client, and family via
	Cognitive	*Media or Modalities*	simulation	written or verbal reports
	Psychosocial	Adapted equipment/	Problem-solving	Discharge
		devices	Audiovisual aids	
		Avocational activities	*Therapeutic approaches*	
		Creative arts	Normal developmental	
		Developmental toys/	sequencing	
		games	Normal activity	
		Educational	sequencing	
		readiness	Task analysis	
		Manual crafts	Graded activity	
		Prevocational/	Adapted activity	
		employment	Consulting	
		preparation tasks	Activity groups	
		Prosthetic/orthotic	Normal environment	
		devices	Adapted environment	
		Self-care tasks	One to one	
		Use of self/groups		

Plan
Client and
therapist deter-
mine short- and
long-range out-
comes based on
needs

Client's → available interest and motivation

→ Availability in clinic or community of equipment, materials, etc.

Determines which media

Figure 25.2. Occupational therapy practice model.

health line. Intervention in a developmental program should stop the decreasing health progression and start a rising one. Intervention through a remediation program should stop the sudden drop in the health line and begin an upward trend toward the preexisting health line. In an environmental adjustment program. the intervention program should stop the plateau line, which is below the normal health line, and begin an upward trend toward the preexisting health line. A health maintenance program should maintain the health line or retard the downward trend for as long as possible.

Figure 25.2 shows the integration of the service programs in occupational therapy with the process of delivering service. When the service programs and processes are combined, the result is a practice model for occupational therapy. The practice of occupational therapy is determined by selecting one or more service models, determining which occupational areas and performance components are to be assessed, deciding the goals and media to be planned, choosing the teaching methods and therapeutic approaches to be used in intervention, and preparing for reassessment and communication. Thus, the practice of occupational therapy has a fixed set of service programs and a process of delivering service but has a great variety of combinations within the service programs and process that can be employed to benefit the client.

The service programs can be summarized by examining each program according to entering level function; program objectives, skills, and techniques used in program planning; implementation; objectives accomplished through instructional strategies; working assumption or rationale; staff relationships; and exit criteria. The following outline summarizes each occupational therapy service program.

PROGRAMS

A. Prevention
   1. Entering level—the individual is currently functioning in the normal community environment to his or her relative satisfaction.
   2. Objectives:
      a. Prevent developmental regression, physical and psychosocial, such as in a pediatric program in a general hospital.
      b. Prevent biogenic disorders, such as in a program for adults with arthritis to prevent deformity and injury to the hands.
      c. Prevent psychogenic disorders, such as in a program for the aged to prevent isolation and depression.
      d. Prevent sociogenic disorders, such as in a program for adolescents to prevent delinquent or criminal behavior.
   3. Skills and techniques used in program planning implementation:
      a. Scheduling and performing activities of daily living.
      b. Instruction in efficient home management.
      c. Recommending change of work situation or job change.

    d. Instruction in the application of behavior modification.

    e. Instruction in the development and use of adapted equipment to prevent deformity or injury.

    f. Programmed activities designed to prevent loss of sensorimotor functions, such as range of motion, coordination, muscle strength, physical tolerance, sensory perception, and integration.

    g. Instruction in work simplification and energy conservation.

    h. Instruction in the elimination of architectural barriers and hazardous furniture and equipment.

    i. Planned activities to make constructive use of leisure time.

4. Objectives accomplished through:

    a. Individual or group lecture, discussion, and demonstration.

    b. Development of illustrated booklets, tapes, and films.

    c. Consultation with community organizations concerned with the health and general welfare of its citizens.

5. Working assumption—loss of functional ability skill (disability) can be prevented by active intervention of therapists to inform citizens of potential dangers to health.

6. Certified Occupational Therapy Assistant (COTA)/OTR relationship—the COTA may collaborate and consult with an OTR or may be supervised by an OTR in providing prevention programs.

B. Development

1. Entering level—the individual has not learned or developed skills/abilities appropriate to age level or life task. The program includes individuals throughout the life cycle.

2. Objectives:

    a. Increase sensorimotor functions to appropriate age level or life task.

    b. Increase cognitive skills to appropriate age level or life task.

    c. Increase psychosocial (behavioral) skills to appropriate age or life task.

    d. Increase ability to perform self-maintenance activities.

    e. Increase ability to perform life tasks, productive or leisure.

3. Skills and techniques:

    a. Instruction in and opportunity to perform skills and activities within the individual developmental level.

    b. Instruction in performing activities of daily living (ADLs).

    c. Programmed activities designed to develop concept of self, interpersonal relationships, and group interaction skills.

4. Objectives accomplished through:

    a. Explanation and demonstration.

    b. Normal developmental sequencing.

    c. Repeated practice.

    d. Behavior modification.

e. Simulation; role playing.
f. Task analysis.
5. Working assumption—developmental disability can be understood in terms of a deviation from normal performance in a profile of skills by measuring what is expected for the person's age with the level of current functioning.
6. COTA/OTR relationship—the COTA assists the OTR in the assessment phase and must be directly supervised by the OTR during the implementation/management phase of the developmental program.

C. Remediation
1. Entering level—the individual has lost skills and ability due to illness or trauma but can be expected to regain at least some skills and relearn some activities through specialized treatment and training.
2. Objectives:
  a. Increase independence in performing activities of daily living.
  b. Increase sensorimotor functions.
  c. Improve home management skills.
  d. Improve work proficiency and task performance.
  e. Improve cognitive functions.
  f. Improve job-related skills.
  g. Improve psychosocial performance.
  h. Prevent deformity.
  i. Prevent extension of disease or trauma pathology.
3. Skills and techniques:
  a. Increase sensorimotor functioning in such areas as range of motion, muscle strengthening, coordination, physical tolerance, sensory discrimination, and cognitive function through planned activities.
  b. Instruction in performing ADLs.
  c. Instruction in selected aspects of home management.
  d. Instruction in specific work-related skills.
  e. Instruction in the development of leisure activities.
  f. Instruction in psychosocial skills.
4. Objectives accomplished through:
  a. Individual or group—planned specific activities.
  b. Environmental control—structured or not structured.
  c. Development of home program.
5. Working assumption—disability can be understood by varying the conditions and task performance.
6. COTA/OTR relationship—the COTA must be directly supervised by an OTR during all phases of the remedial program.

D. Environmental adjustment
1. Entering level—individual's change and recovery have achieved a level of function that can be expected in the immediate or long-range period. Fur-

ther improvement in function can be expected if the external environment is changed to reduce barriers to performance.
2. Objectives:
   a. Further improve sensorimotor functions.
   b. Further improve psychosocial functions.
   c. Further increase ability to perform ADLs.
   d. Further increase ability to perform work/play skills.
3. Skills and techniques:
   a. Modification and instruction in use of equipment.
   b. Construction and instruction in use of splints.
   c. Elimination of architectural barriers.
   d. Reconstruction of physical surroundings.
   e. Instruction in use of prosthetic devices.
4. Objectives accomplished by:
   a. Task analysis.
   b. Explanation and demonstration.
   c. Repeated practice.
   d. Consultation.
5. Working assumption—devices and environments can be developed and applied that will extend, enlarge, and facilitate the behavior (physical and mental) of the handicapped person.
6. COTA/OTR relationship—the COTA may collaborate and consult with an OTR or may be supervised by an OTR in providing an environmental adjustment program.
E. Supportive/health maintenance
1. Entering level—the individual is living in a semiprotected environment, such as a residential home or other institution. A program is usually adopted for a group of persons and is frequently called an "activity program."
2. Objectives:
   a. Maintain general sensorimotor functions of the group.
   b. Maintain or increase psychosocial skills of the group.
   c. Maintain or increase ability to perform life tasks, including ADLs.
   d. Maintain cognitive functions of the group.
3. Skills and techniques:
   a. Instruction in activities designed to encourage individual interaction with others and with the nonhuman environment.
   b. Programmed activities designed to maintain physical and sensory functions within the individual's current level of function.
   c. Selection of and instruction in activities within the individual's ability level that enable the person to make constructive use of available time.
4. Objectives accomplished through:
   a. Group and individual explanation, discussion, and demonstration.

    b. Task analysis of group and individual abilities and task requirements.

    c. Consultation with staff personnel.

5. Working assumption—disability in terms of increased loss of function can be slowed/avoided by active intervention.

6. COTA/OTR relationship—the COTA may collaborate or consult with an OTR or may be supervised by an OTR in providing a supportive/health maintenance program.

The Contextual Base

CHAPTER 26

Development of Professional Organizations

BEGINNING

The national organization for occupational therapy was created in March 1917 when five people gathered in Clifton Springs, New York, to write the Certificate of Incorporation of the National Society for the Promotion of Occupational Therapy, Incorporated (see Appendix E). The objectives of the corporation were "the advancement of occupation as a therapeutic measure; the study of the effect of occupation upon the human being and the scientific dispensation of this knowledge" (1). Officers included George E. Barton, president; Eleanor C. Slagle, vice president; William R. Dunton, treasurer; and Isabel G. Newton, secretary. Membership consisted of those persons interested in occupational therapy and accepted as members by the governing board, which was comprised of five members. The Maryland *Psychiatric Quarterly* was selected as the official journal for the new society, in part because Dr. Dunton was the editor.

In September, the first annual meeting was held in New York. Mr. Barton was unable to attend so Dr. Dunton was elected president. Louis J. Haas became treasurer and Marian R. Taber, secretary. The membership at the end of 1917 was 40 persons strong, but the society had a treasury balance of only $0.51 (2).

THE AMERICAN OCCUPATIONAL THERAPY ASSOCIATION

Until 1920, the Society functioned essentially as the founders envisioned. In 1921, Herbert Hall, then president, suggested that the name of the organization be changed to the "crisper and quite as descriptive" American Occupational Therapy Association (AOTA) (3). This change was accepted by the members and remains the official name of the national organization today. At the same time, a new constitution was adopted that created two governing units, a Board of Management and a policy-making body, the House of Delegates. The Board of Management functioned continuously until 1964, but the House of Delegates did not become a permanent structure until 1939.

In 1922, the new House of Delegates voted to hold the annual conferences of the Association in conjunction with the American Hospital Association. The rationale was that hospital executives would have a chance to become familiar with occupational therapy and therapists could attend some of the AHA meetings (4). This joint arrangement continued until 1938 when the delegates decided that Dallas was too far to travel and chose to meet in Chicago instead.

Another important event in 1922 was the initiation of an official journal devoted to occupational therapy. The new journal was titled *Archives of Occupational Therapy* and was owned and edited by Dr. Dunton (5). Subscription fees were separate from Association membership. In 1925, the name was changed to *Occupational Therapy and Rehabilitation* in an effort to broaden the journal's scope and attract more articles. Also, the journal became an automatic membership benefit. Finally, the Board of Management authorized the secretary-treasurer, Mrs. Eleanor C. Slagle, to secure an office, which she did, at the Terminal Building with the National Health Council at 370 Seventh Avenue in New York City (6). The move was necessary because Mrs. Slagle had been keeping the records in her kitchen and was running out of room.

The major accomplishment of the Association for 1923 was the adoption of minimum standards for training (7). Education and training had been an important concern since 1917, but the membership had not voted on the unified set of standards until the 1923 meeting in Milwaukee. These standards provided for a minimum course length of 12 months, including 3 months of "hospital-practice training."

At the same meeting, an official emblem was adopted, and discussion was held regarding the establishment of a national register of qualified occupational, therapists. In 1926, the House of Delegates voted to take immediate steps to establish such a registry. The task was completed finally in 1932 when the first National Registry of Occupational Therapists was published, consisting of 318 occupational therapists (8).

Another sign of growth for the Association was the decision to relocate the national office. The Association took up residence in the Flatiron Building, Fifth Avenue at 23rd Street, in 600 square feet of space (9). The staff included Mrs. Slagle, who was the Association's elected secretary-treasurer and Idelle Kidder, who was hired in 1926 as the first paid staff secretary.

One other noteworthy event of 1926 was the adoption of the Pledge and Creed. The Pledge and Creed was submitted by the Boston School of Occupational Therapy and remains official today (10). By 1929, membership had increased to 879 members.

In 1931, the Board of Managers asked President Dr. Joseph C. Doane to approach the American Medical Association about the possibility of undertaking the inspection of occupational therapy schools. A resolution supporting the request was adopted in 1933 by the AMA. Inspection began later that year. New standards were developed based on the inspection findings. These standards, which were adopted by the Council on Medical Education and Hospitals and ratified by the House of Delegates of the AMA in 1935, were titled "Essentials of an Acceptable

School of Occupational Therapy" (11). Thus, the AOTA became the first organization to initiate a collaborative accreditation procedure with the AMA. The "Essentials" were revised in 1943, 1949, 1965, 1973, and 1983.

The maintenance of standards continued to be a major concern of the Association. In 1933, an announcement was made that, after December 31, only graduates of accredited schools who had completed 1 year of practical experience—in addition to the hospital practice included in training courses—would be eligible for registration (12). However, accreditation was not completed until 1939. Thus, people who met general education and service requirements were admitted for membership until 1939.

The war years began in 1939. An annual meeting in Toronto was canceled, as were meetings for the years 1942, 1943, 1944, and 1945. The Board of Management and House of Delegates continued to meet, but no membership meetings or conference programs were presented.

Registration became a primary topic again in 1945. This time, registration was tied to the completion of an essay examination for all would-be therapists (13). In 1947, the examination format was changed to the use of multiple choice questions rather than essay. The examination was developed under a grant from the Kellogg Foundation. Furthermore, space at the Flatiron Building was becoming too small; thus, the offices were moved in 1945 to the Aeolian Building, at 33 West 42nd Street (14). The expanded quarters provided 1000 square feet of space.

The year 1946 brought to a close 25 years of service by the journal *Occupational Therapy and Rehabilitation* and its editor, Dr. Dunton (15). Although the journal continued to be published under its title until 1951, the editor was Dr. Sidney Licht, and the journal itself was not the official journal of the AOTA. Instead, the Association had elected to start a journal that would be owned by the Association. This new journal was named the *American Journal of Occupational Therapy*. It began publication in 1947 under the editorship of Charlotte Bone (16).

In 1950, the Association began to recognize, on a regular basis, therapists who had made a significant contribution to the profession. The first Award of Merit was granted to Eva Otto Munzeheimer for her service to the Association in 1950 (17). The first Eleanor Clarke Slagle Lectureship Award was given to Florence Stattel in 1955 (18).

Meanwhile, 1955 marked the move to larger quarters for the national office, which was rapidly expanding as the Association grew. The new office was located in the Fiske Building at 250 West 57th Street and provided 3200 square feet of space (19).

The year 1955 also marked the time for another revision of the Constitution and Bylaws. Among other revisions was the statement of purpose, which was changed to read as follows:

The objects of the Association shall be to promote the use of occupational therapy, to advance the standards of education and training in this field, to promote research, to engage in any other activities that in the future may be considered advantageous to the profession and its members. (20)

The subject of developing standards of training for assistants was discussed in 1956 and led to the adoption of the standards for training and recognition of occupational therapy assistants in psychiatry at the 1958 annual meeting (21). The Certified Occupational Therapy Assistant was to be a person trained in a specialty area, usually in a hospital-based or inservice program.

The Constitution and Bylaws once again became a major topic for discussion in 1964 (22). The discussion led to a major change in organization and structure. The House of Delegates was changed to the Delegate Assembly, and the Board of Management was replaced by the Executive Board. In 1965, there were 39 delegates representing affiliated associations at the first meeting of the Delegate Assembly.

At the 1968 annual meeting, an official definition of occupational therapy was adopted for the first time (23). Other definitions had been used widely but were not adopted by the membership as a whole. During the following year, a Statement on Referral was adopted by the Delegate Assembly to distinguish the circumstances in which an occupational therapist needs a physician's referral from those in which a referral from other than a physician is acceptable (24).

Licensure by individual states became a major concern in the 1970s. A model act for developing licensure bills was adopted in 1969 and revised in 1974 (25). Prior to this time, the Association had been opposed to licensure as restrictive to members and unresponsive to changing techniques and service locations.

Once more, space at the national office had become too small and, in addition, the rent was quite costly. A suggestion was made that the office be moved to the Washington, DC area, because the Association could lobby for legislation favorable to occupational therapy directly from the office. The decision was made in 1972, and the office was moved to the Wilco Building, at 6000 Executive Boulevard, Rockville, Maryland (26). The available space was 6000 square feet.

In 1976, there was another revision of the Bylaws (27). Changes included proportional representation in the Assembly, which was called the Representative Assembly. States that have 5% of the total Association membership are granted one additional representative. Those with 10% are granted two additional representatives. Another change was the requirement that representatives be elected from an election area of national Association members and not just from members of a given state association. Election areas are organized by state boundaries. A third change was the development of specialty sections for members to share information about issues in areas of practice.

The latest changes in headquarters location and bylaws occurred in 1980 and 1981. As rents continued to rise and the space in the Wilco Building seemed to shrink, there was renewed interest in locating additional space, which the Association would own. In early 1980, a building became available which seemed to meet the needs (28). As of June 1980, the Association became the owner of and moved into 1383 Piccard Drive in Rockville, Maryland. The Association occupied part of the building and rented out the additional space until the Association needed the space for its own activities.

THE AMERICAN OCCUPATIONAL THERAPY ASSOCIATION TODAY

The current revision of the Bylaws was adopted in May 1981. Under these Bylaws, the major structures are the Representative Assembly and Executive Board of the Representative Assembly, which are comprised of representatives from each state, the District of Columbia, and Puerto Rico. Representatives are elected on the basis of proportional representation. Those with 5% of total membership get an extra representative. Those with 10% get two extra representatives. Other voting members include the Assembly officers (speaker, vice speaker, and recorder), Association officers (president, vice president, secretary, treasurer), first alternate delegate to the World Federation of Occupational Therapists (see chapter 30), a COTA representative, and the Chair of the Student Committee. The Assembly is responsible for formulating Association policy on such subjects as public issues, legislative matters, internal Association affairs, accreditation, and educational and professional standards. The Assembly also approves the budget.

The Executive Board is comprised of 16 voting members: the Association president, president elect, vice president, secretary, treasurer, treasurer elect, Assembly speaker, vice speaker, recorder, chairs of the Committee of State Association Presidents, Commission on Education, Commission on Practice, Standards and Ethics Commission, Special Interest Section Standing Committee, COTA representative, and delegate to the World Federation of Occupational Therapists. Other members without voting privileges include the Executive Director and liaison from the American Occupational Therapy Foundation. The Student Committee is represented by a member of the Board. The Executive Board is charged to manage the affairs of the Association, to make necessary budget adjustments, and to oversee implementation of policies established by the Assembly.

The Executive Board is responsible also for appointing the executive director of the national office. In turn, the executive director organizes and supervises the staff personnel. The national office contains five divisions and 22 departments. The divisions that report directly to the Executive Director are finance and operations, professional issues and special programs, professional affairs, academic education and practice, and professional development. The organizational chart for the national office is shown in Figure 26.1.

Members of the Association participate by voting for the Association officers and Assembly representatives. Members also may be asked to serve as officers or as Assembly representatives, although only OTR members may serve as national officers. In addition, members may serve on committees at the national, state, or local level. Serving on committees probably is the best way to become familiar with how the national, state, or local associations operate and to become recognized for

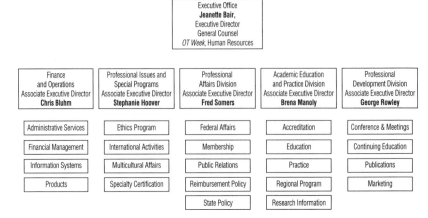

Figure 26.1. AOTA: 1998 National office organization chart.

individual expertise. Finally, members can participate by joining one or more Special Interest Sections when annual dues are paid. Membership is open to all Association members.

Currently there are 11 Special Interest Sections: administration and management, developmental disabilities, education, geriatrics, home and community health, mental health, physical disabilities, school systems, sensory integration, technology, and work programs. The purpose of the sections are to 1) develop knowledge and skills in specific areas of occupational therapy practice, 2) promote continuing education, 3) promote research, 4) promote publication, 5) function as a resource or collaborate with any body of the Association, and 6) respond to emerging issues as they relate to the special interest section.

Other important business of the Association is carried out by three commissions, which report to the Representative Assembly. These commissions are entitled Standards and Ethics, Education, and Practice. The purpose of the Special Interest Section Standing Committee is to coordinate the activities of the other three commissions so that information is shared and activities are done cooperatively whenever tasks require joint efforts.

The Commission on Standards and Ethics is responsible for enforcing all standards and ethics of the Association and recommends and coordinates the development of new standards and ethics that ultimately must be approved by the Representative Assembly. A subcommittee of Standards and Ethics is the Standards Review Committee, which reviews Association documents concerned with standards and ethics to determine if the document is accurate and up-to-date according to Association policy.

The Commission on Education is responsible for promoting quality of education for occupational therapists and occupational therapy assistants relative to educator, student, and consumer needs. Membership includes the chairperson, chairperson elect, five appointed members, and six elected members who represent the fieldwork and academic educators at the technical, professional, and postprofessional levels.

The purpose of the Commission on Practice is to develop standards and guidelines for practice in occupational therapy and to serve as a channel for information relative to practice. Functions include the following: establishing standards for practice, collecting and disseminating current information about practice, developing patterns and alternatives for the delivery of occupational therapy services, identifying and developing practice methodologies, and encouraging and assisting efforts in research.

In addition to the commissions, there are committees of the Representative Assembly and of the Executive Board that are responsible for specific tasks to aid the functioning of the Association. Furthermore, the national office staff has developed advisory committees to provide additional information on specific tasks, such as types of publications or continuing education, which would be useful to consumers as well as to occupational therapists.

There are also several committees, councils, and one board that report to the Executive Board. These are the Committee of State Association Presidents, which provides a channel for communication between the state associations and the national association; the International Committee, which serves practitioners working aboard; the American Student Committee of the Occupational Therapy Association, which serves the interests of students; the Special Interest Section Standing Committee, which coordinates the activities of the Special Interest Sections; the Accreditation Council for Occupational Therapy Education (ACOTE), which is responsible for accrediting all academic programs for the occupational therapist and the occupational therapy assistant; and the Speciality Certification Board, which is responsible for developing and implementing speciality certification programs.

In summary, the AOTA serves its members by promoting the use of occupational therapy by establishing standards for such use and supporting research. Promotion has included the following: publishing a journal and newspaper, printing recruitment literature, making films, publishing monographs, and speaking before congressional committees on bills of interest to the profession. Standards established by the Association have related to setting minimal essentials for educational programs and to establishing standards of practice in various areas of occupational therapy. Also, statements on referrals to occupational therapy, guidelines on policies and procedures, guidelines for fieldwork education, and guidelines for continuing education in occupational therapy have been developed. Research has been promoted by annual conference programs, publication of a professional journal and monographs, and financial support to the American Occupational Therapy Foundation. Furthermore, AOTA has provided a model for other associations in member services, especially in educational standards.

Today, the Association continues to be the primary supporter of occupational therapy. Through the efforts of paid staff in the national office and the voluntary time of many therapists, the Association continues the business of making occupational therapy a viable health care service. It is a major resource for information for professional development and practice. OT BibSys is AOTA's computerized information system for bibliographic information, Association documents, and purchases of publications from the Association. Members may also access all AOTA services and information through a toll-free telephone number (1-800-SAY AOTA). Immediate, hands-on response through FAX service is available (1-301-948-5512). Among the functions of the Association is the monitoring of educational standards through accreditation of educational programs. The national office keeps a record of current members of the Association. Other functions include publishing the *American Journal of Occupational Therapy (AJOT)*, *OT Week*, the Association's weekly news and employment bulletin, and monographs. Publicity and recruitment involve printing brochures, making slide tape presentations, and producing films. Another function is that of providing testimony to the United States Congress on issues of importance to occupational therapy, such as reimbursement for services. Still other functions involve setting standards for practice and ethical behavior. Research continues to be a function that includes collecting statistics on the number of therapists in various areas of practice. Coordination with the state associations is yet another important function.

All these functions deserve the support of occupational therapists. Financial support is provided through annual fees. However, the major support of the Association is achieved when members are involved actively by serving on committees, commissions, and boards. To continue to be strong, the Association must have the support of all its members. A strong Association can continue to promote occupational therapy as a viable health care service.

AMERICAN OCCUPATIONAL THERAPY FOUNDATION

In 1965, the Association established the American Occupational Therapy Foundation to advance the science of occupational therapy and increase the public knowledge and understanding of occupational therapy (29). The rationale for a separate organization was to meet the code of the Internal Revenue Service, which does not approve of Associations operating as business and charitable organizations simultaneously. The Foundation, therefore, is a charitable organization dedicated to research, education, and publication.

Research is supported through grants to occupational therapy researchers, clinical research symposia, and Centers for Scholarship and Research, which began in 1981. The Academy of Research was established in 1982 to recognize exemplary scientific research by occupational therapists (30).

Education is supported through scholarship awards. Money for the awards comes from contributions, including bequests and memorials. Publications include consumer-oriented brochures, such as "Watch Me Grow"; a developmental chart; and "The Child with Minimal Brain Dysfunction," which tells parents about learning disabilities.

Another aspect of the Foundation began in 1980 when the Wilma L. West Library was organized. The Association had a library for many years, but it was never cataloged. These references plus additional donations have been cataloged and indexed for member use and are available through interlibrary loan. The collection includes most of the books written by occupational therapists or about occupational therapy plus many other books of interest. The journal collection includes all volumes of the *Archives of Occupational Therapy* and *Occupational Therapy and Rehabilitation,* 1922–1951, and all volumes of the *American Journal of Occupational Therapy* starting in 1947. There are numerous masters' theses and doctoral dissertations as well. The library should be a useful reference to the student, practitioner, and researcher; it is available 24 hours a day through OT BibSys, AOTA's computerized information system (31).

Members can support the work of the Foundation through donations and by making use of the services provided. Applications for student scholarships and grant requests are available by contacting the Foundation office located at the national office.

STATE ASSOCIATIONS

Each of the 50 states and the District of Columbia and Puerto Rico have state associations recognized by the American Occupational Therapy Association. The primary purpose of a state association is to collaborate with the national association to carry out the objectives of the profession at the local level. Most state associations have more specific objectives, such as providing continuing education to members, promoting the use and understanding of occupational therapy in the state, providing consultation and information to members, and participating in state and local health planning organizations.

The state associations are required to have at least four meetings a year although the executive board may meet more frequently to conduct ongoing business. Usually one meeting per year is designated as the annual meeting and may include special events or programs. Members may participate as officers or as committee members. Issues raised at the state or local level can be brought to the attention of the national association through the state president who sits on the Committee of State Association Presidents or through the representative who sits on the Representative Assembly.

STUDENT ORGANIZATIONS

Each occupational therapy educational program is encouraged to have a student organization or club for occupational therapy students. The specific rules or guidelines for development and continuation of such a student organization is governed by the institution in which the occupational therapy program is located. The American Occupational Therapy Association can offer suggestions and guidance, but each local student organization must first abide by the regulations within the institution.

The purposes of such student organizations vary, but common objectives include providing a forum for discussion of student issues; organizing special programs of interest to the members; and raising funds to attend conferences, such as the national conference of occupational therapists; and contributing books or equipment to the occupational therapy program. Student organizations also may cooperate with the state association on projects of mutual interest, such as student recruitment or public awareness.

STUDENT COMMITTEE

The Student Committee, also called the American Student Committee of the Occupational Therapy Association (ASCOTA), has a permanent or standing committee of the Executive Board. All student members of the Association are members of the Student Committee. The purpose of the Student Committee is to provide an opportunity for student members to have input into decision making and actions of the Association, to promote the well-being of students, and to enhance their knowledge of the structure and functions of the Association.

A representative from each education program is selected to attend the meeting of the student representatives at the annual conference. At the meeting, students discuss issues of concern and make recommendations for actions. The officers are elected by mail ballot and serve not only on the Student Committee but also as liaisons to the Commission on Education, Commission on Practice, Committee of State Association Presidents, and Fiscal Advisory Committee to learn more about how the Association functions and how issues may affect students.

Student members can participate by running for ASCOTA office, serving as a representative, or serving on a local committee. Through participation, students can begin to learn about the issues, problems, and solutions that the American Occupational Therapy Association encounters and achieves.

NATIONAL BOARD FOR CERTIFICATION IN OCCUPATIONAL THERAPY

The American Occupational Therapy Certification Board (AOTCB) was created in 1986 to manage the certification program (32). In 1996 the name was changed to the National Board for Certification in Occupational Therapy (NBCOT). It was an autonomous board, completely separate from the AOTA. The separation is necessary so that the AOTA is not subject to antitrust litigation for running a closed shop—that is, one where the Association controls entry into the profession by controlling both the accreditation of educational programs and the certification of practitioners to serve its own needs. Prior to the separation, the Association both accredited the educational programs and certified occupational therapy personnel. Standards and policies could be adopted that would be viewed as discriminatory in favor of certain values and knowledge. The solution to the problem of control was separation.

The purpose of the NBCOT is to develop and enforce the certification policies and procedures by which persons will be initially certified as occupational therapists and as registered and certified occupational therapy assistants. The NBCOT develops and conducts the certification examinations for occupational therapy personnel. In addition, the NBCOT provides information on certification and certified occupational therapy personnel to the licensure boards in those jurisdictions with licensure laws.

Finally, federal law requires that certification examinations be based on the actual requirements of the work setting. In other words, the examination must test the areas of knowledge, skill, and attitudes needed by an entry-level person to perform as an occupational therapist or assistant. Therefore, a study must be made of those requirements; such a study is called role analysis or role delineation. The NBCOT is responsible for seeing that role analysis studies are conducted to determine the job requirements of entry level positions of occupational therapy personnel. That information, in turn, must be used as the basis for developing questions on the certification examination.

INTERNATIONAL ORGANIZATIONS

Although the United States was the first country to form a national association of occupational therapists, many other countries followed during the 1930s and 1940s. The Canadian Association of Occupational Therapists was chartered in 1934 (33), the Association of Occupational Therapists (England) was formed in 1936 (34), and the Australian Association of Occupational Therapists began in 1945 (35).

Following World War II, there was an intensive effort made to provide rehabilitation services to all countries affected by the war. The exchange of information regarding standards of education and registration became a major concern (36).

Members of the World Congress on the Welfare of Cripples (now the International Society for the Rehabilitation of the Disabled) encouraged occupational therapists in several countries to form an international association. Finally, after several discussion sessions, a meeting was scheduled in Liverpool, England, to develop the World Federation of Occupational Therapists. The founding members were the United States, Canada, Denmark, the United Kingdom, South Africa, Sweden, New Zealand, Australia, Israel, and India. According to the Constitution, the purposes were as follows:

1. To act as the official international organization for the promotion of occupational therapy; to hold international congresses;
2. To promote international cooperation among occupational therapy associations; occupational therapists, and between them and other allied professional groups;
3. To maintain the ethics of the profession and to advance the practice and standards of occupational therapy;
4. To promote internationally recognized standards for the education of occupational therapists;
5. To facilitate the international exchange and placement of therapists and students;
6. To facilitate the exchange of information and publications to promote research. (37)

To fulfill the first purpose, the World Federation holds an international congress every 4 years. The first was held in Edinburgh, Scotland in 1954. Proceedings of each congress are printed and made available for purchase.

The second purpose is achieved by having representatives attend meetings of the international associations of particular importance in the World Health Organization and its various committees. Purposes 3, 4, and 6 are accomplished through the development of and public statements on ethics and functions, educational standards, a brochure on organizing an occupational therapy department, and a brochure on forming an association and an international bibliography. The World Federation also publishes a bulletin twice a year.

The fifth purpose is facilitated through the reciprocity statements between federation members. For example, a therapist who graduated from a school approved by the World Federation may sit for the certification examination for occupational therapists, provided the person is recommended by the school director, is a member of the occupational therapy association in the country of graduation, and is seeking employment as an occupational therapist in this country. No additional education or training requirements are expected.

There are now 48 member countries of the World Federation including the United States (see Table 26.1) (6). The members meet every 2 years to discuss issues of interest and concern. Each country is represented by an elected delegate who serves 4 years. Many countries also have alternates. The delegates and alternates are responsible for reporting information to and from the World Federation regarding council actions, health and medical problems, educational program standards, and information from other health organizations. The delegate from the American Occupational Therapy Association gives a report each year at the annual business meeting. The report also is printed in the Annual Report of the Association.

Although it is difficult to measure the effect of the World Federation on the profession of occupational therapy among nations, numbers of educational programs may give some indication. In 1954, there were 49 schools of occupational therapy in 11 different countries. By 1966, there were 92 schools approved or tentatively approved in 21 countries (36). In 1981, there were 184 schools in 29 countries (38).

Table 26.1.	Members of the World Federation of Occupational Therapists			
Argentina	1970	Jordan	1992
Australia	1952	Kenya	1976
Austria	1978	Luxembourg	1990
Belgium	1968	Malaysia	1990
Bermuda	1996	Malta	1994
Brazil	1994	Netherlands	1960
Canada	1952	New Zealand	1952
Caribbean	1996	Nigeria	1994
Chile	1980	Norway	1958
China	1986	Pakistan	1994
Colombia	1976	Philippines	1968
Cyprus	1996	Portugal	1964
Denmark	1952	Singapore	1976
Finland	1972	South Africa	1952
France	1976	Spain	1972
Germany	1958	Sri Lanka	1976
Greece	1992	Sweden	1952
Hong Kong	1984	Switzerland	1962
Iceland	1986	Thailand	1994
India	1952	Uganda	1996
Ireland	1970	United Kingdom	1952
Israel	1970	USA	1952
Italy	1978	Venezuela	1968
Japan	1972	Zimbabwe	1990

As of 1992, there were 256 approved or tentatively approved schools in 31 countries (39). The United States had the most with 76 (professional programs only). Japan had 29, Germany had 23, and the United Kingdom had 22. There were 12 schools in Canada, 10 in Belgium, 9 in France, 8 in Sweden, and 7 in India and South Africa. Denmark had 6, Australia had 5, and Austria, Finland, Israel, and Switzerland each had 3. There were 2 schools in Ireland, the Netherlands, Norway, Portugal, Puerto Rico, and Venezuela, whereas Chile, China, Columbia, Hong Kong, Kenya, New Zealand, the Philippine Islands, and Spain each had 1 school. Thus, the number of schools of occupational therapy had more than quintupled in 35 years. Certainly, it has become easier to meet an occupational therapist or receive occupational therapy treatment almost anywhere one might travel or live in this world.

MYTHS AND FABLES

Anyone who has played the telephone game at a party knows that, as a message is passed down from one person to another, the message is changed and sometimes no longer resembles the original. The same distortion can happen in a profession as knowledge is passed from one generation of practitioners to another until the message becomes a myth or fable. Although some myths or fables are harmless, others can become the source of embarrassment when the truth is discovered. This section will discuss briefly some nontruths that therapists should know and not continue to repeat to later generations of therapists.

The first myth is attributed to Galen, the well-known Italian physician to the Gladiators. According to the folklore in occupational therapy, Galen is supposed to have said that "employment is nature's best physician." The source of untruth is an article by Reid (40). Unfortunately, her knowledge of Latin or her memory was poor. What Galen actually said was "exercise is nature's best physician." Thus, his words would provide more support to physical therapy than occupational therapy. Licht uncovered the error in translation in 1947, but occupational therapists enjoyed the supposed support of Galen so much that they continue to employ his words even though they do nothing to advance the cause of occupational therapy (41). Because many physicians know Latin, they can trace the phrase to its origin and embarrass the occupational therapy practitioner who relies on the incorrect translation.

A major fable in occupational therapy concerns a federal act requiring occupational therapy services in all general hospitals. The statement usually appears in historical accounts of occupational therapy and reads approximately as follows: *In 1923, the Federal Industrial Rehabilitation Act made it a requirement for every general hospital dealing with industrial accidents or illnesses to adopt occupational therapy as an integral part of its treatment.* Sounds great but there is not a word of truth in the sentence. There is absolutely no 1923 Federal Industrial Rehabilitation Act and there never was. Someone got some wires crossed. There is a 1920 Federal Industrial Rehabilitation Act, as mentioned previously in this chapter. However, it says nothing about occupational therapy because occupational therapy was classified by the government in 1918 as a part of the medical services (42). The Federal Industrial Rehabilitation Act was designed to help disabled civilians learn or relearn a vocation and get a job. The objective was oriented toward education, vocation, and employment. Medical services, which included occupational therapy, were excluded entirely. Not until 1943 were any medical services included in the federal vocational training acts (43). Occupational therapy could not have been provided under the federal vocational acts in the 1920s because such coverage would have been illegal (44). Any vocational or rehabilitation counselor who knows the history of vocational training in this country can quickly identify the errors. Again, using this erroneous statement is asking to be exposed as someone who does not know the subject matter about which he or she is talking. There are enough true facts about occupational therapy to support its existence. Why resort to myths and fables when the truth is just as compelling?

There are other untruths that surface here and there in the literature of occupational therapy. Eleanor Clarke Slagle is the subject of several. She is supposed to have been the first employed person in the national office as the national society's first Executive Secretary or Executive Director. In truth, she was never paid and she was never the Executive Secretary or Executive Director (45) . She was, in fact, an elected officer of the Association and served as the elected, but not paid, secretary and treasurer. The dual role as secretary and treasure did provide Mrs. Slagle with many opportunities to influence the events in the Association. At her recommendation, the two offices were separated after 1937. Elected officers of the Association have never been paid a salary. The first paid person was Idelle Kidder and the first Executive Secretary was Maud Plummer and first person to hold the title of Executive Director was Wilma West (46).

In summary, the development of a profession is sometimes embellished to enhance the image just as occurs in biographies of famous people. George Washington, as a boy, did not cut down a cherry tree and then admit to his father that he could not tell a lie about the deed, but the idea makes a good story so the myth survives without supporting facts.

References

1. Certificate of Incorporation of the National Society for the Promotion of Occupational Therapy, Inc. Then and Now: 1917–1976. Washington, DC: American Occupational Therapy Association, 1967:4–5.
2. Licht S: The founding and founders of the American Occupational Therapy Association. Am J Occup Ther 1967;21:277.
3. American Occupational Therapy Association is the new name. Mod Hosp 1921;17:554.
4. Discuss joint meeting with AMA. Mod Hosp 1922;18:472.
5. The Fifth Annual Meeting of the National Society for the Promotion of Occupational Therapy. Arch Occup Ther 1922;1:71.
6. Meeting of the board and members of the House of Delegates of the American Occupational Therapy Association. Arch Occup Ther 1922;1:340.
7. Kidner TB: Occupational therapy in 1923. Mod Hosp 1924;22:55.
8. History of service of the Registration Committee. Am J Occup Ther 1950;4:189.
9. Report of the Secretary-Treasurer and Board of Management. Occup Ther Rehabil 1927;6:475.
10. Occupational therapists adopt pledge and creed. Mod Hosp 1926;27:88.
11. Essentials of an acceptable school of occupational therapy. JAMA 1935;104:1631–1633.
12. Report of Registration Committee. Occup Ther Rehabil 1933;12:391.
13. Excerpts from minutes of meeting, Education Committee. Occup Ther Rehabil 1945;24:117.
14. Minutes of the meeting of the Board of Management, June 27, 1945, and committee reports. Occup Ther Rehabil 1945;24:212.
15. Licht S. William Rush Denton, Jr. Occup Ther Rehabil 1947;26:47.
16. Official Report of Board and Committee Meeting. Am J Occup Ther 1947;1:182.
17. Meetings of the Board of Management. Am J Occup Ther 1950;4:236.
18. Meetings of the House of Delegates. Am J Occup Ther 1955;9:36.
19. Executive Director's report. Am J Occup Ther 1956;10:20.
20. Constitution and Bylaws of the American Occupational Therapy Association. Am J Occup Ther 1956;10:23–24.

21. The recognition of occupational therapy assistants. Am J Occup Ther 1958;12: 269–275.
22. Bylaws of the American Occupational Therapy Association. Am J Occup Ther 1965; 19:37–41.
23. Minutes of the annual business meeting. Am J Occup Ther 1969;23:185.
24. Statement on occupational therapy referral. Am J Occup Ther 1969;23:530–531.
25. Model Occupational Therapy Practice Act 1969. Revised 1974. Washington, DC: American Occupational Therapy Association.
26. Occupational therapy newspaper. American Occupational Therapy Association. August 1972;1.
27. AOTA Bylaws. Am J Occup Ther 1977;31:111–118.
28. Occupational therapy newspaper. American Occupational Therapy Association 1980; 34:8.
29. Yerxa EJ. The American Occupational Therapy Foundation is born. Am J Occup Ther 1967;21:299–300.
30. Occupational therapy newspaper. American Occupational Therapy Association. December 1982:36.
31. Binderman MS. The Wilma L. West Library goes on line. Am J Occup Ther 1989;43: 269–270.
32. Occupational therapy newspaper. American Occupational Therapy Association. June 1986;40.
33. Driver MF. A philosophic view of the history of occupational therapy in Canada. Can J Occup Ther 1968;35:53–60.
34. Macdonald EM, MacGaul G, Murrey L. Occupational Therapy in Rehabilitation. 3rd ed. London: Balliere Tindall and Cassell, 1970:9.
35. Sims GE. Occupational therapy in Australia—the formative years. Aust Occup Ther J 1967;14:29–44.
36. Spackman CS: The World Federation of Occupational Therapists. Am J Occup Ther 1967;21:301–309.
37. Constitution for a World Organization of Occupational Therapists. Am J Occup Ther 1952;6:274–278.
38. Barker J. Report of the secretary/treasurer. WFOT Bull 1981;8:5.
39. Punwar A. Current trends in international occupational therapy practice. Occup Ther Int 1994;1(1):1–12.
40. Reid EC. Ergotherapy in the treatment of mental disorders. Bost Med Surg J 1914;171:300–303.
41. Licht S. Occupational Therapy Source Book. Baltimore: Williams & Wilkins. 1948:81.
42. The Official Bulletin 1918;2(359)–8.
43. Lassiter RA. History of the rehabilitation movement in America. In: Cull JG, Hardy RE. Vocational Rehabilitation. Springfield, IL: Charles C Thomas, 1972:43.
44. Industrial Rehabilitation. Washington, DC: Federal Board of Vocational Education, 1920, Bulletin #57:31.
45. Editorial. Occup Ther Rehabit 1937;16:64.
46. Report of the Secretary Treasurer. Occup Ther Rehabil 1926;5:452.

CHAPTER 27

Founders and Early Researchers of Occupational Therapy

The group who gathered on March 15, 1917, to found the National Society for the Promotion of Occupational Therapy was a mix of people from a variety of occupational backgrounds. Among the seven founders were a physician, a teacher of art and design, a former social service worker, a secretary, two architects, and a nurse who was not present at the meeting.

GEORGE EDWARD BARTON

One of the two architects was George Barton. He had become interested in the use of occupations as treatment from his own personal experience as a disabled individual. Barton was born in 1871 in Brookline, Massachusetts. Information concerning his early years is unavailable, but he became an architect and traveled to London. There he met William Morris who interested him in social problems, especially in housing. After returning to the United States, he practiced architecture in Boston and became an incorporator and first secretary for the Boston Society of Arts and Crafts. In 1901, he became a member of the Boston Society of Architects and American Institute in Architecture.

Also in 1901, he discovered he had tuberculosis, attacks of which were to recur through out the remainder of his life. During the fourth attack, he moved to Denver and resumed his architectural practice after recuperating. In 1912, he was asked by the governor of Colorado to investigate the extent of the famine that had struck the farmers along the Kansas border. On the survey, his left foot was frozen and then gangrene developed. While recovering from the amputation of his foot, he suffered an hysterical paralysis of the left side of his body, which did not abate. He felt hopelessly "down and out" (1).

At someone's suggestion, he went to see Dr. James G. Mumford who was superintendent of Clifton Springs Sanitarium, a hospital for convalescents in New York. He also encountered Reverend Dr. Elwood Worcester of the Emmanuel Church in Boston who convinced him that life could be worth living if he showed what could be done for others who had similar problems.

With the goal of helping others in mind, he bought a house on Broad Street in Clifton Springs, which he remodeled. On March 7, 1914, he opened Consolation House, a school, workshop, and vocational bureau for convalescents. He wanted to "raise the cry that it is time for humanity to cease regarding the hospital as a door closing upon a life. . . ." (1).

To prepare himself for the job of administering Consolation House, he studied anatomy, surgery, nervous diseases, and drug treatment with various physicians and attended lectures for nursing students at the Clifton Springs Sanitarium Training School. He also began corresponding with other people who used occupations as treatment. Among these persons was Dr. William R. Dunton Jr, a psychiatrist. In a letter dated November 15, 1914, he states he had "discussed and practically decided to call a conference of those actually working in invalid occupations" (2). Although Dr. Dunton replied favorably to the idea, the conference did not convene. However, correspondence continued, and the idea of a conference kept recurring along with various names of possible attendees. Among these names were Susan Tracy, Eleanor Clarke Slagle, and Susan Johnson. Finally, in 1917, the arrangements for the conference were made to Barton's satisfaction and the conference was called for March 15th through the 17th at Consolation House in Clifton Springs, New York. One member was added at the last minute. Thomas B. Kidner, from Canada, was invited to give an international perspective. Miss Tracy was unable to attend, but Isabel G. Newton, Barton's secretary, was included.

At the meeting, Mr. Barton was elected president, but he served for only 6 months. He was unable to attend the first annual meeting held in New York City in September 1917, probably because of his health, and did not attend any further meetings of the National Society for The Promotion of Occupational Therapy.

In addition to calling the founding conference, Barton is responsible for popularizing the term "occupational therapy" in 1914. As stated in Chapter 1, he said, "If there is an occupational disease, why not an occupational therapy?" (3). Barton thought that occupational therapy could provide an occupation that would produce a similar *therapeutical effect to that of every drug* in materia medica. His goal may have been slightly grandiose and perhaps impractical, but the term occupational therapy has prevailed in spite of attempts to replace it with ergotherapy, work cure, and others.

Barton also found a suitable title for the new organization. In November 1915, he suggested that the title be The Society for the Promotion of Occupational Reeducation, but by December 1916, he had changed his mind and favored The National Society for the Promotion of Occupational Therapy. He felt the title suggested SPOT or an ever alert "Johnny."

In 1918, Barton married his secretary, Isabel Newton, and 2 years later they had a son, George Gladwin. Barton continued to run Consolation House and explore activities by trying to do the tasks himself. He became a one-handed gardener and woodworker. When physicians saw the improvement in his own health, they began to refer patients to him to help as he had helped himself.

Lectures, articles, and books on occupations for invalids filled more of his time. The number of lectures and articles is not certain, but he wrote three books. The first, *Occupational Therapy,* is a compilation of previously published articles. The second is *Re-Education: An Analysis of the Institutional System of the United States,* and the third is *Teaching the Sick,* which was the most popular. The last book includes many of the activities that Barton worked out for himself.

George Barton died on April 27, 1923 of tuberculosis. He had succeeded in convincing people that occupations could help patients return to useful work activity. Moreover, he had initiated a national society to promote the use of occupations for therapeutic purposes and had given such application a name, occupational therapy.

SUSAN COX JOHNSON

Of the seven founders, the least is recorded about Susan Cox Johnson. She was born in 1876 in Corsicana, Texas. Sometime later she moved to Berkeley, California, where she taught high school and wrote a textbook on textiles. In 1912, she went to the Philippines where she taught arts and crafts. Upon returning to the United States she took a position in New York State as Director of Occupations, Department of Public Charities in August 1916. This position impressed George Barton. In a letter to Dr. Dunton he says, she "has by all odds the most important job in the world, together with a very level head, a keen insight, good experience and a tremendous interest in the therapeutic side" (2).

At the founding meeting, Isabel Newton describes Miss Johnson as having a strong personality but a quiet, modest manner. Although her role at the meeting is not recorded, she was appointed chairman of the committee on Admissions and Positions. This committee was responsible for determining who should enter schools and get jobs.

In July 1917, Miss Johnson accepted a position at Columbia University in New York City as lecturer in occupation therapy in the Department of Nursing. She also was Director of Occupation at Montefiore Home and Hospitals where she organized the department. Later she directed the Jefferson Needle Craft Shop, a special shop for women who had tuberculosis. In 1925, she became director of the Convalescent Shop of the New York Visiting Committee of the New York State Charities Aid Association. The shop provided sheltered work for mentally ill and disabled persons.

Her work on the Admissions and Positions Committee made her aware of the importance of standards. In 1921, she became chairman of the Committee on Education, which helped to develop the first set of minimal standards for educational programs in occupational therapy.

Miss Johnson wrote five articles that were published in *Modern Hospital.* All were related to the training of personnel to become occupational therapists and the role of occupational therapy in the hospital program. She was very concerned that occupational therapists should have good training and that the relationship between nursing and teaching occupations for therapeutic purposes should be clearly separate functions.

In 1924, Miss Johnson left the Association for reasons not recorded. She continued, however, to help people help themselves by establishing sheltered workshops for convalescing patients. On January 19, 1932, she died of pneumonia.

ISABEL GLADWIN NEWTON BARTON

Isabel Newton was born in Geneva, New York, on July 21, 1891. Her introduction to George Barton began on a note of misunderstanding. Mr. Barton phoned her at home asking if she would be interested in becoming his secretary. Miss Newton did not hear his name and thought he was offering her a job at the Hotel Seneca where he was staying. She did not want to work at the hotel since she already had a job as a bookkeeper in a preserving and canning factory making $11 a week.

That evening while she attended church, a friend asked her if a Mr. Barton of Clifton Springs had contacted her. The friend explained that Barton needed a secretary to help write a book and articles and would pay $15 a week for shorter hours than the bookkeeping job. She wrote Barton immediately expressing her desire to reconsider and was granted an interview.

Barton agreed to hire her on a trial basis, and she began work on August 1, 1916, just 7 months before the founding meeting of the National Society for the Promotion of Occupational Therapy. She was attracted to Barton from the initial interview. Her own account states that he was like no one she had ever seen in her 25 years: "Such a fascinating personality, such a boyish young air, such a sense of humor, all belied with a painful life of bitter experiences he had been through" (4).

Miss Newton commuted daily the 14 miles from Geneva to Clifton Springs by train. She was still commuting when the founders met in March. Her role in the founder's meeting was as a secretary. Barton, however, seemed to think of her role as very important; she was elected secretary of the new organization and was included in the official photograph of the founders.

In May 1918, Barton and Miss Newton were married, and in 1920, they had a son who they named George. Mrs. Barton continued to work with her husband as he prepared his books and continued the activities of Consolation House until 1923 when he died and Consolation House was disbanded.

Mrs. Barton returned to live in Geneva. She participated in the 50-year celebration of the AOTA at which time a plaque commemorating the founding was placed on the house at 16 Broad Street in Clifton Springs, which had been Consolation House.

Mrs. Barton died November 4, 1975, at the age of 84. She had become well acquainted with occupational therapy through her tasks as secretary to George Barton and was the historian of activities at Consolation House, including those that occurred during the founding meeting.

ELEANOR CLARKE SLAGLE

Eleanor Clarke Slagle is the only founder to serve in all offices of the Association. She, more than any other founder, shaped and molded the American Occupational Therapy Association.

According to church records, Mrs. Slagle was born Ella May Clark in Hobart, New York, on October 13, 1870. Her parents were William James and Emmeline Davenport Clark. She probably received her early education in the local school but attended a summer session at Claverack College. Sometime during her childhood she changed her name to Eleanor Mai, added the letter 'e' to Clark, and changed her birthdate to 1876, which was actually the date of her baptism but is the date most often seen in biographical sketches about her. She married Robert E. Slagle, the son of a preacher in 1894 but later divorced him, probably while in Chicago. They had no children. Her brother, John Davenport Clarke, was a Republican representative to the United States Congress from the 34th district. He was killed in an automobile accident. He was born in 1869 but changed his birth date to 1873.

In 1911, at the age of 40, she began studying social service work. While observing patients at the Kankakee State Hospital, she became concerned about the undesirable effects of idleness. On the advice of Julia Lathrop and Jane Addams of Hull House, she enrolled in the Special Course in Curative Occupations and Recreation, which had been developed in 1908 by Miss Lathrop and Rabbi Hirsch as a class for attendants of the insane. The courses were sponsored by the Chicago School of Civics and Philanthropy, another settlement house in Chicago, which was run by Graham Taylor. Mrs. Slagle completed the fourth class in July 1911. She then went to Newberry, Michigan to offer a similar course and returned the following July to conduct the fifth class in Curative Occupations and Recreation at Hull House.

From 1913 to 1914, she followed Dr. Adolph Meyer from Illinois to Johns Hopkins Hospital in Baltimore, Maryland, where she became Director of Occupations at the Henry Phipps Psychiatric Clinic. While at the clinic, she developed her method of treating psychiatric patients, which was called "habit training." Habit training was based on the theory of balanced activities between work, pleasure, and self-care. Also while in Maryland, she became a frequent guest at Dr. William R. Dunton's home and wrote her first paper. In 1915, she returned to Illinois to start the Experimental Station at the Illinois Mental Hygiene Society. The purpose was to help people find occupation who could not because of their various health problems. Initially, the workshop was housed near the Society's office but rapidly outgrew the available space. Hull House offered the use of space until larger quarters could be located.

In 1918, she was asked to become director of the Department of Occupational Therapy for the Illinois Department of Public Welfare while she continued her work as Director of the Henry B. Favill School of Occupations, the new name for the Experimental Station. She continued to train occupational therapists even though she was asked by Dr. Thomas Salmon, a psychiatrist, to become director of Occupational Therapy of the neuropsychiatric division in France during World War I.

At the founding meeting in March 1917, she was elected vice president and appointed chairman of the Committee on Installations and Advice. During the years 1919 to 1920, she served as president and the annual meeting was held at Hull House.

When she moved to New York to care for her ailing mother, the Henry B. Favill School of Occupations closed in 1918. In 1920, she became the executive secretary of the New York Society for Occupational Therapy. She also became the director of the Bureau of Occupational Therapy of the New York State Department of Mental Hygiene on July 1, 1922. Her primary interests were to provide uniform programs in all institutions and to direct services to the "back ward" patients using habit training. The same year, the Association elected her secretary-treasurer. Both offices were held until 1937 when she resigned. Mrs. Franklin D. Roosevelt and Dr. Adolph Meyer attended the farewell banquet given for her by the AOTA. She remained Director of Occupational Therapy in New York State until her death on September 18, 1942.

At the founding meeting, Isabel Newton Barton described Mrs. Slagle as "a person of strong personality, great calm, and a dignity that won instant admiration" (4). Also, Mrs. Barton recalled that Mrs. Slagle had a certain flair for style, which can be observed in the founders' official photograph in which Mrs. Slagle wore the violet corsage given to her at the start of the conference.

Sidney Licht, editor of *Occupational Therapy and Rehabilitation*, following Dr. Dunton, states that Mrs. Slagle "was regally tall and there were those who found that some of her pronouncements were in keeping with her appearance and bearing" (5). An example of such a pronouncement is noted in an article by Florence Cromwell, in which Mrs. Slagle is supposed to have said, upon learning that a therapist would be a day late in giving an annual report: "Who is this Miss that finds it more important to work in the garden with patients than be here to give her report!" (6).

By all accounts, Mrs. Slagle was a capable, energetic person who was dedicated to promoting and improving the practice of occupational therapy. The Association officially recognized her significant contribution in 1953 when the House of Delegates endorsed the concept of an Eleanor Clarke Slagle honorary lectureship. Although occupational therapists were originally elected to receive the award, the process was changed to selection based on nomination by peers. The Eleanor Clarke Slagle lectureship is awarded at one conference, and the awardee presents a lecture at the next annual conference. The first such lectureship was presented by Florence Stattel in 1955. Thus, the influence of Eleanor Clarke Slagle continues to be present as a model of excellence.

SUSAN EDITH TRACY

Susan E. Tracy did not attend the founding meeting in Clifton Springs, but she was accorded "all the rights and privileges of an incorporator" and was named chairman of the Teaching Methods Committee (7). She could not be present because she was teaching a new course in invalid occupations at the Presbyterian Hospital in Chicago.

In 1864, Miss Tracy was born in Lynn, Massachusetts. Mary Barrows, who published Miss Tracy's book, *Studies in Invalid Occupations,* stated that Miss Tracy as a child, learned various "handwork" activities and made gifts and toys for her three siblings instead of buying ones. While Miss Tracy was a nursing student, she became aware that patients who occupied themselves benefited from the activity.

After graduating from nursing at the Massachusetts Homeopathic Hospital in 1898, Miss Tracy was a private duty nurse. Private duty permitted her to study at Teachers College in Home Economics, where she took courses in the Manual Arts Department.

On completion of her studies at Teachers College in 1905, Miss Tracy joined the nursing staff at Adams Nervine Asylum in Jamaica Plain, Massachusetts, and she became superintendent of the training school of nurses in June 1906. That same summer, Miss Tracy began teaching a course on invalid occupations to nursing students in her own apartment because the new occupational treatment building was not complete. The course began as a special summer session but later became a regular subject in which every nurse received 10 lessons. These lessons evolved into the book *Studies in Invalid Occupations,* which was originally printed in 1910 but was reprinted in 1912.

Miss Tracy continued to work at Adams Nervine Asylum until early in 1912. Thereafter, she gave lectures and private instruction and continued writing at her own workshop, known as the Experimental Station for the Study of Invalid Occupations, which opened in March 1912. She was interested in surgery and better care of kidney and obstetrical patients as well as occupations. These articles are recorded in the *Index Medicus* at the rate of one or two a year, from 1906 until her death in September 12, 1928.

Miss Tracy felt that only nurses should be permitted to provide invalid occupations to patients because nurses would be most likely to adapt the occupation to the illness of the patient. In spite of her belief, she became a friend of Eleanor Clarke Slagle and even urged Mrs. Slagle to become the secretary-treasurer of the American Occupational Therapy Association in 1922. Miss Tracy also served on the Board of Managers.

According to Mrs. Slagle, Miss Tracy had a "delightful magnetic personality" and was a very persuasive conversationalist (7). She enjoyed talking about the use of invalid occupations and stressed the use of waste materials, the need to adapt the occupation to the condition, and the selection of an occupation that suited the patient's interest.

Her book was the first occupational therapy textbook to be published and has become a classic in the profession's literature. Miss Tracy may rightfully be called the first occupational therapist of the twentieth century.

THOMAS BESSELL KIDNER

Thomas Bessell Kidner was invited to become a founder because Mr. Barton wanted someone from another country to add an international perspective to the mix. He was a good choice and served the Association he helped found for many years.

Mr. Kidner was born in London in 1866. He received his training as an architect at the Merchant Venturers College in Bristol. In 1900, he went to Canada to establish a technical education program in the Canadian provinces of Nova Scotia and New Brunswick. He was appointed Director of Technical Education for Calgary, Alberta in 1911. In 1915, he was appointed the vocational secretary in the Canadian Military Hospitals Commission located in Ottawa. During his tenure, he developed a system of vocational rehabilitation for disabled veterans in Canada.

One year after the conference at Clifton Springs, in June 1918, Mr. Kidner was asked to become a Special Advisor on Rehabilitation to the United States Federal Board of Vocational Education. In November 1919, he joined the National Tuberculosis Association because of his knowledge of institutional construction and curative occupations. He resigned his position in 1926 to engage in private practice as a consultant in planning medical institutions of all types. He was a consultant to the United States Public Health Service and to the Veteran's Bureau.

In 1923, he was elected president of the Association, for the first of six consecutive terms. He also served temporarily as president in 1930 after President Haviland and Vice President Carr died suddenly. During his term as president, the Association established minimal standards for training occupational therapists, 1923; adopted an emblem, 1923; adopted a pledge and creed, 1926; and initiated the task of establishing a national registry of qualified occupational therapists. The registry was Mr. Kidner's favorite project and he prodded, cajoled, and urged the Association to get the registry completed at every opportunity. The first national registration was completed finally in the year of his death in 1932.

Mr. Kidner is described as a man who wore tailored clothes, spoke clear and correct English, knew parliamentary procedure, and knew how to conduct a meeting. At the same time, he is said to have been witty, a good raconteur, a genial man, and a lover of art, music, and literature. He used his wide knowledge and many affiliations to help the Association whenever he could.

He wrote several articles concerned with development and maintenance of standards for training therapists. He also wrote two books and several articles that were reprinted as pamphlets. Mr. Kidner was an able organizer who knew how to keep an Association on the right track no matter how long the job took to complete. His insistence on quality and attention to detail served the young Association well as it struggled to help occupational therapy become a profession.

He was married and had a daughter, Lilian, and two sons, Arthur W. and Charles E. After his death, his wife and daughter returned to England where he was buried.

WILLIAM RUSH DUNTON JR, MD

William Rush Dunton was the patient prodder of the founders. He kept his head when the others lost theirs and kept the objectives on track when others had lost their sense of purpose. The Association was to feel his steady hand and influence for 50 years.

Dr. Dunton was born July 24, 1868, in Philadelphia, Pennsylvania, and grew up in the wealthy suburb of Chestnut Hill. He was a direct descendent of Benjamin Rush, who signed the Declaration of Independence and wrote the first book on psychiatry in the United States. Although Dr. Dunton himself was named for an uncle, not his father, he was called "junior."

In 1893, Dr. Dunton obtained his medical degree from the University of Pennsylvania after graduating with baccalaureate and master's degrees from Haverford College. He spent 2 years in internship and then accepted a position at Sheppard and Enoch Pratt Hospital in 1895 where he stayed for 30 years. At Sheppard and Enoch Pratt, he began using occupations with patients and began writing about the value of occupations in 1912 after Dr. Edward Brush, the director, put Dr. Dunton in charge of occupation.

His early articles on occupation must have come to the attention of George Barton because, on November 15, 1914, Mr. Barton wrote inviting Dr. Dunton to meet to discuss the use of invalid occupations. Dr. Dunton replied with interest, suggesting that a meeting could be held with the next conference of the American Medico-Psychological Association in 1915. This group had already conducted sessions on using occupations in psychiatric hospitals.

Mr. Barton may have misinterpreted the suggestion as a move on Dr. Dunton's part to take over the unformed organization. On November 30, Mr. Barton replied that he felt the offers from New York citizens were too attractive to call the conference elsewhere. However, no meeting was called. Dr. Dunton, undaunted, continued the correspondence and offered to publish any call for a conference in the *Maryland Psychiatric Quarterly* to give it wider publicity.

In 1916, Mr. Barton had become doubtful that an organization could be formed because most people were doing "craft work" to make articles for sale to monetarily benefit the patient or institution. He complained that such workers had no knowledge of medicine or the therapeutic value of occupations. Dr. Dunton again pressed for initiating an organization on the basis that Mr. Barton's arguments against it were, in fact, arguments in favor. An organization could educate and stimulate craft workers to their real function in a hospital, according to Dr. Dunton's letter of December 7.

Apparently, Dr. Dunton was persuasive enough to enable Mr. Barton to regain his sense of direction. The letters that followed were concerned with the details of organizing, including a notice in the *Maryland Psychiatric Quarterly,* a constitution, a list of incorporators, and a location.

At the founding meeting, Dr. Dunton was elected treasurer. However, at the September annual conference when Mr. Barton was unable to attend, Dr. Dunton was elected president and served for 2 years. Dr. Dunton was also chairman of the Committee on Finance, Publicity and Publication. Finance soon became a separate committee, but he retained his interest in publicity and publications. In 1921, he proposed that a journal be developed for occupational therapy because the Maryland *Psychiatric Quarterly* and *Modern Hospital* could not devote enough space to the growing profession. *The Archives of Occupational Therapy* began publication in 1922 with Dr. Dunton as editor, a position he held until 1947 when he retired. The journal changed to the name *Occupational Therapy and Rehabilitation* in 1925 with volume 4. In addition to editorial duties, he published six books and more than 100 articles although not all dealt with occupational therapy.

Dr. Dunton was described as a "gentle, friendly and team man" by Dr. Sidney Licht who succeeded him as editor of *Occupational Therapy and Rehabilitation.* In private life, he married Edna D. Hogan, a nurse, in 1897. They had four children, but one died in infancy. He had many hobbies, including gardening, writing, and music. His interest in music led to the formation of the Doctor's Orchestra in Baltimore. His wife Edna died in 1935 on October 8. He married Mrs. Jesse Lecra Pollard on August 26, 1942.

Professionally, he remained active for many years. After 19 years at Sheppard and Enoch Pratt Hospital, he opened a small private center called Harlem Lodge in Catonsville, Maryland. In 1939, the lease expired so he went into private practice. He continued to publish and edit and was named associate editor of the *American Journal of Psychiatry* in 1950. His death on December 23, 1966, at the age of 99, meant that one of the most ardent supporters of occupational therapy had died. Although he did not exhibit some of the showmanship that drew attention to Mr. Barton, Mr. Kidner, and Mrs. Slagle, Dr. Dunton was probably the most influential in promoting occupational therapy both to the Association members and to the public.

His tributes from a grateful Association were the right to call himself an Occupational Therapist, Registered, an honorary life board membership in 1947, and the Award of Merit in 1957. He summed up his own feelings in his credo:

> That occupation is as necessary to life as food and drink;
>> That every human being should have both physical and mental occupations;
>> That all should have occupations that they enjoy or hobbies—at least two, one outdoor and one indoor;
>> That sick minds, sick bodies, and sick souls may be healed through occupation. (8)

References

1. Newton IG. Consolation House. Trained Nurse Hosp Rev 1917;59:321.
2. Dunton WR Jr. An historical note. Occup Ther Rehabil 1926;5:428–434.
3. Barton GE. Occupational therapy. Trained Nurse Hosp Rev 1915;54:138.
4. Barton IG. Consolation House: fifty years ago. Am J Occup Ther 1968;22:344–345.
5. Licht S. The founding and founders of the American Occupational Therapy Association. Am J Occup Ther 1967;21:271.
6. Cromwell FC. Eleanor Clarke Slagle, the leader, the woman. Am J Occup Ther 1977;31:647.
7. Slagle EC. Trained Nurse Hosp Rev 1938;100:376–380.
8. Presidents of the American Occupational Therapy Association (1917–1967). Am J Occup Ther 1967;21:271.

BOOKS BY G. E. BARTON

Occupational Therapy. New York: Lakeside Publishing Co., 1916.
Re-education: An Analysis of the Institutional System of the United States. New York: Houghton-Mifflin, 1917.
Convalescent Clubs: A Plan for Rehabilitation. Clifton Springs, NY: Consolation House Convalescent Club, Inc., 1918 (pamphlet).
Teaching the Sick: A Manual of Occupational Therapy and Reeducation. Philadelphia: Saunders, 1919.

ARTICLES BY G. E. BARTON

A view of invalid occupation. Trained Nurse Hosp Rev 1914;52:327–330.
Votes for nurses and the hospital. Trained Nurse Hosp Rev 1914;53:129–132.
Occupational therapy. Trained Nurse Hosp Rev 1915;54:138–140.
Occupational therapy and the war. Trained Nurse Hosp Rev 1916;57:9–10.
Occupation and auto-inoculation in tuberculosis. Trained Nurse Hosp Rev 1916;57: 129–133,189–193.
Inoculation of the bacillus of work. Mod Hosp 1917;8:399–403.
The movies and the microscope. Trained Nurse Hasp Rev 58:193–197, 1917.
Hamlet with Hamlet left out. Proceedings of the Third Annual Meeting of the National Society for the Promotion of Occupational Therapy, Chicago 1919;3:126–132.
What occupational therapy may mean to nursing. Trained Nurse Hosp Rev 1920;64: 304–310.
The existing hospital system and reconstruction. Trained Nurse Hosp Rev 1922;69: 317–320.

REFERENCES ABOUT G. E. BARTON

Barton IG. Consolation House. Fifty years ago. Am J Occup Ther 1968;22:340–345.
Editorial. George Edward Barton. Arch Occup Ther 1923;2:409–410.
Newton IG. Consolation House. Trained Nurse Hosp Rev 1917;59:321–326.

BOOK BY S. C. JOHNSON

Textile Studies. Berkeley, CA: W. R. Morris, 1912.

ARTICLES BY S.C. JOHNSON

Occupational therapy in New York City institutions. Mod Hosp 1917;8:414–415.

The teacher in occupational therapy. Proceedings of the First Annual Meeting of the National Society for the Promotion of Occupational Therapy, New York. 1917;1:45–51.

Educational aspects of occupational therapy. Proceedings of the Second Annual Meeting of the National Society for the Promotion of Occupational Therapy, New York. 1918;2:44–49.

Practical results of a year's work at Montefiore. Proceedings of the Third Annual Meeting of the National Society for the Promotion of Occupational Therapy, Chicago. 1919;3: 119–125.

Occupation therapy. Mod Hosp 1919;12:221–223, 1919.

Instruction in handcrafts and design for hospital patients. Mod Hosp 1920;15:69–72, 1920.

Training of teachers for occupational therapy. J Outdoor Life 1920;17:341,344.

Should there be separate O.T. schools? Mod Hosp 1921;17:362–363.

Occupational therapy and post-hospital employment. Mod Hosp 1924;22:196–197.

REFERENCE ABOUT S.C. JOHNSON

Obituary. Susan C. Johnson. Occup Ther Rehabil 1932;11:152–153.

BOOKS BY E.C. SLAGLE

Robeson HA. Syllabus for Training of Nurses in Occupational Therapy. Utica, NY: The State Hospitals Press, 1923, 1925, 1933, and 1941.

Games and Field Day Program. Utica, NY: State Hospitals Press, 1933.

ARTICLES BY E.C. SLAGLE

History of the development of occupation for the insane. Md Psychiair Q 1914;4:14–20.

Something to do: the new medicine. Survey 1917;37:431–432.

The training of teachers of occupational therapy. Proceedings of the Second Annual Meeting of the National Society for the Promotion of Occupational Therapy, New York (abstract) 1918;2:52.

The department of occupational therapy. Inst Q 1919;10:29–32

Occupational therapy. NY State Conf Charities Corrections 1919;19:121–130.

To organize an "OT" department. Hosp Management 1921;15:43–45,80; Occup Ther Rehabil 1927;6:125–130.

Training aids for mental patients. State Hosp Q 7:167–174, 1922, and Arch Occup Ther 1922;1:11–17.

A year's development of occupational therapy in New York State Hospital. State Hosp Q 1923;8:590–603;Mod Hosp 1924;22:98–104.

Handicrafts used as treatment. Handicrafter 1928;1:26–27.

Occupational therapy. Soc Work Yearbook 1929;1:289–300; 1933;2:328–330; 1935;3: 297–298; 1937;4:298–300.

The training of occupational therapists. Psychiair Q 1931;5:12–20.

Occupational therapy: recent methods and advances in the U.S. Occup Ther Rehabil 1934;13:289–298.

The occupational therapy program in the state of New York. J Ment Sci 1934;80:639–649.

Editorial. From the heart. Occup Ther Rehabil 1937;16:343–345.

Occupational therapy. Trained Nurse Hosp Rev 1938;100:375–382.
The training of a therapist for work with mental patients. In: Moulton FR, Komora PO. Mental Health. Lancaster, PA: Science Press, 1939:408–415.

REFERENCES ABOUT E. C. SLAGLE
Eleanor Clarke Slagle. Psychiair Q January 1938;12(Suppl.):8–15.
Loomis B, Wade BD. Occupational Therapy Beginnings. Hull House, The Henry B. Favill School of Occupations and Eleanor Clarke Slagle. Chicago, University of Illinois (USPHS AH 50579–01), 1973.
Cromwell FS. Eleanor Clarke Slagle, the leader, the woman. Am J Occup Ther 1977;31: 645–648.
Editorial. Eleanor Clarke Slagle. Occup Ther Rehabil 1942;21:373–374.
Robeson HA. Eleanor Clarke Slagle. J Occup Ther Trial Issue P3–4, September 1937.
Pollack HM. In memoriam. Eleanor Clarke Slagle. Am J Psychiatry 1942–1943;99:473–474.
Komora P. Eleanor Clarke Slagle. Ment Hyg 1943;27:122–125.
Smith P. Memorial tribute to Mrs. Slagle, Psychiatric Quarterly Supplement 1943;17:43–45.
Eleanor Clarke Slagle. In: James ET, James JW, Boyer PS. Notable American Women 1607–1950. Cambridge: Belknap Press, 1971:296–298.

BOOKS BY S. E. TRACY
Studies in Invalid Occupation. Boston: Whitcomb & Barrows, 1910.
Rake Knitting and Its Special Adaptation to Invalid Workers. Boston: Whitcomb & Barrows, 1916.

ARTICLES BY S. E. TRACY
Some profitable occupations for invalids. Am J Nurs 1907–1908;8:172–177.
Occupational treatment for sick children. Pedagologic Semin 1909;16:457–458.
The place of invalid occupation in the general hospital. Mod Hosp 1914;2:386–387.
A three months' test of invalid occupations in a large general hospital. Md Psychiair Q 1916–1917;6:54–56.
The influence of hospital architecture on methods of occupational teaching. Proceedings of the First Annual Meeting of the National Society for the Promotion of Occupational Therapy, New York 1917;1:42–44 (plus 14 pgs of drawings).
Twenty-five suggested mental tests derived from invalid occupations. Md Psychiatr Q 1918;8:15–18.
Power versus money in occupational therapy. Trained Nurse Hosp Rev 1921;66:120–122.
Development of occupational therapy in the Grace Hospital. Trained Nurse Hosp Rev 1921;66:401–403.
Two practical suggestions for occupying desperate cases. Occup Ther Rehabil 1925;4: 181–183.
Getting started in occupational therapy. Trained Nurse Hosp Rev 1921;67:397–399.
Treatment of disease by employment at St. Elizabeth's Hospital. Mod Hosp 1923;20: 198–200.

REFERENCES ABOUT S. E. TRACY
Barrows M. Susan E. Tracy. R.N. Md Psychiair Q 1916–1917;6:57–62.
Parson SE. Miss Tracy's work in general hospitals. Md Psychiair Q 1916–1917;6:63–64.

Cameron RG. An interview with Miss Susan Tracy. Md Psychiatr Q 1916–1917;6:65.
Personalities from the past. Trained Nurse Hosp Rev 1928;1:582.
Brainerd W. The evolution of an occupational therapy department in a general hospital. Occup Ther Rehabil 1932;1:33–40.
Editorial. Susan E. Tracy. Occup Ther Rehabil 1929;8:63–65.
Shoe EC. Occupational therapy. Trained Nurse Hosp Rev 1938;100:375–382.

BOOKS BY T. B. KIDNER
Educational handwork. Toronto: Educational Book Co., 1910.
Notes on the tuberculosis sanatorium planning. Washington, DC: Government Printing Office (Public Health Reports no. 667), 1921.
Selecting a site for a tuberculosis sanatorium, with some remarks on plot plans. New York: National Tuberculosis Association, Technical series, no. 2, 1925.
Hamilton SW Buildings for the Tuberculous Insane. New York: National Tuberculosis Association, Technical series, no. 4, 1925.
Hamilton WI, Kidner TB. Advising the Tuberculosis About Employment. Baltimore: Williams & Wilkins, 1926.
Planning a Tuberculosis Sanatorium. New York, National Tuberculosis Association, 1926.
Frankel E, Kidner TB. The Care and Treatment of Nervous and Mental Patients in General Hospital. Trenton, NJ: Department of Institutions and Agencies, 1929.
Room, Ward and Porch Design and Equipment for Tuberculosis Hospitals and Sanatoria. New York: National Tuberculosis Association, 1929.
Occupational Therapy. The Science of Prescribed Workforce. Stuttgart, Germany: Invah & Kohihammer, 1930.

ARTICLES BY T. B. KIDNER
Vocational reeducation of the handicapped and incapacitated in Canada. Bull Nat Soc Vocat Educ 1918;27:39–46.
The vocational re-education of Canadian soldiers. American Industries 1917;18:16–20.
The return of the Canadian soldier to civil life. Conference of Social Work, 45th Annual Meeting 1918;45:10–17.
Vocational reeducation of the handicapped and incapacitated in Canada. Bulletin, National Society for Vocation Education 1918;27:39–46.
Guiding the disabled to a new job. Carry On 1918;1:17–21.
Vocational re-education of the handicapped and incapacitated in Canada. Bulletin of the National Society for Vocation Education 1918;27:39–46.
Notes on tuberculosis sanatorium planning. Public Health Reports 1921;36:1371–1395.
Accommodation for occupational therapy in federal tuberculosis sanatoriums. Mod Hosp 1922;18:292,294.
The relation of occupational therapy to vocational rehabilitation. Bulletin (Presbyterian Hospital, Chicago) 1922;49:8–12.
Work for the tuberculous during and after the cure. Arch Occup Ther 1922;1:363–376; 1924;3:169–193.
Occupational therapy in 1922. Mod Hosp 1923;20:43–45.
President's address. Arch Occup Ther 1923;2:415–424.

Planning for occupational therapy. Mod Hosp 1923;21:414–428; Am Architec 1923;123: 291–299.

Editorial. American Occupational Therapy Association. Arch Occup Ther 1922;1:499–502.

Reconstruction schemes in hospitals for mental and nervous diseases. State Hosp Q 1923;9:221–275; Arch Occup Ther 1924;3:117–120.

President's Address. Arch Occup Ther 1924;3:423–432.

Occupational therapy in 1923. Mod Hosp 1924;22:55–57.

Therapeutic versus selling value of occupational therapy work. Mod Hosp 1924;23:96,98.

The relation of occupational therapy to vocational rehabilitation. J Am Inst Homeopath 1924;17:577.

The hospital pre-industrial shop. Occup Ther Rehabit 1925;4:187–194; State Hosp Q 1925;10:445–453.

President's Address. Occup Ther Rehabil 1925;4:407–416.

Tendencies in sanatorium planning. Hospital Management 1925;19:30–33.

President's Address. Occup Ther Rehabil 1926;5:400–405.

Hamilton WI, Kidner TB: Vocational advisement and guidance. Occup Ther Rehabil 1926;5:267–276.

President's Address. Occup Ther Rehabil 1927;6:421–430.

Occupations for the tuberculous insane. Psychiatric Q 1927;1:344–351.

Professional training in occupational therapy. Psychiatr Q 1928;2:184–188.

President's Address. Occup Ther Rehabil 1929;8:1–10.

Standards in occupational therapy. Occup Ther Rehabil 1929;8:243–248.

Address to graduates. Occup Ther Rehabil 1929;8:379–386.

Importance of "refresher" work for individual and professional advancement. Psychiair Q 1929;3:389–403.

Presidential Address. Occup Ther Rehabil 1930;9:315–322.

Occupational therapy: its development, scope and possibilities. Occup Ther Rehabil 1931;10:1–12.

Occupational therapy and its relation to social service. Hosp Soc Serv 1931;24:311.

Aims and developments of occupational therapy. Occup Ther Rehabil 1932;11:233–239; Proceedings of the Annual Congress of Medical Education 1932;119–121.

Sanatorium planning. In: B Goldberg. Procedures in Tuberculosis Control, for the Dispensary, Home and Sanatorium. 2nd ed. Philadelphia: F.A. Davis Co., 1934.

REFERENCES ABOUT T. B. KIDNER

Addresses made at the memorial meeting for Thomas Bessell Kidner. Occup Ther Rehabil 1932;11:435–445.

Dunton WR Jr. Thomas Bessell Kidner. Am J Psychiatry 1932;89:194–196.

The late Thomas Bessell Kidner. Can Med Assoc J 1932;27:296–297.

Obituary. Occup Ther Rehabil 1932;11:321–323.

BOOKS BY W. R. DUNTON JR

Occupation Therapy: A Manual for Nurses. Philadelphia: Saunders, 1915.

Reconstruction Therapy. Philadelphia: Saunders, 1918.

Prescribing Occupational Therapy. Springfield, IL: Charles C Thomas, 1928 (revised 1945).

Dunion WR Jr, Licht S. Occupational Therapy. Principles and Practice. Springfield, IL: Charles C Thomas, 1950 (revised 1957).

ARTICLES BY W.R. DUNTON JR

A nurses' occupation course. Selected Proc Am Medico-Psychol Assoc 1912;19:269–278.

Occupation as a therapeutic measure. Med Rec 1913;83:388–389.

Should there be a recreation schedule? Proc Am Medico-Psychol Assoc 1915;22:337–342.

Occupation as a part of the nurses' training course. Md Psychiatr Q 1916;6:44–46.

The training of occupation teachers and directors. Md Psychiatr Q 1917;7:8–23.

History of occupational therapy. Mod Hosp 1917;8:380–382.

A plan for the organization of the re-educational facilities of a community. Proceedings of the First Annual Meeting National Society for the Promotion of Occupational Therapy 1917;1:52.

Rehabilitation of crippled soldiers and sailors—a review. Md Psychiatr Q 1918;7:85–102.

The principles of occupational therapy. Proceedings of the Second Annual Meeting National Society for the Promotion of Occupational Therapy 1918;2:26.

The principles of occupational therapy. Pub Health Nurse 1918;10:316–321.

Occupational therapy and tuberculosis. Med Rec 1919;95:941–944.

Problems in occupational therapy. Md Psychiair Q 1919;9:37.

Occupational therapy in state hospitals. Mod Hosp 1920;15:322–325.

The development of reconstruction therapy. Trained Nurse Hosp Rev 1921;67:16–21.

The passing of the Henry B. Faville School. Md Psychiair Q 1921;10:77–78.

Attendants for convalescents. Trained Nurse Hosp Rev 1922;69:301.

Educational possibilities of occupational therapy in state hospitals. Arch Occup Ther 1922;1:403–409.

Toy making as a therapeutic occupation. Arch Occup Ther 1923;2:39–42.

Financial charts. Arch Occup Ther 1923;2:198–202.

Round table on crafts best suited for the mental and nervous. Arch Occup Ther 1923;2:221–223.

Address delivered at the opening of the new assembly hall at Manhattan State Hospital, December 15, 1923. Arch Occup Ther 1924;3:21–33.

Occupational therapy for the general practitioner. Arch Occup Ther 1924;3:205–210.

Music cataloging. With Helen F. Carleton. Arch Occup Ther 1924;3:289–294.

The need for and the value of research in occupational therapy. Occup Ther Rehabil 1934;13:325–328.

Relationship of occupational therapy and physical therapy. Arch Phys Ther 1935;16:19–22.

Economic studies of crafts. Occup Ther Rehabil 1925;4:219,441; 1926;5:135,293.

An historical note. Occup Ther Rehabil 1926;5:427–439.

How mental patients react to color and a homelike atmosphere. Mod Hosp 1927;28:106.

The "three R's" of occupational therapy. Occup Ther Rehabil 1928;7:345; Bull Mass Assoc Occup Ther September 1928.

Museum meanderings. I, Occup Ther Rehabil 1930;9:103; VI, 1930;9:153; VII 1930; 9:293; X, 1931;10:343; XI, 1931;10:393.

Quilts and quilting. With Edna H. Dunton. Occup Ther Rehabil 1930;9:159.

The tale of a hooked rug. Hosp Soc Serv 1930;22:87.

Occupational Therapy: Read at meeting of the Mississippi Valley Sanatorium Assoc., Oct. 14, 1930. Occup Ther Rehabil 1930;4:343.

Occupational Therapy: Read before Annual Congress on Medical Education, Licensure and Hospitals, Chicago, Ill., Feb. 1931;16–18; Occup Ther Rehabil 1931;10:113–121; JAMA 1931;96:1879.

Convalescence. Hosp Soc Serv 1931;24:232; reprinted in Ir Nurs News October. 1931.

Occupational therapy. In: Pemberton R. Hagerstown, MD: Principles and Practice of Physical Therapy Prior Co., 1935:1–48.

Coordination of rehabilitation processes for the physically and mentally handicapped. Occup Ther Rehabil 1934;13:175.

Progress in occupational therapy. Hospitals 1936;10:89.

Quilt making as a socializing measure. Address before 12th Institute of Chief Occupational Ther apists, N.Y. State Dept. Mental Hygiene, March 3, 1937; Western N.Y. O.T. Assn., May 28, 1937. Occup Ther Rehabil 1937;16:275.

Occupational therapy in private sanitaria of the United States. 2me Congress des Maisons de Sante Prives, Paris, July 12–17, 1937.

Evaluation of occupational therapy. Occup Ther Rehabil 1937;16:315.

The Craftmart of Baltimore. Occup Ther Rehabil 1938;17:159.

Occupational therapy. Therapeutics of Internal Diseases. New York, Appleton-Century Co., 1940:389–433.

Occupational therapy. In: Modem Medical Therapy in General Practice. Baltimore: Williams & Wilkins, 1940:695–710.

Round table at Cincinnati. Occup Ther Rehabil 1940;19:265.

Round table at Richmond, Va. Occup Ther Rehabil 1941;20:259.

How I got that way. Occup Ther Rehabil 1943;22:244.

Scrapbooks. Occup Ther Rehabil 1945;24:97.

Chintz work. Occup Ther Rehabil 1946;25:14.

Old Quilts. Published by the author, 1946.

Editorial. Specialization. Am J Occup Ther 1952;6:215.

Editorial. Terminology. Am J Occup Ther 1953;7:177.

Today's principles, reflected in early literature. Am J Occup Ther 9:17–18, 1955.

REFERENCES ABOUT W.R. DUNTON JR

Licht S. William Rush Dunton, Jr. Occup Ther Rehabil 1947;26:47–52.

Tribute to Dr. Dunton. Am J Occup Ther 1958;12:150–151.

A tribute to William Rush Dunton Jr, MD. Am J Occup Ther 1960;14:140–149.

Bing RK. William Rush Dunton, Jr., American psychiatrist and occupational therapist. Am J Occup Ther 1967;21:172–175.

Occupational Therapy
and Society

EARLY INPATIENT SERVICES—1906–1916

Occupational therapy got its current impetus in the early part of the twentieth century when workers in long-term care facilities, such as state psychiatric hospitals and tuberculosis sanitariums, observed that patients engaging in some occupation or activity were less restless and seemed to do better than when they were lying or sitting with nothing to do. Among these observers were a nurse, Susan E. Tracy; a social work student, Eleanor Clarke Slagle; and a psychiatrist, William R. Dunton Jr.

Miss Tracy began using occupations in conjunction with nursing in 1905 when she started working at Adams Nervine Asylum, a psychiatric facility. She stressed the need for occupations to be selected individually for each patient based on the patient's condition and interest. Furthermore, she believed that all use of occupations should be ordered by a physician and carried out by a qualified person (1).

Mrs. Slagle became interested in the use of occupations while observing patients in Kankakee State Hospital, a mental institution, as a social work trainee at the Chicago School of Civics and Philanthropy. Two of her instructors, Jane Addams, who founded Hull House, and Julia Lathrop, encouraged her to attend a summer course in occupations for hospital attendants in 1911. Two years later, in 1913, Dr. Adolph Meyer, a psychiatrist, asked her to accompany him to the new Phipps Psychiatric Clinic at Johns Hopkins Hospital in Baltimore. There she developed her own technique of occupational therapy called "habit training," which was most successful with chronic regressed schizophrenics (2). Because drugs such as tranquilizers were unknown and electric shock was not used until the 1940s, treatment for schizophrenics consisted of locking the patients on the wards and using hydrotherapy, in which water was heated to body temperature and the patient submerged to the neck. Mrs. Slagle suggested that a regressed patient should be placed on a 24-hour schedule of planned activities in which self-care was stressed. Each patient was required to get up, toilet, wash, dress, eat using proper table manners, clean up the ward, make beds, do basic craft activities such as tearing rags or winding yarn, and go for walks. The aim was to stimulate the patient toward resuming and maintaining contact with the environment.

As the patient improved, ward occupations, such as weaving, sewing, embroidery, and wood and leather work, were begun for the purpose of winning social approval and discharging emotion into constructive activity. In the third step, the patient went to the occupational therapy center or clinic, where a greater variety of projects and equipment was available. The purpose was to continue socialization and emotional control while discovering aptitudes and interests. Finally, the patient moved to the preindustrial or prevocational area, where work attitudes and tolerance were assessed as well as the aims.

The technique was successful in getting many patients out of the "back wards" for "hopeless" patients in the state hospitals of New York. Habit training continued to be popular until the 1940s when other treatment techniques, such as electric shock and the drug reserpine, became popular. In many ways, the milieu therapy and group-living drug treatment approaches use the concept of a graded habit training program.

Dr. William R. Dunton Jr was a young psychiatrist at Sheppard and Enoch Pratt Hospital when he began exploring the use of occupations with patients under the direction of the superintendent, Dr. Edward N. Brush. First, a printing press was installed and then basketry, metal work, and card games were added. In 1908, a teacher, Miss Grace Fields, was hired to provide instruction in occupational therapy. After she resigned for health reasons, Dr. Dunton began a course of instruction for nurses in the fall of 1911. Instruction was given in the use of games, string work, paper folding and cutting, binding, crepe paper, basketry, embroidery, leather, wood, and metal. This instructional sequence is presented in detail in the book *Occupation Therapy,* published in 1915.

Dr. Dunton believed that in addition to instructing nurses, physicians should become aware of occupational therapy. Beginning in 1912, he helped organize a sectional meeting of members of the American Medico-Psychological Association to discuss the use of occupations and training courses in mental institutions. Also, as an editor for the Maryland *Psychiatric Quarterly,* he began a department entitled "Occupations and Amusements" to "discuss, gossip or talk" about the various forms of occupation and amusement.

Dr. Dunton also was concerned that occupational therapy had become a more exact science and had proven its efficacy as a treatment for both mental and physical disabilities. Therefore, he began to formulate the first principles of occupational therapy. The nine principles are as follows:

1. That work should be carried on with cure as the main object;
2. That work must be interesting;
3. The patient should be carefully studied;
4. That one form of occupation should not be carried to the point of fatigue;
5. That it should have some useful end;
6. That it preferably should lead to an increase in the patient's knowledge;

7. That it should be carried on with others;
8. That possible encouragement should be given to the worker; and
9. That work resulting in a poor or useless product is better than idleness. (3)

These principles are still valid today, although they could be updated to reflect greater knowledge and the modem approach:

1. The occupations (activities) should be selected to achieve the goals and objectives of the management plan.
2. The occupations should be selected with the client's interest in mind.
3. The client should be thoroughly assessed at the beginning and throughout the program.
4. Precautions, such as fatigue, should be observed at all times and occupations stopped whenever precautions indicate.
5. All occupations should be purposeful and result in a useful end product when possible.
6. Occupations should be selected that will increase the client's knowledge, ability, and skill.
7. Participation in group activity should be encouraged.
8. Clients should be given encouragement and praise throughout their program.
9. The quality of the end product is not as important as the person's willingness to try.

EARLY OUTPATIENT SERVICES—1906–1916

Not all persons interested in the use of occupations were interested in inpatient programs. Dr. Herbert J. Hall, a general practitioner, and George Barton, an architect with tuberculosis, set up workshops for convalescents, which might be called the first sheltered workshops.

Dr. Hall received a grant of $31,000 from the Proctor fund of Harvard University in 1906 "to assist in the study of the treatment of neurasthenia by progressive and graded manual occupation" (4). Neurasthenia was a general term applied to cases of nervous exhaustion. With the fund money, Dr. Hall started a workshop and Devereux Mansion in Marblehead, Massachusetts. Here he used handweaving, woodcarving, metal work, and pottery as the major occupations. Of the first 100 cases, he reported that 59 had improved, 27 were much improved, and 14 had no relief. His guiding ideas were to teach the patient "to economize strength-to do deliberately and without undue excitement what simple manual work may be deemed advisable" and to divide the "twenty-four hours into changeable periods of work, rest and recreation, plenty of air, wholesome food, wise suggestions and such medical treatment as may be indicated" (4). Dr. Hall understood the concepts of work efficiency and a balanced schedule of activity.

Dr. Hall later wrote three books about his knowledge and use of occupational therapy. These books are: *The Work of our Hands*, 1915; *Handicrafts for the Handicapped*, 1916; and *O.T.: A New Profession*, 1923.

Mr. Barton, whose life and work is described in Chapter 28, was the founder of Consolation House located in Clifton Springs, New York. He started the workshop in 1914 after he had been at the Clifton Spring Sanatorium as a tuberculosis patient. Consolation House was described as a school, workshop, and vocational bureau for the convalescents who wanted to be away from the hospital and, at the same time, learn something of value (5). Mr. Barton worked out most of the therapy ideas himself using his own disability as a teaching situation. The major occupations he used were gardening, woodworking, and drawing plans for projects.

Patients came as Mr. Barton's medical friends observed the improvement in his own health. They stayed upstairs in the house and went to a converted barn behind the house for woodworking. The garden was next door. Consolation House existed until Mr. Barton's death in 1923.

In summary, these early leaders did much to advance the cause and concept of occupational therapy. Each worked largely in isolation, however, until Mr. Barton called them together in March 1917. Thereafter, more coordination and sharing of information was possible through the annual meetings that provided a forum for presenting papers and encouraged visits to other facilities where occupational therapy was being practiced. Also, there was a rapid expansion of printed information about occupational therapy in books and through articles in the *Maryland Psychiatric Quarterly, Modem Hospital, Trained Nurse and Hospital Review* and others.

RECONSTRUCTION AIDES—1918

In March 1918, four women sailed to France to help the sick soldiers get back on their feet and back to fighting the war. These women had no rank in the Army, no uniform, and no specific duties. They went as civilian aides, a classification for scrub women because the Army authorities could not comprehend what occupational therapy was, according to Dr. Frankwood E. Williams (6). They made their own uniforms of brightly colored smocks and took many of their own supplies and equipment. Only one could have been said to have some occupational therapy training. Mrs. Clyde Myers had studied several arts and crafts at Columbia University and worked for a few months in the occupational therapy department at Bloomingdale Hospital, a New York state psychiatric facility. The other three people included Laura LaForce, a nurse who had taught basketry and weaving in the New York City Hospital for children; Corrine Dezellor, from Columbia University, who had taught woodworking in special education class in New York; and Amy Drenenstredt, who taught art history at Hunter College and was skilled in design and color (6).

These four women were assigned to Base Hospital 117 near the Voges Mountains near La Frauche, France. The hospital treated war neurosis and "shell shock" victims who could not adjust to military situations. Treatment of such cases was fairly new in military history and Dr. Sidney L. Schwab, the medical director of Base 117, says that "an attempt was made to treat them with all the methods that were in vogue" (7). Occupational therapy just barely qualified as being "in vogue." If a few physicians had not pushed, the Army would not have sought the women at all.

The women set up their clinic in a barracks 20 × 100 feet. Two other tenants were installed already. A Red Cross Supervisor of Gardens had one end and the hospital carpenter had the other. Occupational therapy got the center. The women started scrubbing to clean the area and set up their equipment. Male patients watched but soon began to help by solving problems such as how to get work benches and chairs and a furnace without military requisitions that might never come. The answers came from the dump heaps of old French beds and tin cans from the kitchen. The beds made work benches and the cans lined salvaged bricks for the furnace. The tin cans also were used to make candle holders, toys, decorate bookends, and other projects. All patients were treated equally and were not allowed to "pull rank" in the clinic. A democratic environment prevailed. The clinic was a success in helping return soldiers' concentration and confidence in their ability to perform. Within a few weeks, Dr. Salmon, chief of the psychiatric division in France, asked for more aides. Finally, the surgeon general of the A.E.F., under General Pershing's signature said, "Send over a thousand of these aides as soon as you can get them ready" (6). This request came as a result of the work done at Base 117.

When the United States entered the war, the field of reconstruction aides was created officially. These aides included both physiotherapists and occupational therapists. An announcement appeared in the September 1918 issue of Carry On, a military publication stating the qualifications and asking for 2000 more aides to go abroad (8). Applicants in occupational therapy were divided into three classes. Class A included expertise in social work, library service, or academic subjects. Class B was for teachers or craftsmen of arts and crafts. Class C was a general category of information on administrative procedures and programs. Applicants were to have unusual strength of character, be able to do hard and serious work, be willing to spend long hours working if necessary, to forego luxuries of normal life, to subordinate personal interests to the good of the service, and to cooperate with other medical personnel. Personal qualifications listed were knowledge and skill of occupation, attractive and forceful personality, teaching ability, sympathy, tact, judgment, industry ingenuity, and cleverness in adapting work to prevailing conditions. All of these qualifications would seem to be as necessary today as during World War I.

In reality, many occupational therapy recruits did not serve abroad because the war ended in November 1918, and most soldiers were sent home. Only 116 arrived in France before the armistice was signed. Some had little previous training, according to Mrs. Myers, but they did the best they could.

Other reconstruction aides served in the Army hospitals in the United States. They built up the knowledge and skills of occupational therapy in physical disabilities as well as psychiatry and tuberculosis.

Walter Reed General Hospital started an occupational therapy department in February 1918 under the direction of Bird T. Baldwin, a psychologist. Mr. Baldwin learned quickly about occupational therapy and gives a good account of his understanding of occupational therapy in spite of his lack of specific training. He states that the purpose of occupational therapy "is to help each patient find himself and function again as a complete man, physically, socially, educationally and economically . . ." (9). Furthermore, occupational therapy "is based on the principle that the best type of remedial exercise is that which requires a series of specific voluntary movements involved in the ordinary trades or occupations, physical training, play, or the daily routine activities of life" (9). Mr. Baldwin set as a goal: to isolate, classify, and standardize the type of movements involved in particular occupational and recreational activities.

Dr. Wilson H. Henderson at Fort McHenry, Maryland, also pioneered in applying occupational therapy to physical disabilities. He felt that occupations for disabled men should require technical rather than physical strength, mental activity should be greater than physical, and the occupation should afford some exercise needed by a particular patient to stimulate recovery (10).

The reconstruction aides who worked for these men and others helped develop occupational therapy as a treatment for traumatic injuries. Their techniques were sound according to modern knowledge, but the practice of occupational therapy in physical disabilities did not flourish much beyond the war. The problem was not so much a fault of occupational therapy as of medicine, which had not developed the techniques to save the lives of polio victims or seriously injured patients, such as spinal cord–injured patients. Life-saving techniques for polio and spinal cord injuries would not be known until World War II. In civilian life, after World War I, there were not enough fractures, amputations, or peripheral nerve injuries to require many hospitals to hire occupational therapists for those with physical disabilities. A summary of occupational therapy practice as late as spring 1937 by the American Medical Association showed that 36 occupational therapists were employed in orthopedic facilities and 456 in general hospitals whereas 809 were employed in mental hospitals (11).

EARLY SCHOOLS OF OCCUPATIONAL THERAPY—1906–1920

The first courses in occupational therapy probably were little more than the equivalent of a two-credit or three-credit college laboratory course with a one-credit lecture course. According to the chronological record provided by Dr. Dunton, Susan Tracy is credited with offering the first of these courses in the summer of 1906 to nursing students (12). The course consisted of 10 lessons, each involving a different case study for which the nurse was to think of a suitable activity and make a sample. These lessons, which are summarized in her book *Studies in Invalid Occupations,* could make good learning sessions if used today.

The next course of record was offered by Julia Lathrop and Rabbi Hirsch at the Chicago School of Civics and Philanthropy, an institution for training social workers that was founded by Graham Taylor. This first course was given from July 7 to August 7 in 1908, with the assistance of state funds, to attendants of psychiatric facilities. Attendants were to learn how to "re-stimulate by occupation instruction and amusement" (13). Mrs. Slagle recorded that the students were not particularly enthusiastic because nursing was their primary interest. Even when social service workers were added to the student body the next year, interest was not keen. Finally, when technically trained persons enrolled—persons who had insight into social economics and philanthropy and a desire to serve—then interest increased (14).

Dr. William R. Dunton gave a course at Sheppard and Enoch Pratt Hospital in Towson, Maryland, in the fall of 1911 (12). He, just as Tracy, also had 10 lesson plans. However, his were concerned with specific media, not case studies. The media included games, string work, paper folding and cutting, book binding, crepe paper work, reed basketry, embroidery, leather work, woodwork, and metal work. The other course was given by Reba G. Cameron, Superintendent of Nurses at Taunton State Hospital. No information on the course itself is available.

The first course to be given in a university was offered the same year at Teacher's College, Columbia University (15). The course was called Invalid Occupations and was a nursing elective given for 3 hours each week. There were lectures, practical work, and demonstrations. The first teacher was Evelyn Collins, a kindergarten teacher with postgraduate training in manual and industrial arts and experience in working with psychiatric patients. In 1916, Susan C. Johnson, a founding member of the AOTA, started lecturing.

Probably the first real course of study in occupational therapy was given at the Henry B. Favill School of Occupations in Chicago.

HENRY B. FAVILL SCHOOL OF OCCUPATIONS

The Henry B. Favill School of Occupations of the Illinois Society for Mental Hygiene was stared in 1914 but was renamed for Dr. Favill in 1917 (16). Dr. Favill was a Chicago physician interested in social issues. The department was started "to serve as a clearinghouse for cases of doubtful insanity which the courts considered as showing promise of return to usefulness if given a proper environment and trade" (16). In 1918, a program of study titled Special Courses in Curative Occupations and Recreation was offered by the Chicago School of Civics and Philanthropy in cooperation with the School (17). Each course of study ran 6 months, covering two terms. Technical work was offered in the mornings at Hull House where Mrs. Slagle was also general superintendent of occupational therapy. Lectures were given in the afternoon at the Chicago

School of Civics and Philanthropy. Technical courses included kinesiology, department organization, folk dancing, gymnastics, games, and handwork (crafts). Lectures related to the administration of institutions, principles of case work, psychology of play, and others. Students had 33 hours of class per week plus 2 to 3 hours of practice work.

The school provided many of the reconstruction aides for World War I as well as occupational therapists for the Midwest area. After the war, there was a drop in enrollment. Mrs. Slagle took a position as executive secretary for the New York Society for Occupational Therapy in early 1920 (18). The school was then moved to the state hospital in Dunning but was never reopened.

OTHER PIONEER SCHOOLS

The founding of the National Society for the Promotion of Occupational Therapy and World War I provided the impetus for more schools to open. In 1918, four schools started that were to play an important role in training occupational therapists. Two are still active today in Boston and St. Louis. These schools were located at Milwaukee Downer College, the Philadelphia School of Occupational Therapy, the Boston School of Occupational Therapy, and the St. Louis School of Occupational Therapy. The school at Milwaukee Downer College, founded in September 1918 by Elizabeth Upham Davis and Charlotte R. Partridge, developed a model program for occupational therapy as others moved into colleges and universities (19, 20). In 1931, Milwaukee Downer offered the first baccalaureate degree in occupational therapy (21). Discontinued in 1972, the program at Milwaukee Downer was moved to Lawrence University in Appleton, Wisconsin; this was eventually discontinued in 1975.

The Philadelphia School of Occupational Therapy was started by Florence Willsman Fulton (22). It was incorporated in 1923 as a nonprofit organization. However, students took some courses at the University of Pennsylvania. Finally, in 1950, the school was accepted into the university. Helen Willard was the director for many years. She and Clare Spackman coauthored the first comprehensive textbook on occupational therapy in 1947 (23). The school was among the first group accredited by the AMA and the AOTA in 1938; nonetheless, the school was discontinued in 1981.

The Boston School of Occupational Therapy began in April 1918 to give 12-week classes in occupational therapy as part of the war emergency program (24). It was incorporated in 1921 and later became affiliated with Tufts University. The first principals were Marjorie B. Green and Ruth Wigglesworth, both of whom served as chairpersons of the AOTA Committee on Teaching Methods. Dr. Herbert J. Hall helped plan the school with Dr. John D. Adams. However, in 1986, Tufts phased out the undergraduate program. The graduate program continues.

The St. Louis School of Occupational and Recreational Therapy began in December 1918 under the direction of the Missouri Association of Occupational

Therapy. Alice H. Dean, a graduate of the Henry B. Favill School of Occupations, was the director (25). The school was affiliated with the Washington University School of Medicine from the beginning. It was accredited in 1938. Many other schools came and went. At least 29 schools were known in addition to the ones cited here (26).

INDUSTRIAL REHABILITATION ACT—1920

In 1920, Congress passed the Industrial Rehabilitation Act, also called the Smith Bankhead or Smith Fess Act (27). The purpose of the act was to promote vocational rehabilitation of persons disabled in industry. Within a year, 23 states established services under this act (28).

The act helped occupational therapy by recognizing the value of rehabilitation services and promoting the use of prevocational training as part of rehabilitation. Occupational therapy services could not be paid for specifically under the act, but occupational therapists could work in programs. There is no record of how many occupational therapists were employed through the act, but Mr. Kidner acknowledged the contribution in his report of 1923 (29). He stated that the impetus given by this act had led to the study of the possibilities of curative work by many officers in state departments. The veterans' hospitals and other federal institutions also used the provisions of the act to develop or expand their occupational therapy personnel.

THE 1930s

The Depression—1930–1939

During the Depression from 1930 through the start of World War II in 1939, the development of occupational therapy slowed down. Membership in the Association leveled off to approximately 860 to 960. The number of schools decreased from 17 in 1926 to 11 in 1935 (29, 30).

The Depression caused many departments to close or to lay off therapists. Money for supplies and equipment became more scarce. Use of recycled and waste materials became the rule. Because accurate records were not kept, the real impact of the Depression cannot be measured, but some well-known facilities closed the doors of the occupational therapy departments. Presbyterian Hospital in Chicago, whose occupational therapy department was started by Susan Tracy, closed in 1932.

However, the Depression did not stop all activity. In 1932, the registration of occupational therapists was begun (31). There were 318 names in the main registry. In 1935, accreditation of occupational therapy training programs was started, with five programs in the United States being accredited in 1938 (32). These were the Boston School of Occupational Therapy, Milwaukee Downer College, Philadelphia School of Occupational Therapy, St. Louis School of Occupational Therapy and Recreational Therapy, and Kalamazoo State Hospital School of Occupational Therapy. Both the registration of occupational therapists and the accreditation of educational programs increased the visibility of occupational therapy in society as a recognized discipline and developing profession. The next surge of activity would be the result of World War II.

THE 1940s

World War II—1940–1947

When the United States entered World War II, occupational therapy personnel in the military were in very short supply. Occupational therapists had elected not to seek military status after WWI because they could earn more money as civilians and had more freedom (33). As civilians, they were paid by a special fund under the control of each military hospital's post commander. During the Depression, most of the positions in occupational therapy were discontinued; thus, only 12 occupational therapists were working in the Army hospitals in December 1941 (34). Probably fewer were working in Navy hospitals and none were employed in the Air Force. Army personnel were classified as subprofessionals under the division of Trades and Industries. People were hired on the basis of their knowledge of arts and crafts. No educational requirements or certification standards were needed (33).

When the United States entered the war, the War Department did establish requirements for occupational therapists to be graduates of accredited schools of occupational therapy. However, the demand for occupational therapists was greater than the supply. Educational requirements took 21 months to complete, which was too long to wait for the therapists to be of assistance (35). Therefore, War Emergency Courses (WECs) were established to meet the demand. Students for WECs were required to have a baccalaureate degree in industrial art, education, home economics, or fine arts. They received 4 months' academic training and 8 months' fieldwork experience in the Army (36). Approximately 600 to 700 persons were trained by July 1946 in eight accredited schools. There were 375 occupational therapists employed in 85 Army hospitals (37).

The Navy did not provide any shortened courses. All occupational therapists were graduates of regular courses. Approximately 75 occupational therapists were employed as reserve officers in the WAVES (34).

Both the Army and Navy trained assistants to work with the occupational therapists (37). These people became the group to give impetus to the development and creation of the certified occupational therapy assistant.

In 1947, the Army, Navy, and Air Force granted permanent status to occupational therapists and other allied health personnel to ensure that personnel would be available to work with enlisted and retired service people (38). The Army established the Women's Medical Specialist Corps, the Navy created a Medical Service Corp, and the Air Force enacted a Women's Medical Specialist Corp. These Armed Service Units continue to employ occupational therapists today.

Veterans' Administration Hospitals

Although the Veterans' Administration hospitals had employed occupational therapists since before the beginning of the VA system in 1921, most had been in psychiatric or tuberculosis units (39). After World War II, departments of Physical Medicine and Rehabilitation (PM and R) were created. Occupational therapists were employed in PM and R to provide services to service veterans physically. Also, many veterans' administration (VA) hospitals began accepting fieldwork students for physical dysfunction rotations. Attractive salaries and federal benefits also encouraged occupational therapists to in VA facilities (34).

Physical Rehabilitation in the 1940s

In 1941, Elizabeth Kenny, an Australian nurse, demonstrated her methods of treating persons with infectious poliomyelitis, which is also called infantile paralysis or polio. Initially, her methods were scorned by the American Medical Association, but a year later, the *Journal of the American Medical Association* endorsed her system (40). Facilities began adopting and modifying the Kenny method. Interest in rehabilitation grew and, in turn, attention was focused on physical and occupational therapy. Soon thereafter, money from the National Foundation for Infantile Paralysis was available to train therapists under Kenny's direction in Minneapolis. Partly as a result of Kenny's insistence that careful records be kept of muscle strength and joint range, many new evaluation and recording methods were begun (41). The public interest in polio, which was heightened during the polio epidemic, further augmented the support and interest of the treatment of persons with physical disabilities. Thus, polio treatment contributed to the maintained interest in physical disabilities after the war injuries had been treated and the service people were sent home.

Sidney Licht, a physician and editor of *Occupational Therapy and Rehabilitation,* probably helped recognition of the treatment of physical disabilities by suggesting the terms kinetic treatment and metric occupational therapy (42). Kinetic treatment included muscle strengthening, joint mobilization, and coordination training. These were the principal aims in the treatment of polio. Metric treatment included increasing the amount of work completed in a unit of time or the number of times an activity was completed in a calendar unit. These terms became part of the classification of occupational therapy in most VA hospitals.

Another diagnosis that gained considerable attention in the 1940s was cerebral palsy. Winthrop M. Phelps, a physician, developed a method of treatment that stressed teaching children to perform activities of daily living independently to develop a dominant preferred hand (43). As a result, occupational therapists became more skilled in analyzing the steps in the sequence of an activity—such as self-feeding—and in making adaptations of the equipment—such as bending a spoon handle to decrease its angle and tilt in relation to the bowl of the spoon.

The attention to developing dominance initiated the exploration of adapted equipment for typing and writing. Guards were developed to place on the keys and the space bar to prevent unwanted keys from being depressed. Games were adapted to develop shoulder and hand coordination, such as enlarging a checkerboard and making handles for the checkers.

All of these developments in occupational therapy practice helped enlarge the image of occupational therapy as being more than just arts and crafts. The scope of occupational therapy was seen as more than diversified. Unfortunately, the public still saw the arts and crafts products for sale, and the number of hospitals with occupational therapy departments was only 13% (44).

More School—1939–1949

The largest expansion in occupational therapy during the 1940s was in the number of schools. In 1939, there were 5 but by 1945, there were 17 accredited schools and 3 awaiting accreditation (37). Enrollment in the accredited schools was 1410, and in the new schools, 153. By 1949, there were 25 accredited schools in 17 different states (34). Most of the programs were in the New England, upper north central, or far western states. Only two southern states, Virginia and Texas, were represented. Minnesota, Iowa, and Colorado were as far west as the schools were located until the states of California and Washington were reached. Thus, the sources of occupational therapy personnel were unequally distributed at best. Where schools were established, the practice of occupational therapy increased. Where no schools existed, the practice of occupational therapy was usually spotty, and frequently, facilities went for many years without an occupational therapist.

THE 1950s

Plastics and Bioengineering

The treatment of physical dysfunction problems improved greatly when new plastics, fiberglass, and lighter weight metals became available. Flexible plastics permitted the early development of temporary orthotic devices, such as splints for the forearm, wrist, and hand (45). However, the plastics had to be heated to high temperatures and were brittle, which caused breakage. Getting a good fit to the hand was also a problem because the plastic was too hot to place flesh against.

Fiberglass was also used to make splints (46). The fiberglass resin was embedded into a special cardboard to strengthen and hold the cardboard into the desired shape. The process produced an elastic splint. A better fit could be obtained, which was an improvement. However, the fiberglass resin produced very toxic fumes and was flammable. Usually, clients could not be in the room during the time a splint was being made. Furthermore, the splint needed to dry for 24 hours before the resin had set enough to permit the splint to be worn.

Metals such as stainless steel and aluminum were used to make more permanent forms of splints and various adapted devices. Persons with a chronic hand disability could have a hand splint that would last for several years (47). Upper extremity braces were developed also to assist in eating and other daily life tasks (48).

Neuroleptic Drugs

In 1952, the drugs known as tranquilizers were used to treat mental disorders (49). These psychotropic drugs brought about a fundamental change in psychiatric treatment. First tested in the Veterans' Administration Hospitals, the acceptance of tranquilizers or phenothiazine drugs started and rapid development of drug therapy as a means of changing or altering behavior. Drugs made possible the concept of chemical restraints on behavior instead of mechanical and physical restraints. For the first time, large numbers of institutionalized psychiatric patients could be housed on open wards instead of closed, locked wards. Also, many patients could be released to other facilities or to home communities. The result was a dramatic decrease in the number of patients in state institutions and a corresponding decrease in the length of time patients were confined. No longer was the state psychiatric institution a lifelong sentence for people with mental health problems.

However, the drugs did not provide the answer for all mental health problems. Not all patients could make the transition from institution to community. They did not have the life skills to function independently in the community. Some patients may have never developed the tasks and others lost skills or had not updated their skills to modern times. For example, one person may have never learned to drive a car whereas another may have never driven on a modern freeway, which may require a right-hand turn to go left. Such lack of living skills cannot be corrected by drugs alone. The person must learn the skills to function in society.

Polio Vaccine

In 1954 and 1955, Jonas Salk and Albert Sabin perfected vaccines that prevented poliomyelitis epidemics (50). After the epidemics were over, the interest in rehabilitation again decreased because public attention was diverted to other vaccines for childhood diseases that did not require rehabilitation services. In clinics today, acute cases of polio are rarely seen. Postpolio patients may be seen for continuing problems in adjustment to disability or for problems not related to polio, such as strokes.

Prevocational Exploration and Training

Another byproduct of the polio era was the large number of persons who needed different vocations or jobs because of changes in functional ability. In partial response to the need, occupational therapists as well as vocational counselors began to provide simulated work environments, work samples, and on-the-job training situations. Tests were developed also to measure speed and accuracy of performance as well as to compare handicapped performance to normal performance.

Simulated work environments could be provided in the occupational therapy clinic itself. The stress was in performing an assigned task with acceptable work habits (51). Attendance, promptness, ability to follow directions, interactions with coworkers, length of time worked, and speed and accuracy could be assessed. Such information was helpful to the individual in measuring performance potential and could be forwarded to a vocational counselor as general information.

Work samples were used by occupational therapists to determine specific job skill potential. The TOWER system was developed by the Institute for the Crippled and Disabled in New York City. The test consisted of 13 different occupational work samples, including drafting, electronics assembly, mail clerking, performing receptionist duties, and welding (52). Based on the performance on the work sample, clients could be referred to vocational training centers.

On-the-job training situations were easy to provide in large institutions. Clients could gain work experience in skills, such as housekeeping, dietary, maintenance, clerical, secretarial, librarian, accounting, and messenger service while still in the facility (53). Sometimes such on-the-job experience led to a job in the community or provided a good work reference. Other times the on-the-job training provided a basic training situation that would lead to more specific work training in a vocational training center.

Prevocational exploration and training became the glamour area of practice in the later 1950s and early 1960s. Workshops on prevocational issues were well attended and most clinics set up some type of prevocational program. No specific issue diminished the interest in prevocational practice, but as health care swung toward acute and short-term care there simply was not time to provide prevocational exploration and training.

THE 1960s

Group Process and Community Mental Health

In 1953, a British psychiatrist, Maxwell Jones, wrote a book about treating psychiatric patients as a therapeutic community in which the group was used as a behavioral change unit (54). Near the same time, the National Training Laboratory in Bethel, Maine began training professionals to lead groups of patients in activity tasks rather than as talk groups only. Occupational therapists became interested in the activity group approach to mental health problems in the

1960s. Groups were used extensively as a treatment modality with psychiatric patients to increase interpersonal skills, reality orientation, and functional independence (55). Some groups of clients with physical disabilities were used also to increase participation in basic exercise programs and support speech communication.

Grouping patients together was not new to occupational therapy. Occupational therapists had been used to having several people together in the clinic for many years. What was new was the use of a group itself as a therapeutic agent. Such use required that the size of the group be limited to approsimately 8 to 12 people, that the dynamic interactions of the members to recognized and explored, and that a task or activity be involved (55). The problems were the rapid change of patients in the acute settings, which reduced the stability of group interaction, and the institutions' administrators who wanted occupational therapists to see all patients without concern for individualizing the program.

In spite of the problems, group process workshops became popular during the 1960s and a class in group process soon became required subject matter for all occupational therapy students. Interest in task groups also increased the visibility of occupational therapists practicing in mental health and psychiatry.

A second approach that held promise for occupational therapists in psychiatry was the move to treat mental health problems in the home community rather than in large institutions located many miles away. In 1963, the Community Mental Health and Mental Retardation Act was passed by Congress. The purpose was to provide community-based treatment centers. The concept of community mental centers appealed to occupational therapists because functional occupations and skills could be developed, improved, or restored in the person's living arena (56). Simulation would be performed as well as real events.

Unfortunately, the community mental health approach did not work as well for occupational therapist as had been hoped. Community mental health centers did not employ many professionals but preferred paraprofessionals and became more concerned with dispensing drugs than in providing activity programs.

Medicare/Medicaid Legislation

In 1965, Titles 18 and 19 were added to the Social Security Administration Act. The popular titles were Medicare and Medicaid. Medicare is a federally sponsored and administered insurance program for persons 65 years of age or older. Medicaid is a federally sponsored health care program but administered by the states for needy persons with low income.

Occupational therapy is a covered service under Medicare for inpatients when treatment is part of a total program prescribed by a physician (57). Outpatient coverage was available if nursing, physical therapy, or speech pathology was needed also (57). Medicare thus provided expanded opportunities for occupational therapists to service the elderly, especially those who had had strokes, atherosclerosis, and other chronic disorders. The primary problem was the emphasis on acute inpatient care, which frequently meant that long-term rehabilitation was not provided. Also, occupational therapy as an outpatient service could not be ordered alone. These limitations would change in 1980s.

Coverage for occupational therapy under Medicaid was and is dependent on individual states. Some states provide good coverage whereas others provide no coverage at all. Thus, the impact of Medicaid has been more varied than Medicare.

Social Concern for People

The 1960s ushered in a decade of social concern for people's lives. The government, under John F. Kennedy and Lyndon B. Johnson's Great Society legislation, funded many social and health programs. Young people became aware of the increased attention to social programming and began to gain interest in the helping professions. By the late 1960s, occupational therapy had become a popular major with more applicants than positions in educational programs. Even an increase in the number of schools from 32 in 1960 to 38 in 1970 did not keep pace with the demand (58, 59). Other professions that work with disabled persons experienced a similar growth pattern.

Improvements in Plastics for Splinting

Splint making was refined further by the improvement of plastics. Royalite and Bakelite became popular. These plastics were more pliable and less brittle than the early acrylic and nitrocellulose plastics. They did, however, require a high temperature, 300 to 350°F, to become workable and were hard to fit to the person because the high temperature could burn the skin (60).

In the later 1960s, prenyl and Orthoplast became popular (61, 62). These plastics were the beginning of the low temperature splinting materials that could be molded at temperatures less than 200°F.

THE 1970s

Neurophysiology

Advances in the understanding of how the neuromuscular system works brought about significant changes in the approach to treating physical dysfunction. Prior to the information discovered in the 1950s and 1960s, treatment for such disorders as cerebral palsy and stroke and other upper motor neuron disorders was directed primarily to teaching skills through repeated practice, helping the person compensate for disability by substituting other movement patterns, or providing adapted devices and equipment (63). When therapists began to understand that the neuromuscular system could be assisted toward normalization of postural tone, sensorimotor integration, and finally, of function, the concept of treatment shifted (64). Emphasis was on developing or redeveloping the normal motor actions and encouraging normal function without substituting other movement patterns. Adapted devices and equipment were used to aid the normalizing process rather than in place of normal function. For example, long leg braces had been used extensively to assist children with cerebral palsy to walk prior to 1970. Increasingly under new treatment techniques, long leg braces have been discarded because they interfere with normal muscle action and development.

Legislation for the Disabled

In 1975, the United States Congress passed the Education Handicapped Act, PL 94–142. The purpose of the act was to provide public education opportunities to all children, regardless of type or degree of disability. Prior to the passage of the Act, some states and school districts had refused to permit children who were considered to be uneducable or too difficult to manage in school. Occupational therapy was included as one of the related services. As a result, many school systems began hiring occupational therapists in large numbers to work with children who had developmental disabilities in an effort to help the children participate more effectively in the educational programs (65).

Lightweight, Low-temperature Plastics

During the 1970s, more low temperature plastics were developed, including Aquaplast, K-splint, and Polyform. These plastics become pliable at 140–170 °F and can be molded and shaped directly on the person, making splint making easier, faster, and more accurate. Furthermore, the plastics can be remolded as changes occur in the person's body part. Remolding reduces the need to make several splints for the same person. The polymolecular plastics have facilitated the treatment of hand injuries and hand deformities.

Quality Care and Health Planning

The concern for providing quality care and good health planning always has been important in the delivery of health services. During the 1970s, the concern became nationwide after the enactment of the Professional Standards Review Organization (PSRO) (PL 92–603) and National Health Planning and Resources Development Act (PL 93–641). PSROs require that medical care be examined through an audit procedure to determine if the care was needed according to specified norms, standards, and criteria. Occupational therapists are affected by the PSRO because of the fiscal implications related to payment, the need to develop audit procedures on occupational therapy, and the potential for serving on advisory groups or program review groups of the PSRO (66).

The National Health Planning Act was designed to help make health care more accessible by requiring states to designate health service areas (67). Health Systems Agencies (HSA) in the areas were to plan for the development and expansion of health care services in each area. The HSAs are responsible for making a yearly plan for future health care priorities. Policy making and implementation of the health plans are under the direction of a State Health Coordinating Council (SHCC). Administration of the plan is under the control of the State Health Planning and Development Agency.

Occupational therapists can participate as members of HSA or SHCC governing bodies, serve on ad hoc or advisory committees, communicate needs to the HSA regarding development of services, or contribute information to the data-gathering activities (68). The effect on occupational therapy may be to increase the number of services using occupational therapists and also to increase the recognition of occupational therapy as a health care service that can function in many different settings.

THE 1980s

Prospective Payment System

The prospective payment system became law in 1983. It was designed to curb the rapid growth in Medicare hospital costs by paying for services based on a preset rate of payment for the kind of illness treated. Rates are based on a unit of payment called Diagnosis Related Group (DRG). Each of the 470 DRGs is constructed from 1) statistical and clinical analysis of all cases treated, 2) patient age and sex, 3) treatment procedure, and 4) specific diagnosis (69). Medicare will pay only the DRG rate and beneficiaries cannot be billed beyond that level. If hospitals provide treatment at a lower cost than the DRG rate, they make a profit; if hospitals provide treatment at a higher cost than the DRG rate, they suffer a loss.

A study by Gray found that occupational therapists were adjusting well to the changes caused by DRGs (70). In acute hospitals, there had been an increase in the number of referrals to occupational therapy, the referrals were being made earlier, and the length of stay in occupational therapy was decreasing. Therapists were marketing their services more and physicians seemed to be more aware of the needs. At the same time, therapists had to streamline their services so that assessments were done quickly and a program of intervention started immediately.

DRGs will not solve the problem of costs for all diseases or disorders. Some diseases and disorders do not proceed in a predictable course of recovery or death. Examples include many psychiatric disorders, mental retardation, head injuries, multiple problems seen in aged persons, and some genetic disorders, such as cystic fibrosis. For these, other health plans must be devised.

Medicare Amendments

Occupational therapy always has been a covered service under Medicare for hospitalized beneficiaries but other types of coverage for outpatient services have been limited or nonexistent. As part of the budget deficit reduction legislation of 1986, coverage for occupational therapy was expanded. In skilled nursing facilities, occupational therapy services are covered under both Part A and Part B. In rehabilitation centers, such as an Easter Seal center, a public health department, or outpatient physical and occupational therapy clinic, coverage is available without restrictions requiring concurrent use of physical or speech therapy. Finally, coverage has been extended to provide for the services of an occupational therapist in private practice who can become an independent provider and bill directly to Medicare for services rendered to beneficiaries. These additions to the Medicare program should increase the use and availability of occupational therapy to more consumers and provide additional evidence of the value of occupational therapy services in assisting the client to obtain functional independence.

Home Health Care

With many elderly patients being discharged directly home after stabilization of an acute illness, occupational therapy treatment in the patient's home has been an increasingly more common practice site. Therapists delivering this type of care are either in private practice or are working in an acute care hospital that has a home health component to its occupational therapy or rehabilitation department.

Private Practice

With the advent of changes in the Medicare program and the Education for All Handicapped Act, private practice has become a more common option. Therapists have formed corporations to do such diverse functions as treat individual patients in the patient's home, consult with a nursing home, contract with one school or an entire district to provide treatment to its eligible children, or contract with an industry to assess prospective employees for body mechanics/work capacity potential. This type of practice is expected to continue to increase throughout the 1990s (71).

Acquired Immune Deficiency Syndrome (AIDS)

A new, fatal disease syndrome, AIDS, was identified in the 1980s. Because there is no known cure for the syndrome, occupational therapists emphasized universal blood and body fluid precautions with all patients who have the potential for carrying the human immunodeficiency virus (HIV). Therapists working in hospice settings found a shift in caseload from patients with cancer to an increase in patients with AIDS. As the number of new cases is expected to increase markedly (72), occupational therapists may find that more patients with AIDS will require occupational therapy services to help them maintain independence as long as possible (73).

Biomedical Devices

The rapid development of technology in the area of biomedical devices has had a significant impact on occupational therapy services. Dynamic splints and braces powered by miniature transistors assist or substitute for normal motions in paralyzed or severely weakened limbs. Transistors can substitute for flexion, extension, and opposition. Myoelectric prosthetics allow amputees to open and close the hand or flex and extend the wrist and elbow by transistors that pick up impulses from muscles in the stump (74).

Computers

Computers, especially microcomputers, have made possible many new innovations in practice. Programs are available for standardized assessment and can be developed for new evaluations. Computer-assisted therapy can expand the types of programs offered in a clinic setting or at home. Programs are available to teach basic skills that require repetitive practice, advanced skills in creative thinking, or judgment skills in simulated situations. Computers do not run out of patience at the end of a long day and can repeat the same instructions 99 times in exactly the same words if necessary. Computers do not notice how many mistakes are made or how long a task has taken unless programmed to do so. If the client has a compatible computer at home, instructions can be developed for a home program. Use of a bulletin board can permit the client and therapist to communicate regularly without the limitations of the telephone. The client can send a question in the evening for the therapist to read the next morning and answer before the client has finished breakfast. Records, reports, accounts, and budgets all can be kept on computer. Progress notes can be written on a word processing program instead of typed or handwritten in illegible scribble.

THE 1990s

The Americans With Disabilities Act

The passage of the American with Disabilities Act (PL 101–336) in July 1990 provided occupational therapy practitioners with many opportunities to act as advocates for person with disabilities. The Act also changed the vocabulary used by many people. The term "disability" superseded the term "handicapped" in the lexicon. School and work settings needed help in figuring ways to accommodate persons with disabilities without expensive modifications. Public areas encountered similar problems. More cities began making curb cuts for wheelchairs and providing public transportation.

Problems remain in spite of the gains. Changing the physical aspects of the work setting is easier to do than changing the work habits of other workers and the hiring practices of personnel managers. People with disabilities are still underemployed. Public transportation is available but often requires much planning in advance for persons in wheelchairs or those with other special needs. Such persons cannot spontaneously decide to go to the movies or even to a shopping mall.

Gerontics

The increased number and percentage of persons who are 65 years of age or older living in society has continued to influence the practice of occupational therapy. The role of older people is changing. Workers are not required to retire at 65 years of age but may continue to work well into their seventies. Occupational therapists have had to assist older workers as advocates to show employers that older workers can be productive when jobs are designed to reduce the fatigue and stress on them.

Health problems have shifted slowly also. Whereas stroke and heart disease have been common problems seen in occupational therapy, there has been a shift to cancer and other diseases of aging, such as osteoporosis and Alzheimer's disease. Changing roles and health problems will necessitate changes in the goals, intervention techniques, and modalities selected by occupational therapy.

Finally, occupational therapy practitioners have had to develop more programs to prevent chronic illness from robbing older people of their health and their life's savings years before they actually die. Programs have stressed enabling people to continue to function independently so they do not need to be institutionalized or become dependent on their children. A focus on maintaining health, not overcoming the problems of illness, has become important. Industries, churches, and colleges have been used as places where groups of people are gathered to learn about patterns of occupation that prevent loss of health and maintain functional living skills for persons who are 80, 90, or even 100 years of age. The knowledge is available but must continue to be organized into effective programs that occupational therapy practitioners promote and implement.

Adult Day Care

As the population ages and as more people survive catastrophic illnesses or birth trauma, there has been an increase in the numbers of individuals who do not need the intensity of institution care, but who are unable to be alone for all or parts of a day. For financial or other reasons, grown children have choosen to have frail elderly parents live with them, yet both husband and wife must work outside the home. Also, a severely physically or mentally disabled individual may have lived at home and attended public school until 21 years of age, but is not able to function in even limited employment at 22 years of age or older. The need for adult day care centers that provide supervision, nutrition, activity, and therapy for adults of all ages with various limitations has continued to increase.

Infant and Preschool Programs

Public Law 99–457, or the Early Intervention Act, mandated services for disabled preschoolers 3 to 5 years of age in the school year 1990/91, and emphasized services for disabled children from birth through 2 years of age (74). The focus for this age group will be for a more family centered approach rather than just a child-centered treatment. This law, along with the reauthorized Individual Disability Education Act (formerly the Education for all Handicapped), has greatly increase the need for more occupational therapists, and especially for more to enter pediatric practice.

Manpower Needs

The profession has had a personnel shortage for many years, and the demand for occupational therapists is expected to grow well into the twenty-first century (76). As the population increases and the number of elderly people within the population increases, as new diseases appear and disabling conditions increase in incidence, so have the number of persons with limitations that require the services of an occupational therapist. The problem is especially acute in rural areas and in states with no educational programs at either the occupational therapist or occupational therapy assistant level.

Education

As the average age of students attending college gets older, occupational therapy educational programs have been forced to offer courses in more nontraditional ways. An increased number of older individuals has returned to school to pursue a second career. Women who stayed home until their children were raised are now attending college for the first time. With the cost of education increasing, many students have had to work to support themselves while they attend school so they are unable to carry a full course load each term. Not all individuals who could be excellent occupational therapists live in areas with colleges that offer occupational therapy programs, and for any number of reasons, are unable to uproot families to move to a college community for 1 to 4 years. Occupational therapy educational programs have become more innovative in course offerings to fit these nontraditional students. Evening courses; weekend classes; 3-day, 4-day, or 5-day seminars; computerized instruction; and interactive television are some of the options that have been used.

LOOKING INTO THE TWENTY-FIRST CENTURY

Person Power

For the first time in the history of occupational therapy the numbers of practitioners may be closing in on the number needed to serve the consumer population. The number of educational programs needed in states such as New York and Pennsylvania may also have reached or overreached the saturation point. The question is: How many practitioners is enough? Because the profession of occupational therapy has always had a shortage, the subject of too many has received little attention. Another question is: How can institutions of higher education be discouraged from starting more occupational therapy education programs in areas that already have enough? Can the AOTA work with the Bureau of Labor to recast some the forecasts about the need for large numbers of occupational therapy practitioners? Numbers of needed workers is potential dollars to higher education institutions looking for more students.

The Internet

The Internet already has become popular among some occupational therapy practitioners. E-mail, LISTSERVs, and chat groups seem to be the most popular means of communicating. However, the Internet offers more potential. Students could be taking the Certification Examination over the Internet from their home or a local library instead of having to travel to a site. More courses could be available via the World Wide Web. An entire academic program could be offered via the Internet. Speciality Certification examinations, including those with case studies, could be taken via the Internet.

The down side to the Internet is the lack of control. Inaccurate information on occupational therapy already exists and is likely to get worse. Can the misinformation be identified and attempts to correct such information be made? Who will do this?

Continuing Competency and Recertification

Both continuing competency and recertification are fighting words for many practitioners. These practitioners were educated with the understanding that once they finished their basic education and passed the certification examination, there would be no more tests to take—ever. Then, some state licensure boards began requiring continuing education credits and finally the issue of "not certified for life" became a reality. How will the reality be dealt with? Will reexamination become a fact of life? Will tests be added to continuing education courses? How else could a person demonstrate continued competency?

National Health Insurance

Will national health insurance become a reality in the first decade of the twenty-first century? What types and range of coverage will be included for occupational therapy services? If the coverage is limited to in-service rehabilitation and mental health treatment, occupational therapy may be severely curtailed. However, if coverage is based on a continuum of care from prevention to maximum recovery and adjustment, then occupational therapy services probably will be expanded. Further considerations that will affect the role of occupational therapy include the extent of coverage for mental health problems, adaptive devices and equipment home health benefits, nursing home benefits, adult day care benefits, and community-based programs.

At the same time, occupational therapy will be required to provide more and better documentation that services are needed and that those services have been provided as efficiently and effectively as possible. The work done to develop audit procedures and performance criteria should provide a good foundation for justifying reimbursement under a national health insurance program.

Marketing

Marketing involves identifying an existing demand and developing a program to satisfy that demand. The critical element is identifying the demand. To identify the demand, one must survey, study, and analyze the marketplace. Then, when a demand is identified, the occupational therapist must determine what other suppliers (competition) can meet the demand, what costs would be incurred if occupational therapy enters the marketplace with a service, and whether occupational therapy has the expertise required to fulfill the demand. These steps are what distinguish marketing from selling. Selling, a subset of marketing, is a process of attempting to create a demand for an existing service whereas marketing analyzes what the consumer wants and builds programs to satisfy those wants.

Health care services traditionally have not been marketed. They have been established and then wait for consumers to come to the door. The result is overuse of some services and little use of others. Inefficiency and high costs were the result. Rising costs have forced health care delivery systems to take a different approach. Competition for consumers has become reality. Occupational therapists cannot assume that occupational therapy is inherently good and, therefore, consumers will want it. The consumer must see occupational therapy as meeting an existing demand that the consumer has at a price the consumer can afford to pay. An excellent program for failure-to-thrive infants probably will not be successful in a community of retired persons because there may be very few, if any, infants available. In a retirement community, the demand will be for services to older individuals. Perhaps a gerontics program would be more likely to meet an existing demand. Older people might want to come to the occupational therapy center if they could learn more about maintaining their health and prolonging their independence. In other words, occupational therapists must learn how to "package" the knowledge and skills of occupational therapy into programs of service that consumers want and demand at a cost that is affordable.

Managed Care and Unmanaged Health

Attempts to manage the dollars spent on health care became a major theme in the 1990s. Insurance carriers of all types were instituting managed care plans. Limitations on what health care services were covered and how much money could be spent became common place. Waste and fat in health care delivery were to be eliminated. Largely the objective of controlling health costs was attained. Better health, however, did not necessary follow.

Occupational therapy is sometimes considered a luxury that cannot be afforded. Other times the complaint is that there is no proven value. Only occupational therapy practitioners and researchers can show the need for and value of occupational therapy services. Practitioners and researchers need to join forces more often to engage in studies that show occupational therapy makes a difference in people's lives that is cost-ffective, occupationally important, and health wise.

SUMMARY

In summary, society influences occupational therapy in many ways. Changes and advances in knowledge lead to new techniques. Developments in materials and equipment make possible new devices or modifications in old ones. Politics influence the passage of laws that control the reimbursement of services and direct the kinds of service to be supported in the future. Demographics alter the practice of occupational therapy through the changing patterns of problems and needs that people experience. Disease profiles change as one disease is cured, controlled, or prevented and new or other diseases emerge.

Occupational therapists can influence the direction and quality of occupational therapy services by being aware of the social changes taking place and by devising new approaches to meet the changing demands. An example is developing strategies to help implement the Americans With Disabilities Act passed in July 1990. As long as occupational therapists understand the society in which they live, define the needs of persons for occupations, and provide intervention techniques to help meet the needs, occupational therapy will continue to have a positive future in the years ahead.

References

1. Tracy SE. Some profitable occupations for invalids. Am J Nurs 1907–1908;8:176.
2. Slagle EC. Training aides for mental patients. Arch Occup Ther 1922;1:11–17; State Hosp Q 1922;7:167–174.
3. Dunton WR Jr. The principles of occupational therapy. Pub Health Nurse 1918;10:320.
4. Hall HJ. Work cure. JAMA 1910;54:12–13.
5. Newton IG. Consolation House. Trained Nurse Hosp Rev 1917;59:324–325.
6. Myers CM. Pioneer occupational therapists in World War 1. Am J Occup Ther 1948;12:208–209.
7. Schwab SI. The experiment in occupational therapy at Base Hospital 117, A.E.F. Ment Hyg 1919;3:580.
8. Haggerty ME. Where can a woman serve? Carry On 1918;1:26–29.
9. Baldwin BT. Occupational therapy. Am J Care Cripples 1919;8:447–449.
10. Henderson WH. Occupational therapy in army hospitals. Mod Hosp 1920;15:325.
11. Statistics. JAMA 1937;108:1046.
12. Dunton WR Jr. The training of occupational teachers and directors. Md Psychiair Q 1917;7:9.
13. 20th Biennial Report of the Board of Public Charities of the State of Illinois, Springfield, IL, 1909:55–58.
14. Slagle EC. The training of occupational therapists. Psychiair Q 1931;5:12.
15. Johnson SC. Practical results of a year's work at Montefiore. In: Proceedings of the Third Annual Meeting of the National Society for the Promotion of Occupational Therapy, Towson, MD, 1919:120.
16. Favill J. Henry Baird Favill. Chicago: Rand McNally, 1917:87.
17. Special courses in curative occupations and recreation. Chicago School of Civics and Philanthropy, Special Bulletin, December, 1917.
18. Lermit GR. Vale. Md Psychiatr Q 1921;10:80.
19. Upham EG. A training course for occupational experts. Mod Hosp 1917;9:458–459.
20. Partridge CP. Milwaukee-Downer College gives O.T. course. Mod Hosp 1921;17:64–65.
21. A forward step in the education of occupational therapists. Occup Ther Rehabil 1931;10:204–206.
22. Fulton FW. The Philadelphia School of Occupational Therapy. Mod Hosp 1921;16:572–574.
23. Willard H, Spackman C. Occupational Therapy. Principles and Practices. Philadelphia: Lippincott, 1947.
24. Greene MB, Wigglesworth R. Boston School of Occupational Therapy Inc. Mod Hosp 1921;16:568,570.
25. Kidder L. St. Louis School of Occupational Therapy. Mod Hosp 1921;17:65–67.
26. Then and Now: 1917–1967. New York: American Occupational Therapy Association, 1967:12.
27. Rehabilitation. Social Work Yearbook. New York: Russell Sage Foundation, 1933:431.
28. Kidner TB. Occupational therapy in 1923. Mod Hosp 1924;22:55.

29. Montgomery A. Report of the Methods of Teaching Committee. Occup Ther Rehabil 1927;6:65.
30. Report of the Council on Medical Education and Hospitals. JAMA 1935;104:1631.
31. Occupational Therapy Yearbook. New York: American Occupational Therapy Association, 1932.
32. Approved schools of occupational therapy. JAMA 1938;110:979–980.
33. West W. The future of occupational therapy in the Army. Am J Occup Ther 1947;1:155.
34. Franciscus ML. Opportunities in Occupational Therapy, N.Y. Vocational Guidance Manuals 1952:2, 54–55,108–109.
35. Report of Education Committee. Occup Ther Rehabil 1944;23:36.
36. Occupational Therapy. Bull US Army Med Dept 1945;4:18–20.
37. Excerpts from minutes of meeting, Committee on Education, American Occupational Therapy Association. Occup Ther Rehabil 1945;24:115–116,218,220.
38. Messick HE. The new Women's Medical Specialist Corps. Am J Occup Ther 1947;1:298.
39. Kefauver HG. Vocational aspects of occupational therapy. US Veterans' Bur Med Bull 1926;2:118.
40. Thompson CG. Occupational therapy and the Kenny method. Occup Ther 1943;221:270.
41. Hurt S. Occupational therapy with orthopedic and surgical conditions. Occup Ther Rehabil 1941;20:154–155.
42. Licht S. The objectives of occupational therapy. Occup Ther Rehabil 1947;26:17.
43. Phelps WM. The correlation of physical therapy and occupational therapy in cerebral palsy. Arch Phys Ther 1941;22:587–590.
44. Stern E. The work cure. Surv Graphic 1939;38:285.
45. Bovee MH. Plastic splints. Am J Occup Ther 1952;6:203–207.
46. Wood MK. A functional handsplint. Am J Occup Ther 1959;13:22.
47. Doescher M, Werssowitz D. Training in the use of the functional assist for the flail hand. Am J Occup Ther 1955;9:115–117.
48. Holser P. Upper extremity control braces. Am J Occup Ther 1966;13:165.
49. Alexander FG, Selesnick ST. The History of Psychiatry. New York, Harper & Row, 1955:288.
50. Hammond Almanac of a Million Facts, Records, Forecasts. 10th ed. Maplewood, NJ: Hammond Almanac, 1979:277.
51. Ayres AJ. A pilot study on the relationship between work habits and workshop production. Am J Occup Ther 1955;9:264–267,297.
52. Rosenburg B. Vocational evaluation-TOWER-rehabilitation center. In: Jones M. Work Adjustment as a Function of Occupational Therapy. Dubuque, IA: Kendall-Hunt, 1963.
53. Forrer GR. Work therapy program at Northville State Hospital. Am J Occup Ther 1955;9:154–155,183.
54. Jones M The Therapeutic Community: A New Treatment Method in Psychiatry. New York: Basic Books, 1953.
55. German SA. A group approach. Am J Occup Ther 1964;18:209–214.
56. Howe M, Dippy K. The role of occupational therapy in community mental health. Am J Occup Ther 1968;22:521–524.

57. Medicare coverage for occupational therapy services. Am J Occup Ther 1974;28:9,110.
58. Schools offering courses in occupational therapy. Am J Occup Ther 1960;14:back cover.
59. Occupational therapy curricula. Am J Occup Ther 1970;24:144–145.
60. Koepke GH, Feallock B, Feller I. Splinting the severely burned hand. Am J Occup Ther 1963;17:147–150.
61. Kester DL. New product makes splinting easier. Am J Occup Ther 1966;20:43.
62. Willis B. The use of Orthoplast Isoprene splints in the treatment of the acutely burned child: preliminary report. Am J Occup Ther 1969;23:57–61.
63. Marmo NA. Brain damaged adult. Am J Occup Ther 1974;28:201.
64. Carisen PN. Comparison of two occupational therapy approaches for treating the young cerebral palsied child. Am J Occup Ther 1975;29:268.
65. Jantzen J. The current profile of occupational therapy and future—professional or vocational? In: Occupational Therapy. 2001 AD. Rockville, MD: American Occupational Therapy Association, 1979.
66. Ostrow PC. PSRO and quality assurance: what is the occupational therapist's role? Am J Occup Ther 1975;29:333–340.
67. Meredith S, Meredith G. The Health Systems Agency: a new bureacracy. Am J Occup Ther 1977;31:388–390.
68. Meredith G. Perspectives on occupational therapy's role in Health Systems Agency activities. Am J Occup Ther 1977;1:354–355.
69. HCFA Fact Sheet. Washington, Dept of Health and Human Services, Health Care Financing Administration, August, 1983.
70. Gray MS. Occupational therapy use rises under PPS. Hospitals, 1985:60,62.
71. Occupational Therapy newspaper. American Occupational Therapy Association. Vol 42. January 1988.
72. Occupational Therapy newspaper. American Occupational Therapy Association. Vol 43. January 1989.
73. Occupational Therapy newspaper. American Occupational Therapy Association. Vol 42. February 1988.
74. OT Week, national weekly bulletin. American Occupational Therapy Association. Vol 3. No 45, November 16, 1989.
75. Occupational Therapy newspaper. American Occupational Therapy Association. Vol 40. December 1986.
76. Occupational Therapy Manpower: A Plan For Progress. American Occupational Therapy Association, April 1985.

Professional Literature Base

CHAPTER 29

Sources of
Professional Literature

Information is an important resource in learning about a profession and in maintaining competence as a practicing professional. Literature is one means of providing such information. Professional literature can include documentation of practice, issues in practice, theories on which practice is based, current trends in practice, and the history of practice. In addition, professional literature records the activities of professional organizations and the people who were active in shaping the profession. Literature has the advantage of being relatively permanent whereas workshops, conferences, meetings, and other continuing education events do not create a permanent record unless proceedings are published. Without a permanent record, the details of presentations become blurred or lost. Finally, professional literature provides a significant means of conveying the essence of a profession to other professionals, to financial intermediaries who pay for services, and to consumers.

The founders of occupational therapy understood the value of creating professional literature. From the beginning, efforts were made to record the activities and events of the formation of occupational therapy as a recognized discipline and the documentation of practice as it evolved. Prior to the founding meeting of occupational therapy, Dr. Dunton offered to include information and announcements about occupational therapy in the *Maryland Psychiatric Quarterly,* which he edited (1). The proceedings of the founding meeting in Clifton Springs were published in the journal *Modern Hospital* (2). Proceedings of the next four conferences, 1917–1920, were published separately. In 1921, Dr. Dunton suggested that a journal devoted to occupational therapy be published (3). Thus, in 1922, the first journal of occupational therapy appeared; it was titled *Archives of Occupational Therapy* and was published by Williams & Wilkins. In 1925, the title was changed to *Occupational Therapy and Rehabilitation* in hopes of broadening the journal's appeal to more subscribers and contributors (4). The journal continued to be the official journal of the American Occupational Therapy Association through 1946.

Beginning in February 1947, the Association began publishing its own journal, *American Journal of Occupational Therapy,* which continues today. The advantage of the Association owning the journal was more control over its format and content (5).

From 1947–1951, two journals of occupational therapy were published: *Occupational Therapy and Rehabilitation* and the *American Journal of Occupational Therapy*. However, in 1952, the title of *Occupational Therapy and Rehabilitation* was changed to the *American Journal of Physical Medicine,* and the focus of the content was directed away from occupational therapy (6). Thus, beginning in 1952, occupational therapy was again dependent on one journal to carry the word about occupational therapy to its own practitioners as well as to publicize the profession to others. The only other means of conveying information nationally was a newsletter begun in 1939, which today is called *OT News.* It has grown from one 8½ × 11 page to a multipaged newspaper. From 1939–1989, it was mailed separately to members of the AOTA. However, its purpose was not to record activities of the Association but to alert members to upcoming events and report items of interest. Thus, the newsletter-turned-newspaper was not intended to be a permanent record and was not systematically saved by libraries. Therefore, few complete sets exist in libraries.

Finally, in 1980, the first journal of occupational therapy appeared that was not related to the professional organization. *Occupational Therapy in Mental Health* (OTMH) is owned and published by the Haworth Press. Subsequently, three more titles were started by Haworth including *Physical and Occupational Therapy in Pediatrics* (POTP, 1981), *Physical and Occupational Therapy in Geriatrics* (POTG, 1981), and *Occupational Therapy in Health Care* (OTHC, 1984). In addition, Hanley and Belfus began publishing the *Journal of Hand Therapy* in 1987 and Aspen Publishing Company began publishing *Occupational Therapy Practice* in 1989 but terminated publication in 1994. In 1993, new, internationally focused journals came into being with the *Journal of Occupational Science: Australia* from the University of South Australia. The following year saw the publication of the *Scandinavian Journal of Occupational Therapy* by the Scandinavian University Press and *Occupational Therapy International* by Whurr Publishers. These journals have increased significantly the ability of the profession to communicate with its own practitioners as well as to others outside the field.

Communications was further improved when the American Occupational Therapy Foundation began publishing the *Occupational Therapy Journal of Research* in 1981. As the name implies, research activities and studies are the major focus of the journal, thus separating itself from journals that focus primarily on practice issues.

Journals published by international associations should be considered as sources of occupational therapy literature as well. Three, in particular, may be useful. These are the *Canadian Journal of Occupational Therapy, British Journal of Occupational Therapy,* and *Australian Occupational Therapy Journal.* OT-Bib-Sys also indexed the *Israel Journal of Occupational Therapy* and the *New Zealand Journal of Occupational Therapy.*

Journals on occupational therapy are not the only source of information about the profession. Other journals have published articles on occupational therapy as well. A few journal titles are *Archives of Physical Medicine and Rehabilitation, American Journal of Physical Medicine and Rehabilitation, Developmental Medicine and Child Neurology, Journal of Allied Health, Journal of Hand Surgery*, and *Physical Therapy*. Since 1900, more than 3500 articles have appeared in journals that are not concerned primarily with occupational therapy. There is a rich heritage of literature available to the student or therapist who is willing to take the time and effort to locate the many articles in other journals.

Books have contributed to the literature on occupational therapy also. Probably the first textbook on occupational therapy was printed in 1910; it was titled *Invalid Occupations* and was by Susan Tracy (7). She wrote about the activities she used to work with various types of patients she saw in her practice as a nurse. Dunton, Hall, Barton, Baldwin, Slagle, Haas, and Kidner also wrote early textbooks on occupational therapy. These books are listed at the end of Chapter 27.

From 1933–1946, no new occupational therapy textbooks were published in the United States; however, two were published in Great Britain (22, 23). In 1947, Helen Willard and Clare Spackman wrote and edited the first comprehensive textbook of occupational therapy titled *Principles of Occupational Therapy* (24). Although the text has been revised several times and has two new sets of editors, Helen L. Hopkins and Helen D. Smith for the 6th through 8th editions and Maureen E. Neistadt and Elizabeth Crepeau for the 9th, it remains the best-known text on occupational therapy.

In 1951, the American Occupational Therapy Association began publishing literature on occupational therapy. The *Manual on Administration* (1951) and *Objectives and Functions* (1958) are two of the more well known publications. These and others were printed and distributed by William C. Brown Publishing Company, later named Kendall/Hunt, in Dubuque, Iowa.

Beginning in the 1970s, the number of books on occupational therapy and related subjects began to increase rapidly. Today there are more than 500 books and monographs written about occupational therapy. Many, however, were published in very small quantities and thus are not readily available in most libraries. Most are available, however, through the Wilma L. West Library in the American Occupational Therapy Foundation office.

Audiovisual material and other nonprint media also have played a role in documenting the development of occupational therapy. Traveling exhibits, consisting of craft items and photographs, were used by the national association and hospital departments of occupational therapy to show physicians and hospital administrators what occupational therapists did (25). In 1964, the first film was sponsored by the national association and was titled *To Pick a Life* (26). Four video tapes and six television spot commercials were developed in the same year. All were aimed at the recruitment of students. Films, slide series, and videotapes are available on numerous topics from the national association and a few commercial vendors. Most are concerned with issues in practice, such as how to make a type of splint or use of occupational therapy with a particular type of client.

LOCATING LITERATURE ON OCCUPATIONAL THERAPY

To be useful, information must be located. Obviously, the journals published by the professional organization and by Haworth are a good source of information about occupational therapy. However, topics on occupational therapy and of interest to occupational therapists appear in other journals as well. Locating literature on occupational therapy in journals not specific to occupational therapy can be a challenge. Occupational therapy makes use of and is used by a variety of disciplines, which includes biological, social and applied sciences (see Fig . 19.1) Thus, journals serving a variety of interests may include articles that occupational therapists want to locate. Titles might be directed to schools, special education, psychiatry, nursing, rehabilitation medicine, abnormal psychology, hospitals, nursing homes, business administration, and more.

Students and therapists should become familiar with tools used in most libraries to locate information about occupational therapy. These tools include printed bibliographic indexes, online (computer) bibliographic databases, and CD-ROM (Compact Disk-Read Only Memory) bibliographic databases. A bibliographic citation usually provides the author, title, and source of an article or book. Other information, such as price, number of pages, and language of publication, may be included. Standard print sources of literature relevant to occupational therapy are listed in Table 29.1, online sources are listed in Table 29.2, and CD-ROM sources are listed in Table 29.3. Most medical libraries will have copies of all the print indexes in their reference sections and access to the online sources. Hospital libraries, however, may have only a few indexes and limited access to selected online sources.

Use of print indexes and CD-ROMS usually is free of cost, but online searches may be available only on a fee-for-service basis. All online databases are available to individual users for a fee. However, the individual searcher must sign up for the service, get a user number, and learn the computer language and its commands in order to access the information. Librarians know how to access the databases; thus, students and practitioners may prefer to have the librarians do the online searching.

When using online databases, one should be aware that journal literature is available only from 1966 (MEDLINE) at the earliest. Most databases were developed in the 1970s. Therefore, if journal articles are desired before the 1970s, the searcher must consult the printed indexes. Also important is the knowledge that various databases include a different group of journal titles. MEDLINE shows which databases include which occupational therapy journals in their database. Note that the Cumulative *Index to Nursing and Allied Health Literature* (NAHL) and *Psychological Abstracts* (Psyc-INFO) include the most occupational therapy journals.

In contrast, most book titles are available online. The reason is simple. Books were cataloged in card catalogs that could be converted relatively easily to the computer. Also, there are fewer books than journal articles. The National Library of

Table 29.1. Print Indexes Useful in Locating Occupational Therapy Literature

Index Medicus (title varies) 1879–present
Excerpta Medica 1956–present
Cumulative Index to Nursing and Allied Health Literature (CINAHL)
Cumulative Index of Hospital Literature 1950–1994
Rehabilitation Literature 1950–1986
Educational Resources Information Center (ERIC) 1966–present
Exceptional Child Education Resources 1966–1994
Education Index 1929–present
Psychological Abstracts 1929–present
Dissertation Abstracts 1860–present

Medicine produces Catline (Catalog Online), which lists its holdings. The Library of Congress holdings are available on the database titled LC MARC, which details 1968 to the present. Earlier books can be located on REMARC. Audiovisual materials held by the National Library of Medicine are listed on Avline (Audiovisual Online). The holdings are not as complete as the serials or books. Many audiovisual titles must be located through catalogs. Again, a librarian may be helpful in identifying possible catalog sources.

ACCESSING THE LITERATURE

After the citation is found, the next step is finding the article, book, or audiovisual. If the desired item is available in the library, the library staff will be able to locate it. However, no library is able to acquire a copy of every journal, book, or audiovisual published today. The estimated number of biomedical journals worldwide is between 14,000 and 16,000 (27). Publication of books and production of audiovisual materials has also increased; therefore, the volume of published works is too large, costs too much, and takes up too much space. All library collections are limited and may not include the item needed at a particular time. Thus, libraries have developed a sharing network known as interlibrary loan.

The largest loan service for books is OCLC (originally Ohio College Library Center, now Online Computer Library Center, Incorporated). For journal articles on health and medical subjects, the National Library of Medicine organized Docline. One of the services of these computerized systems is a list of member library holdings. These holdings can be viewed online or on microfiche so that other libraries can determine what is available and request the item. Lending is done only from one library to another to provide continuity of service and maintain accountability. Usually, the library patron fills out a form stating what item is desired. The patron's library requests the item from another library, such as the Wilma L. West Library; then, the item or a photocopy is sent to the patron's li-

Table 29.2.   Sources of Occupational Therapy Journal Literature Online

MEDLINE 1966–present (NLM, Dialog, Ovid)
   Source: National Library of Medicine
HealthSTAR (formerly Health Planning and Administration) 1975–present (NLM, Dialog, Ovid)
   Source: National Library of Medicine
Embase 1974–present (Dialog, Ovid)
   Source: Elsevier Publishing Co.
Cumulative Index to Nursing and Allied Health Literature (CINAHL)
1983–present (Dialog, Ovid)
   Source: General Adventist Medical Center
Educational Resources Information Center (ERIC) 1966–present (Dialog, Ovid)
   Source: Educational Resources Information Clearinghouse
Psyc-Info 1967–present (Dialog, Ovid)
   Source: Psychological Association
Dissertation Abstracts Online (Dialog, Ovid)
   Source: University Microfilms International
Mental Health Abstracts 1969–present (Dialog)
   Source: National Clearinghouse for Mental Health
Ageline 1978–present (Dialog, Ovid)
   Source: American Association of Retired Persons
Health and PsychoSocial Instruments (Ovid)
   Behavioral Measurement Database Services
BioethicsLine (Ovid)
   Kennedy Institute of Ethics
NTIS (Dialog, Ovid) Government sponsored research reports and studies
   Source: National Technical Information Service

Vendors which include the database in their system.

brary, and the patron picks up the item at the library. The same system is available at many hospital and public libraries. However, most students probably will be using a campus or academic library so the example is based on that experience. Also, other interlibrary loan systems exist but all work similarly.

CHOOSING AN ARTICLE VERSUS A BOOK VERSUS AN AUDIOVISUAL

Students and therapists may be tempted to use the first item of information located on a topic so that the term paper or article can be written quickly because it is due tomorrow. So much for planning ahead! The instructor or journal editor is more likely to be pleased with the paper that has a variety of references cited in the bibliography and at least a few current (within the last 5 years) citations. Even history gets revised and reinterpreted; therefore, the careful student or therapist will look for sources of information in both journals and books. Comprehensive reviews of the literature will include audiovisual materials as well.

Table 29.3. CD-ROMs Useful in Locating Occupational Therapy Literature	
Name	**Source of CD-ROM Product**
MEDLINE	Available from many sources
CINAHL	Silver Platter
PsycLIT	Silver Platter
HealthStar	Silver Platter
ERIC	Silver Platter
ECER (Exceptional Child Education Resource)	Silver Platter
NTIS	Silver Platter
Biological Abstracts	Silver Platter
Dissertation Abstracts	University Microfilm
Abledata	Trace

The student or therapist should be aware that the most current information in health and medicine is contained in journals, not books. The reason is that journals are printed more frequently and articles are published on specific aspects of a disease or health problem. In contrast, books take longer to publish on the average and present a more comprehensive coverage of the subject matter. To use journals and books to best advantage, the student or therapist may want to begin with a recently published textbook (check the copyright date on the back of the title page) to get an overview of the subject. Then, current journal articles should be located for print indexes or online databases. Most articles have a reference list on the last page of the article that can be used to locate additional sources.

If the student or therapist is having difficulty locating books or articles on a topic of interest, the assistance of a reference librarian should be sought. Reference librarians are skilled in looking for information sources and may be helpful in identifying other concepts or words that can be used to identify sources. For example, the term architectural barriers may appear in the print indexes under accessibility or barrier-free design. Students and therapists do not always think of the many possible terms that might be used to describe a subject of interest.

Another method of identifying alternate terms or concepts is to consult a thesaurus or list of controlled vocabulary. Indexes and databases use controlled vocabulary as a means of bringing the literature together. The thesaurus for *Index Medicus* is called *Medical Subject Headings* and appears every year with the January issue of *Index Medicus*. For MEDLINE, the thesaurus comes in three parts: the *Medical Subject Headings—Annotated Alphabetic List, Medical Subject Headings—Tree Structures,* and *Permuted MESH.* The latter is helpful in locating alternate terms. *Psychological Abstracts and* ERIC also have excellent thesauruses. A few minutes with a thesaurus can save hours of unproductive search time.

INTERNET

The Internet has become a favorite of many for locating information. There is a lot of information to be located, if it can be located. Search engines are one of best methods of locating sites. Table 29.4 lists some of the more well known search engines. Using search engines requires learning the format of the search engine. For single word searches, there is rarely a problem. However, almost any single word search will return thousands of hits (websites). To get a fewer hits but of better quality requires learning how the search engine works. Always check the Help button for details of how to make sure the terms desired are found and to learn how to eliminate those not wanted. For example, the biggest number of websites on occupational therapy concern educational programs to become a therapist. If information on education is not needed, it is helpful to eliminate college and university sites from the search results. Often the search engine can eliminate a term by using the minus sign. One possible search strategy would then be: +occupational +therapy −university −college. The search engine has been instructed to find sites containing both occupational and therapy but to eliminate those with the word university or the word college.

Another concern on the Internet is the quality and reliability. Because anyone can write an e-mail or create a web page, anyone can decide what to say or display. There may be as much false information as true. Misinformation about occupational therapy can be easily documented. Thus, it follows that other misinformation is on the World Wide Web also. Therefore, it is important to examine the source of the information. Generally speaking, certain criteria can be helpful. Know who is most likely to provide reliable information on the topic of interest. Usually, but not always, universities and colleges, government, large medical and research centers, and large organizations are more likely to be reliable. Individuals are the least reliable. Always double-check the information using independent sites if possible. Remember that anyone can link one web page to another so often the same misinformation becomes available on several different web pages. An even better idea is to check information found on the web with information from

Table 29.4. Major Search Engines	
Alta Vista	atlavista.digital.com/
Excite	www.excite.com/
HotBot	www.hotbot.com/
Infoseek	guide.infoseek.com/
Lycos	www.lycos.com/
Opentext	www.opentext.com/
Webcrawler	www.webcrawler.com/
Yahoo!	www.yahoo.com/ (by subject)

a book or journal article. Also be suspicious of information on a web page that does not provide a source and date. Contacting the webmaster who developed the page may help clarify the accuracy of the information. Unfortunately, advertising has become part of the web culture and advertising is not always truthful, as most people have learned. Advertising on the web has the same credibility as in a magazine or on the television. So, know the source and judge accordingly.

SUMMARY

Occupational therapy students and practitioners need information to build their knowledge, improve their skills, and maintain their competence. Professional literature is one source of information that is available to everyone who has access to a library and knows how to use it. This chapter has provided a few tips on accessing occupational therapy literature available through print indexes, online databases, interlibrary loan, and the Internet. Students who develop skills in using the library will find that they are able to locate sources of information as practitioners. Information on occupational therapy and related aspects is available but one must know how to identify where it exists and how to get access to it.

References

1. Dunton WR. An historical note. Arch Occup Ther 1926;5:427–439.
2. Modem Hospital. 1917;8:380–419 (Paper read at the founding conference of the National Society for the Promotion of Occupational Therapy).
3. National Society for the Promotion of Occupational Therapy. Fifth annual meeting of the NSPOT. Arch Occup Ther 1922;1:51–85.
4. Dunton WR. Editorial. Occup Ther Rehabil 1925;4:227–228.
5. Bone CD. Origins of the American Journal of Occupational Therapy: 1947–1949. Am J Occup Ther 1971;25:48–52.
6. Licht S. Editorial. Am J Phys Med 1952;31:1.
7. Tracy SE. Studies in Invalid Occupation: A Manual for Nurses and Attendants. Boston: Whitcomb& Barrows, 1910.
8. Dunton WR. Occupational Therapy: A Manual for Nurses. Philadelphia: Saunders, 1915.
9. Dunton WR. Reconstruction Therapy. Philadelphia: Saunders, 1919.
10. Dunton WR. Prescribing Occupational Therapy. Springfield, IL: Charles C Thomas, 1928.
11. Hall HJ, Buck MMC. The Work of Our Hands. New York: Moffart Yard & Co., 1915.
12. Hall HJ. Buck MMC. Handicrafts for the Handicapped. New York: Moffart Yard & Co., 1916 (revised in 1928).
13. Hall HJ. Bedside and Wheelchair Occupations. New York: Red Cross Institute for Crippled, 1919.
14. Hall HJ. 0. T.: A New Profession. Concord, MA: Rumford Press, 1923.
15. Barton GE. Occupational Therapy. New York: Lakeside Press, 1917.
16. Barton GE. Re-education: An Analysis of the Institutional System of the United States. New York: Houghton Mifflin, 1918.

17. Barton GE. Teaching the Sick: A Manual of Occupational Therapy and Reeducation. Philadelphia: Saunders, 1919.
18. Baldwin BT. Occupational Therapy Applied to Restoration of Movement. Washington, DC: Walter Reed General Hospital, 1919.
19. Slagle EC. A Syllabus for the Training of Nurses in Occupational Therapy. New York: Utica State Press, 1923 (revised in 1925, 1933; reprinted in 1941).
20. Haas L. Occupational Therapy for Mentally and Nervously Ill. Milwaukee: Bruce Publ., 1925.
21. Kidner TB. Occupational Therapy: The Science of Prescribed Work for Invalids. Stuttgart Germany: Kohthammer. Also in Nosokomeion (Quarterly Hospital Review) 1930;1:265–311.
22. Haworth NA, MacDonald EM. Theory of Occupational Therapy for Students and Nurses. London: Balliere, Tindall & Cox, 1941.
23. Colson JHC. The Rehabilitation of the Injured: Occupational Therapy. London: Cassell & Co. Ltd. 1944 (revised in 1945).
24. Willard HS, Spackman CS. Principles of Occupational Therapy. Philadelphia: JB Lippincott, 1947 (revised 1954).
25. The occupational therapy exhibit. Maryland Psychiatr Q 1921;11:19.
26. Executive Director. Annual Report to the Membership. New York: American Occupational Therapy Association, 1964:11.
27. Policing the page. The Economist. June 1989;3:83.

Case Studies and
Discussion Questions

CHAPTER 30

Case Studies

This chapter includes three case studies which may be used to explore the models presented in Chapters 17 and 18. A basic analysis is provided as a starting point.

Occupational therapists may be helpful in assisting persons with a variety of problems. These problems may be grouped into four major areas: biological, psychological, social, and occupational. These areas are interrelated and cross over into each other. The overlapping is a result of the manner in which humans function, namely, as integrated beings. Thus, the areas serve the purpose of permitting classification and analysis of problems. In reality, problem areas must be considered together because each area influences and affects the other. This interrelationship and overlapping is illustrated in Figure 30. 1.

Biological problems are delineated most frequently by medical terms for disease, disorders, or trauma. The primary body systems involved are the neuromuscular skeletal system, cardiopulmonary system, and major sensory systems. Occupational therapists work to undo the limitations and damage done to the systems regarding activity and function. Occupational therapy does little to eliminate the cause or to reverse the course of disease. The kinds of limitations can be listed as follows:

Neuromuscular weakness or loss
Joint limitation or loss
Loss or limitation of vital capacity, cardiac reserve, and endurance
Loss or limitation of sight, touch, sound, taste, or smell
Limitation of development and growth
Increased pain

Psychological problems involve the effects of disorders of orientation, attention, affect, memory and thinking, and the motor aspects of feelings or emotions. Psychological problems may be listed as mental illness and treated as diseases but may not always actually be diseases. Examples include the following:

Loss of reality orientation
Lack of self-identity or self-concept
Lack of self-worth or self-esteem

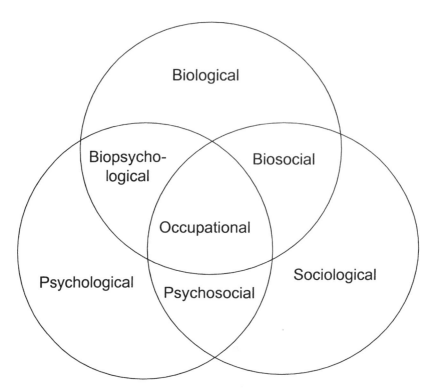

Figure 30.1. Diagram of the health/occupational problems seen by occupational therapists.

 Inability to concentrate attention
 Loss of motivation or initiative
 Lack of self-control
 Lack of judgment of personal safety

Sociological problems involve interactions with other people and the environment. Such interactions may be verbal or nonverbal but must include a person or object other than the self. Problems in this area include the following:

 Environmental changes
 Poor interpersonal skills
 Inability to function in groups
 Lack of communication skills
 Antisocial behaviors
 Withdrawal
 Lack of knowledge about the community

Problems in occupations involve failure or difficulty in combining the biological, psychological, and social areas, including:

Loss or lack of work skills
Inability to perform daily self-maintenance tasks
Failure to learn skills
Difficulty in learning and skills
Limitations of growth and development

The interaction of the areas and overlapping of problems can be illustrated by the person who has lost a job or an occupational skill. Loss of job may lower the person's self-esteem and result in an identity crisis. These are psychological problems. The loss of health benefits from employment may result in failure to treat diabetes, which leads to stroke, both biological problems. The loss of income may force the person to move to a new area in which less is known about the community and few friends are easily made. These are sociological problems. Occupational problems may arise if no employment is available to the person unless he or she obtains more training and education. Thus, the person has multiple problems, as illustrated in the following hypothetical case studies.

C A S E   S T U D Y   I

JOHN BRANDON

The 37-year-old Mr. Brandon is an aviation engineer who lost his job when a federal contract was not awarded to his company, forcing massive layoffs. The Brandons were living in a middle to upper class neighborhood of one-family dwellings in the suburb of a large metropolitan community. He is married and has three children, two girls and a boy, who are 8, 11, and 13 years of age. After the layoff, the family's income decreased from $5300 a month to $1350, including unemployment insurance. Later, the income was reduced further when unemployment insurance discontinued and savings were depleted. In addition, the company health insurance benefit was lost because individual rate payments were too costly for the Brandons to pay.

Mr. Brandon tried to find work with other aviation companies, but owing to the lack of openings, was unable to find employment. Some engineering firms wanted special skills that he did not have and that would require 1 year of training and education. Firms with jobs in the area felt he was overqualified and wanted someone trainable who would accept a lesser salary. Employers with odd jobs would not hire him because they said he would leave as soon as something better came along, causing more employee turnovers.

continued

With no job and little chance of getting a job, Mr. Brandon began to feel depressed; his self-concept as a worthwhile, capable person began to crumble, and his identity as a good provider suffered. His health suffered, too. He began to eat irregularly and to forget to take insulin for his diabetes. Then, he decided the insulin was too expensive and tried to manage with only one shot every other day.

His family life was getting worse as well. He did not like the idea of his wife looking for work and felt that moving to an apartment closer to the city would cut expenses. The cost was less, but the loss of friends, changes in school for the children, and increased noise of nearby neighbors increased family tensions. His wife was considering a divorce.

Finally, Mr. Brandon's health became worse, and he had a stroke that left him with weakness on the right side of his body. He was improving physically with therapy and better medical care, but his feelings of helplessness and hopelessness about himself were hindering his progress.

Occupational therapy can help in all of the major areas of Mr. Brandon's problems although other services are needed. The major problems are as follows:

Biological/Medical
Muscle weakness—right upper extremity and hand
Diminished tactile sensation—right upper extremity
Homonymous hemianopsia (visual—seeing right field of vision only)

Psychological
Depressed (little hope that the situation will improve)
Diminished self-concept (provider to dependent)
Changed self-identity (capable to helpless)

Social
Wife may leave him
Children avoid him
Friends have been lost
Unfamiliar with new neighborhood
Difficulty speaking (aphasia)

Occupational
Inability to dress, bathe, groom, or eat without assistance
Unable to write, print, or draw
Lack of marketable job skills
Inability to engage in leisure activities that require hand function, balance, and body coordination

Further evaluation would pinpoint the exact problems and degree of difficulty as outlined in the chapter on direct services.

C A S E   S T U D Y   I I

DELA FARLEY

Dela is a 56-year-old woman living alone in a third-floor walk-up apartment in the inner city of a metropolitan community. She has had rheumatoid arthritis since she was 27 years old but has managed without assistance. Six months ago, she began having difficulty walking because of the pain in her knees and the swelling in her ankles. Also, her hands have become very deviated toward her little finger (ulnar deviation), which makes it difficult for her to grasp objects firmly, including the staircase bannister. Last month, she had cataract surgery.

Although the surgery was successful, her daughter Gladys feels that her mother cannot live alone any longer. According to Gladys, the apartment is a mess. Newspapers are everywhere. The refrigerator is full of spoiled food. Clothes have not been cleaned. Furthermore, her mother does not answer the phone when she calls and seems to be confused when Gladys comes to visit. Gladys says Dela called her granddaughter Sara by the wrong name and did not even seem to notice. Sara did not appreciate being called by her male cousin's name, Jeffrey, who is the son of Gladys' brother, Josh. Gladys feels that her mother should go to a nice nursing home where people will look after her needs. Dela thinks Gladys just wants to get rid of the "old lady" and is an ungrateful daughter. After all, it was she, Dela, who raised the two children by herself after Charlie, her husband, was struck and killed by a truck. Dela says she has been taking care of herself for 30 years and has no intention of going to a nursing home anytime soon. However, it does bother her that she is no longer able to help with the church socials because her legs get too tired and she cannot see well.

The occupational therapist would be of most assistance in dealing with the following problems:

Biological/Medical
Pain and swelling of lower extremities
Reduced hand grasp—ulnar deviation
Visual loss—cataract surgery
Lack of mobility due to arthritis and visual problems

Psychological
Confusion because of visual problems
Determined to be self-reliant
Diminished self-respect because she is unable to keep house and shop for
   groceries and basic supplies

continued

CASE STUDY II

Social
Daughter fears for mother's safety
Conflict between mother and daughter regarding living arrangements
Difficulty in recognizing people because of poor vision
Limited social contacts because of problems in mobility

Occupational
Difficulty performing self-maintenance activities, including eating, dressing, grooming, and bathing, because of weak hand grip
Difficulty performing home management tasks, such as meal preparation, cleaning, doing laundry, writing checks, and shopping, because of problems using her hands
Lack of leisure interest and activities that have been either adapted for limitations of hand grasp or that do not require fine motor skills

CASE STUDY III

CRISTINA JERADO

Cristina—or Crissy, as her parents called her—is the daughter of a self-employed mechanic from a small town. When she was born, she had a hole between the chambers of her heart that was surgically corrected when she was 3 days old. Crissy's Apgar score was 6 on a 10-point scale because her breathing was poor, heart rate was irregular, and skin color was bluish. At 5 months old, she was diagnosed as a failure-to-thrive baby. Crissy could not hold her head up and could not roll over. Her cry was weak, and she barely seemed to be aware of visual stimuli. She did respond to auditory sounds. Her weight was 8 pounds, which was 1 lb more than her birth weight. Her sucking was weak, and she did not seem to be eating enough. In addition, her growth was stymied.

A cardiologist discovered that Crissy had two additional holes between the chambers of her heart that had gone undetected during the initial diagnosis. Surgery was recommended and performed when she was 7 months old. During the surgery, she went into cardiac arrest for 5½ minutes. After surgery, she had to be placed on a respirator because she was too weak to breathe on her own. Recovery was slow. She caught colds easily and had a difficult time fighting the infections. Her illnesses always seemed to reverse whatever gains had been made.

continued

A neurologist has told Crissy's mother that her child's nervous system is abnormal and her movements are "jerky." Crissy's mother has been concerned that her child would die, but she now worries that she will never be able to do anything. Mrs. Jerado has heard about children who were little more than "vegetables" and is afraid Crissy will become one. She is also concerned that the grandparents will not even hold Crissy because she seems so delicate.

At 2 years of age, Crissy is able to roll over, can bare weight on her hands and knees, and creeps on all fours for short distances. Sitting balance is good with her hands used as support, but she loses her balance if she tries to grasp a toy. She can stand with support but is unable to walk. Her vision is poor: she can see light and shadows but has no focal vision and cannot track objects. Hearing is excellent; however, she does not speak. Tactile responses are normal, and she anticipates being picked up by lifting her head. After 15 minutes of evaluation, she was tired. Her skin was blushed and her breathing was labored.

The occupational therapist should note the following problems:

Biological/Medical
Low body weight—feeding difficulties
Low physical endurance
Subject to respiratory infections
Developmental delay in balance reactions
Developmental delay in motor skills
Poor vision
Poor visual perception

Psychological
Mother worries child will die or be a "vegetable"
Child tries to please adults but cannot because of delayed development
Curiosity and motivation are limited by health factors

Social
People are afraid to touch or hold her because she looks fragile; therefore, they tend to avoid her
No speech, limited communication skills
Few social skills caused by developmental delays
Little opportunity to interact with the physical environment because of developmental delays

Occupational
Inability to feed self or assist in dressing and grooming
Lack of play skills including exploration and imitation

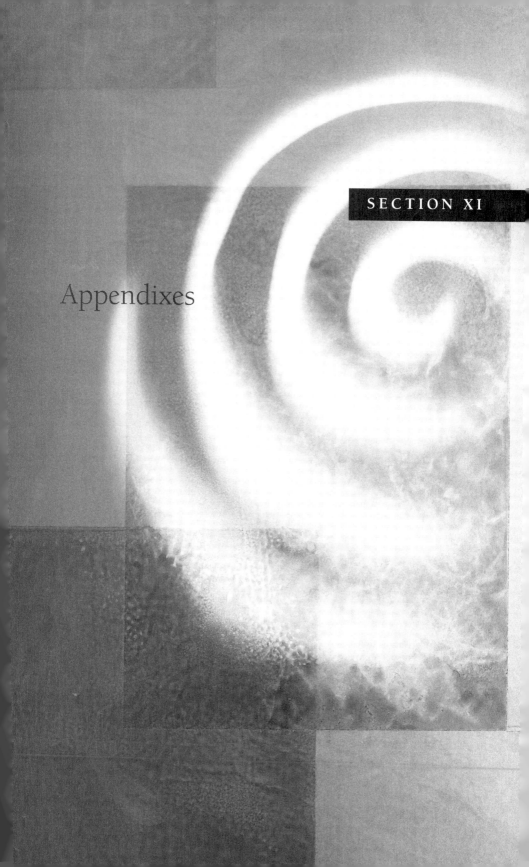

SECTION XI

Appendixes

Other Concepts Related to Organismic and Mechanistic Models

QUALITATIVE VERSUS QUANTITATIVE CHANGE (1–3)

Qualitative changes based on the organismic model are characterized as stages or levels of development, which are defined or delineated unique behaviors occurring at each state or level. Quantitative changes based on the mechanistic model examine the cumulative effects of specific behaviors within periods of the life span. In other words, the changes are in the operational efficiency but not in the structure or formation of the organism. An example of qualitative changes can be found in Piaget's stages of cognitive adaptation. The sensorimotor, concrete operation, and formal operation periods are all characterized by specific subperiods of behavior that are unique to that period. An example of the quantitative process is the process of learning as proposed by behaviorists. Basically, learning is the same process throughout life, but the accumulated experience enables the learner to become more efficient in responding to the environment and thus learn a more complex sequence of behavioral responses.

END POINT VERSUS NO END POINT (1, 2)

In the organismic model, there is an end point to the progression of change. The end point provides an identifiable goal, purpose, and direction to the change. The most common end point is some type of maturity. For example, in Piagetian theory, the formal operations stage is the end point. In Erickson's theory, the eighth and final stage of ego integrity versus despair is the end point.

On the other hand, the mechanistic model has no end point. Behavior is considered to be a function of the situation; thus the goal, purpose, and direction may change, depending on the environmental conditions present at the time. Again, behaviorists' theories such as those of Skinner, Bijou, and Watson are examples.

STRUCTURE–FUNCTION VERSUS ANTECEDENT–CONSEQUENT ANALYSIS (1–3)

Structure–function is basically the assumption that a person has functions, objectives, or a general purpose that is carried out or contained within a structure. Thus, the functions are enumerated and a structure is identified, and both serve the function. The results delineate the process by which functions can occur and achievement can be obtained.

Antecedent–consequent proponents assume that behavior is a function of altering the events that occur before a response or changing the events that occur after a response. Thus, no specific structure is needed because the generating force leading to behavior is external to the individual.

STRUCTURAL CHANGE VERSUS BEHAVIOR CHANGE (1–3)

The organismic model is based on the assumption that change occurs in the form, structure, or organization of the individual and that the changes are directed toward an end state, purpose, or goal. Actual change may or may not be observable to others. In some cases, the person's word must be accepted because changes in thinking processes, values, beliefs, or attitudes are difficult to observe and must be measured indirectly.

In contrast, the mechanistic model is based on the assumption that change is evident through behavioral responses; therefore, change can be observed and measured by others. Change has occurred when the individual responds differently to the situations or events in the environment. Change is measured by the degree of difference in a response from a person's previous behavior.

AGE RESTRICTIONS VERSUS NO AGE RESTRICTION (1, 2)

Models developed from the organismic model often make use of chronological age as a restriction, limit, or boundary for stages and levels. The assumption is that chronological age is a guide to the determining of structural changes within the individual. In contrast, the mechanistic model does not consider age as a change agent because it can be reduced to time, and time simply provides more opportunity for the environment to change behavioral responses.

UNIVERSALITY VERSUS RELATIVITY (1, 2)

Universality is based on the assumption that some behavior or activity is common to all human beings or at least to all biologically intact human beings. Universality is supported by genetic inheritance, which may be common or similar to all humans living or yet to be born. The inheritance includes a number of preprogramed units that provide the basic set of behavior or outline the parameters. On the other hand, relativity is based on the assumption that behavior depends on environmental conditions. The rationale would be that similar environmental conditions exist to which similar responses are given. The same reasoning suggests that individual differences occur because different environmental conditions exist for each individual.

RATIONALISM VERSUS EMPIRICISM (5, 6)

Models based on the organismic model assume that reason and intuition are the primary sources of knowledge. Rationalism permits the individual to know reality independent of experience. In other words, the intellect is the true source of reality rather than the senses. Through the use of reason and intuition, a person has the authority and ability to determine his or her own course of action.

In contrast, the mechanistic model is based on empiricism in which all knowledge is assumed to come from experience and observation. Thus, the senses are the source of knowledge and truth, and the brain is blank tablet (tabula rasa), which must depend on external information for its knowledge.

STEADY STATE VERSUS EQUILIBRIUM (4)

A steady state is achieved by reaching a constant internal and external balance while continuously exchanging and using component materials. Thus, the individual is able to maintain the self in spite of building up and breaking down and importing and exporting nutrients and information. In the organismic model, the individual is viewed as able to maintain the integrity of the self while continuously seeking to interact with the environment.

Equilibrium, on the other hand, is the process of maintaining a balance among bodily processes. When equilibrium mechanisms are working, changes in the internal or external environment stimulate other processes to counteract those changes through a feedback system that leads to the restoration of balance. The mechanistic model is based on the assumption that the individual will seek equilibrium and only interacts with the environment to achieve the elements needed to restore the balance. Homeostasis is an example of equilibrium, and it has been applied to the biomedical model.

EQUIFINALITY VERSUS FINALITY (4)

Equifinality is the capacity of the individual organism to reach the same goal from different starting points and in different ways. The organismic model is based on the assumption that the individual has the capacity to organize the self in a number of different ways that will all reach the same or similar end point. Many of the approaches in occupational therapy are based on the concept of equifinality. Substitution and compensation are two examples.

In contrast, finality is an assumption in the mechanistic model which suggests that the end point, final state, or outcome is determined by the initial conditions. Thus, the individual has no real capacity to alter or change either the direction or the end point that will be achieved. In the biomedical model, the nature of the pathology is assumed to determine the end state. Disease is assumed to lead to a negative or undesired outcome. The idea that it is possible to live with disease does not compute.

NEGENTROPY VERSUS ENTROPY (4)

In the process of negentropy or negative entropy, the system is able to take in more energy than is needed to convert the energy source into a usable energy form. Thus, the individual has a net gain in energy resources, which can be used to build the system a well as maintain it. The organismic model has adopted the assumption that each individual is capable of achieving negentropy and is therefore able to progress through maturation and learning to higher levels of organization and differentiation. An example is Herbert Dunn's concept of high-level wellness.

In contrast, the mechanistic model follows the assumption that the body has a relatively fixed quantity of energy available. As the energy is used, the amount of entropy (conversion of energy) increases, which in turn increases the amount of disorder over time. Thus, the body continues to function until it breaks down, but it cannot expand or improve because limited energy is originally available.

AUTONOMOUS VERSUS DIRECTED ACTIVITY (4)

Basic to the organismic model is the assumption that humans are capable of performing autonomous behavior—behavior initiated within the individual. This assumption of self-initiated and self-directed action permits the individual to take charge of the self and be responsible for the actions taken.

On the other hand, the mechanistic model is based on the assumption that all activity is caused by events external to the individual; thus, the individual is responding to rather than initiating action. There is little need for initiating action because the environment provides the necessary stimulation to produce the behavior needed.

MORAL VALUES VERSUS AMORAL VALUES (5, 6, 8)

Within the organismic model moral values are considered essential and part of the person's responsibility. Moral values include a sense of ethics that describes right and wrong actions. Both right and wrong actions are theoretically possible, but the ethical responsibility will enable the person to choose the right action.

In contrast, the mechanism model has no scope of values or ethics because none are needed. Humans are not considered to be making choices but responding according to learned behavior. If the behavior is rewarded, it will be continued: if not, it will be extinguished. Teaching a person the "right thing to do" is simply a case of rewarding the desirable behavior so the person will continue to perform that behavior.

SYMBOLIC VERSUS NONSYMBOLIC ACTIVITY (4)

The organismic model includes the assumption that humans use symbols to convey their activity and that much of activity in which humans engage is at the symbolic level. After the basic physiological and psychological needs are met, the individual engages in symbolic behavior. This engagement may continue without any observable or known cause other than simply for the pleasure of involvement.

By comparison, the mechanistic model does not recognize symbolic activity. What appears as symbolic activity can be understood at a lower level. What appears as "activity for its own sake" is simply behavior for which the cause is unclear or unidentified at this time. All behavior has a cause because all behavior follows the natural laws of cause and effect.

CRITICAL PERIODS VERSUS NONCRITICAL PERIODS (7)

Critical periods as an assumption of the organismic model states that there are certain times in an individual's life that are optimal for learning specific adaptive behaviors. Therefore, if the critical period age is past, optimal learning will not occur and may never occur. Providing opportunities for learning adaptive behaviors during the critical period is important for achieving maximum results.

In contrast, the mechanistic model is based on the assumption that the individual is plastic and malleable. Therefore, the individual can learn behaviors at any given chronological age. The important factor is the amount of reinforcement provided. Sufficient reinforcement will produce the desired adaptive behavior no matter when the learning occurs during the natural history of the individual.

EMOTIONALISM VERSUS UNEMOTIONALISM (6)

Feelings, affect, and mood are considered to impact the thoughts and reasoning processes, according to the organismic model. Thus, emotion is an integral assumption in which the individual's behavior might be affected by the emotion content. In contrast, the assumption of the mechanistic model is that individuals, like machines, are affected by observable physical forces. An individual can be understood entirely from the outside by observing behavior without referring to inner states, such as feelings or emotions.

SUBJECTISM VERSUS OBJECTISM (8)

The organismic model is based on the assumption that the organism is the sphere of concern. Thinking and reasoning as action potentials are subjective or difficult to discern with the senses. Thus, much of the focus of the individual must be inferred from observation or obtained through interview. Generalizations from one person to the next are risky at best.

In contrast, the mechanistic model operated on the premise that external actions are the major sphere of concern. What can be verified through the senses is what is important. Sensory-based data can be observed, quantified, and measured empirically. Generalizations of behavior can be obtained by using the mathematically derived normal course of distribution and standard deviations.

TENSION SEEKING VERSUS TENSION REDUCTION (9)

Tension seeking involves the active exploration of the environment in an attempt to learn about and master the unknown. In tension-seeking behavior, the person deliberately accepts and consciously risks some degree of potential harm or displeasure in order to gain greater satisfaction. Tension-seeking behavior is a concept of the organismic model because the individual is an active agent in the process.

In contrast, tension reduction is directed toward decreasing the scope of interaction with the environment so as to reduce a designated drive, such as hunger, safety, or belonging. Activity is focused on the target, and when the objective is obtained, behavior ceases and does not usually reappear until the drive reappears. Tension reduction is a concept of the mechanistic model.

On the other hand, tension-seeking behavior such as learning a new skill may lead to further expansion of behavior to learn yet another skill or to perfect the first one. Tension-seeking behavior thus expands the behavioral repertoire whereas tension-reducing behavior tends to become stereotyped and limited.

FLUID DIMENSION VERSUS FIXED DIMENSION OF TIME AND SPACE (8, 10)

The organismic view recognizes that time and space have psychological and sociocultural dimensions as well as physical dimensions. Such dimension may change, depending on the situation and interpretation by the individual. Time may appear to go by slowly if little activity is occurring or rapidly if the person is busily involved. For younger people, the present is all-important, whereas for the older person, the past may be more easily remembered.

In contrast, the mechanistic view states that time and space are absolute quantities and values. Failure to adhere to the values is evidence of loss of reality or failure to understand reality. The person is expected to conform to the values of time and space as stated by the physical senses. Such a view persists in mechanistic philosophy even though experiments have illustrated the fallacy in such logic.

PULL MOTIVATION VERSUS PUSH MOTIVATION (1)

The organismic view includes ideas related to purpose, value, or need as the motivational forces that direct human action. Kelly, a psychologist, calls these "carrot" theories because they depend on the person's willingness to seek out action and "go for" the carrot on the stick.

On the other hand, there are concepts that are described as drives or stimuli. These concepts are associated with the mechanistic view that a person must incur a external force from the environment in order to become active. Kelly describes such theories as "pitchfork" models because the source of energy seems to push a person from behind to get moving.

UNIDIRECTIONAL DEVELOPMENT VERSUS ALTERNATING DIRECTIONAL DEVELOPMENT (1, 2)

The organismic view asserts that developmental change is unidirectional and irreversible. Through the process of development, the organism expands and increases in complexity. As the change occurs, the organism progresses in only one direction, forward and onward. Behavior that appears to be from a younger period is described as caused by temporary instability, especially in times of stress during which older patterns of behavior are more dependable or reliable to the individual.

In contrast, the mechanistic philosophy states that behavior change can be progress forward or backward. Behavior may regress to a more primitive behavior or immature form that the person supposedly had "outgrown." Such behavior is most likely to appear in situations of anxiety or crisis. In psychoanalytic literature, such regression is a mechanism available to the ego whenever it is unable to cope with the present situation.

PRESENT, FUTURE-ORIENTED VERSUS PAST-ORIENTED (2)

Models based in the organismic framework tend to view the present and future time frames as most important when viewing an individual's situation. The focus is on what the person can do and has potential for doing. Thus, the past may or may not be indicative of the person's total being. Therefore, use of the past history should be interpreted with caution because it may be irrelevant or misleading. Instead, much more useful information may be obtained by discovering how a person views the current situation and what plans or interests the person has for the future.

The opposite position is that the past is all-important because infancy and early experience shape the total potential and significantly influence all later action. Just as the machine, a person is able to do only what the person was "built" to do. The building blocks were set in early life. The objective of later life is to understand and use what was built in early childhood.

References

1. Looft WR. Socialization and personality throughout the life span: an examination of contemporary psychological approaches. In: Baltes PB, Schaie KW. Life Span Developmental Psychology. New York: Academic Press, 1973:25–82.

2. Friedrich D. A Primer for Developmental Methodology. Minneapolis: Burgess Publishing, 1972:3–8.
3. Reese HW, Overton WF. Models of development and theories of development. In: Goulet LR, Battes PB. Life Span Developmental Psychology. New York: Academic Press, 1970:115–145.
4. Bertalanffy LV. General Systems Theory. New York: Braziller, 1968.
5. Solomon RC. Introducing Philosophy: Problems and Perspectives. 2nd ed. New York: Harcourt, Brace, Jovanovich, 1981.
6. Blackham HJ. Humanism. 2nd ed. New York: International Publications Service, 1976.
7. Thomas RM. Comparing Theories of Child Development. Belmont, CA: Wadsworth Publishing, 1979:29.
8. Lamont C. The Philosophy of Humanism. 6th ed. New York: Frederick Ungar Publishing 1982:12–14.
9. Hergenhahn BR. An Introduction to Theories of Personality. Englewood Cliffs, NJ: Prentice-Hall, 1980.
10. Capra F. The Turning Point: Science, Society and the Rising Culture. New York: Simon and Schuster, 1982.

Certificate of Incorporation of the National Society for the Promotion of Occupational Therapy, Inc.

We, The Undersigned, All being persons of full age, and all being citizens of the United States, desiring to form a corporation, pursuant to Sub-Chapter 3 of Chapter 18, of the Code of Law for the District of Columbia, do hereby make, sign and acknowledge this Certificate as follows:

FIRST: The name of the Corporation is to be "THE NATIONAL SOCIETY FOR THE PROMOTION OF OCCUPATIONAL THERAPY, INC."

SECOND: The particular objects for which the corporation is formed are as follows: The advancement of occupation as a therapeutic measure; for the study of the effect of occupation upon the human being; and for the scientific dispensation of this knowledge.

THIRD: The territory in which its operations are to be principally conducted is the United States of America.

FOURTH: Its principal business office is to be located in the Village of Clifton Springs, County of Ontario and State of New York.

FIFTH: The number of its directors is to be five.

SIXTH: The names and places of residence of persons to be its directors until its first annual meeting are as follows:

William R. Dunton Jr, MD of Sheppard and Enoch Pratt Hospital of Towson, Maryland.
Susan C. Johnson, of 350 West 85th Street, New York City, New York.
Eleanor Clarke Slagle, of the Hotel Alexandria, Chicago, Illinois.
Susan E. Tracy, of Jamaica Plain, Massachusetts; and
George Edward Barton, of Consolation House, Clifton Springs, New York.

SEVENTH: The time for holding its annual meeting is on the first Monday of September in each year.

IN WITNESS WHEREOF: We have made, signed and acknowledged this certificate in duplicate.
Dated. Clifton Springs, Ontario County, New York, this fifteenth day of
March A.D. 1917.

William R. Dunton, Jr.
Susan C. Johnson
Eleanor Clarke Slagle
George Edward Barton
Isabel G. Newton
T.B. Kidner

STATE OF NEW YORK
COUNTY OF ONTARIO: SS
On this fifteenth day of March, 1917, before me personally came W.R. Dunton, Jr., Susan C. Johnson, Eleanor Clarke Slagle, George Edward Barton, Isabel G. Newton and T.B. Kidner, to me known and known to me to be the same persons described in and who executed the foregoing certificate and they severally duly acknowledged to me that they executed the same.

James A. Rolfe,
Notary Public

(NOTARIAL SEAL)

Index